Designing Bodies

Models of Human Anatomy from Wax to Plastics

Edited by
Elizabeth Hallam

Designing Bodies: Models of Human Anatomy from Wax to Plastics

First edition printed in 2015 in the United Kingdom.

British Library Cataloguing in Publication Data.
A catalogue record for this book is available from the British Library.

ISBN 978-1-904096-25-2

Published by The Royal College of Surgeons of England
35–43 Lincoln's Inn Fields
London WC2A 3PE
www.rcseng.ac.uk

Printed in the United Kingdom by Advent Colour Ltd.
This work is printed on FSC accredited paper.

EDIT, DESIGN AND TYPESET
RCS Publishing

Contents

2 Acknowledgements

4 Bodies, materials, design: hands-on models in anatomy and surgery, 1920 to now
Elizabeth Hallam

HISTORICAL CONTEXT

47 Models and materials in Europe, 1650–1890
Anna Maerker

63 Medical models in Britain, 1750–1920
Samuel JMM Alberti

MODELS

81 Corrosion casts: David Hugh Tompsett

167 Model limbs: John Herbert Hicks

201 Modelled Anatomical Replica for Training Young Neurosurgeons (MARTYN)

232 Further reading

234 Notes on contributors

235 Visual index

Acknowledgements

Elizabeth Hallam

This book arises out of a collaborative exhibition – *Designing Bodies: Models of Human Anatomy from 1945 to Now* – at The Royal College of Surgeons of England (RCS) from 24 November 2015 to 20 February 2016. As guest curator of the exhibition, I have enjoyed the privilege of researching and working with fascinating museum and archival collections, along with immensely talented and dedicated staff at the RCS. Having previously studied and written about some of the models in this exhibition, the invitation to curate them for display in a public gallery has opened up many new and unexpected perspectives on these compelling yet under-researched material objects. This volume builds on the work carried out for the exhibition, and places the RCS' significant collection of models in wider historical and cultural context.

Sam Alberti's expertise has been crucial for both exhibition and book; without his considerable museum insight, scholarly generosity and continued enthusiasm, the project would not have come to fruition. Martyn Cooke has been kind enough to offer me unprecedented access to the production process involved in making the RCS' innovative Modelled Anatomical Replica for Training Young Neurosurgeons (MARTYN). As a skillful model designer and exhibition builder, Martyn has been essential to this project.

Research for *Designing Bodies* has involved fresh identification and interpretation of models at the RCS. Many of the objects relating to MARTYN were considered working objects (for example, moulds and materials for making models), rather than conventional 'museum objects' for exhibiting and long-term preservation. By displaying items involved in the process of manufacturing MARTYN, instead of just the 'finished' model, the exhibition responds to the challenge of displaying the hands-on practice of model design. For making this approach to the exhibition possible in practical terms, I would like to thank Martyn, who has devised and prepared models and other exhibits specifically for *Designing Bodies*, as has model-maker Clare Rangeley, whom I also thank for her expert work.

A number of RCS models produced by John Herbert Hicks in the 1950s have also been reinterpreted through research for the exhibition. For example, Hicks' models of feet – and, in particular, the windlass mechanism in the arch of the foot – have been identified here for the first time since the RCS' acquisition of the collection in 2003. Helping with this identification, Susan Standring, Geoffrey Hooper and Roop Tandon have given invaluable anatomical insights.

I have benefited enormously from the help of RCS Museums and Archives staff, especially Jane Hughes, Louise King, Hayley Kruger, Jyotishree Nath, Geraldine O'Driscoll, Sarah Pearson, Carina Phillips, Krit Poonyth and Bruce Simpson. Without them, the models and original documents in this book would not have made it onto the gallery walls. For their hard work and distinctive visual flair, I am also very grateful to the RCS Publishing staff, especially Matthew Whitaker, Kim Lewry and Vivienne Button. Without them, the same models would not have made it onto these pages.

Photography for the book and exhibition has been specially commissioned, and provides creative insight into aspects of the RCS' collections published here for the first time. I thank John Carr at the RCS and independent photographer Michael Frank, not only for their inspiring images but also for helping me to see models of anatomy in different and surprising ways during this project's intensive photography sessions. Photographer John McIntosh, in Aberdeen, has skilfully produced many images of models during my ongoing research with anatomical collections elsewhere in Britain, images from which I have learnt so much.

For helpfully supplying diagrams, photographs of models and supporting documentation from further collections, thanks to medical artist Francesca Corra; Subhadra Das at the University College London Teaching and Research Collections; Joanna Ebenstein at Morbid Anatomy; William Edwards at the Gordon Museum of Pathology, Guy's Campus, King's College London; Ryan Jefferies, curator at the Harry Brookes Allen Museum of Anatomy and Pathology, University of Melbourne; Graham Nisbet at the Hunterian Museum, University of Glasgow; and the Wellcome Library, London. Permission to publish images relating to Somso® models made in Germany, and access to their company's archival material, was kindly provided by Jenny Whitebread and Michael Whitebread at Adam,Rouilly. Keystone Press Agency also granted permission to reproduce two photographs.

Colleagues and friends at the University of Aberdeen have given support and encouragement from which my work always benefits. My thanks go to the Department of Anthropology, especially to Tim Ingold, Nancy Wachowich and Neil Curtis; and to Anatomy in the School of Medicine and Dentistry, especially Simon Parson and Lucy Watson. At the University of Oxford, the School of Anthropology and Museum Ethnography provides an ever-stimulating environment for my research, and I thank especially Marcus Banks, Clare Harris and Laura Peers. Also in Oxford, Ian Maclachlan has been an endless source of invaluable ideas and advice.

Finally, I gratefully acknowledge the support for this project from The Royal College of Surgeons of England, B Braun, the Henry Moore Foundation, and The Strauss Charitable Trust.

Bodies, materials, design: hands-on models in anatomy and surgery, 1920 to now

Elizabeth Hallam

Three-dimensional (3D) models are designed by anatomists and surgeons to improve medical education and to train students in the latest surgical skills. How are these models devised and made, and how does this work help to enhance knowledge of the body and the practice of surgery? Focusing on model materials and design from 1920 to the present, this chapter explores how human bodies – living and dead – are investigated, fabricated and treated, for just as all medical facilities and equipment are designed – from hospitals to laboratories and from surgical instruments to body implants and pharmaceuticals – so are bodies that are modelled in medical work.

The design of 20th-century and present-day models held at The Royal College of Surgeons of England (RCS), London, is examined here for the first time, in association with the exhibition *Designing Bodies: Models of Human Anatomy from 1945 to Now* (see Acknowledgements). Three collections held at the RCS are particularly significant in terms of medical modelling in

FIGURE 1 (OPPOSITE)
Wax model of the portal venous system, including veins, liver, stomach and intestines, around 1921, by N Rouppert (successor to Maison Tramond), Paris.
University of Aberdeen, Anatomy Museum. Photograph by John McIntosh.

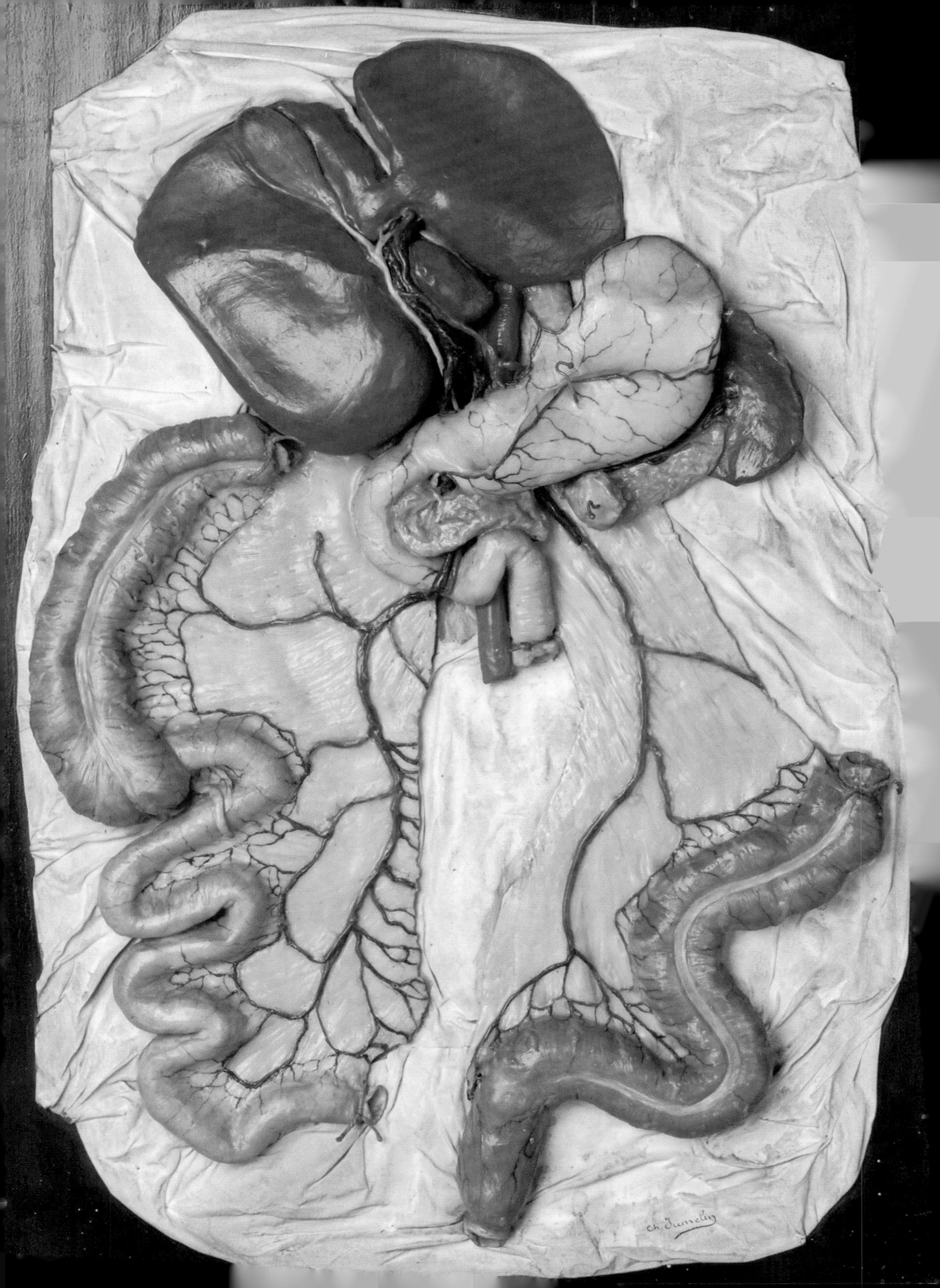

Britain throughout the past century. First, perhaps the world's best (and possibly largest) collection of corrosion cast vessels – tubes and cavities that carry vital fluids and air in the body – was produced by David Hugh Tompsett (1910–1991) during his 30-year appointment as prosector at the RCS from 1945, where he prepared and dissected human and animal bodies for anatomical teaching [see Cat. 1–42]. Second is a comprehensive set of models of the leg and foot created in the 1950s and 1960s by John Herbert Hicks (1915–1992), an orthopaedic surgeon at Birmingham Accident Hospital, to interpret and demonstrate function and movement. This set, along with Hicks' models of bone-fracture repair and his extensive archive of notes and sketches, was gifted to the RCS in 2003 [see Cat. 43–60]. More recently, further innovative models have been developed at the College, including the Modelled Anatomical Replica for Training Young Neurosurgeons (MARTYN). Subsequent generations of this model, with tailored features for training in surgical procedures on the skull and brain, continue to evolve today [see Cat. 61–76].

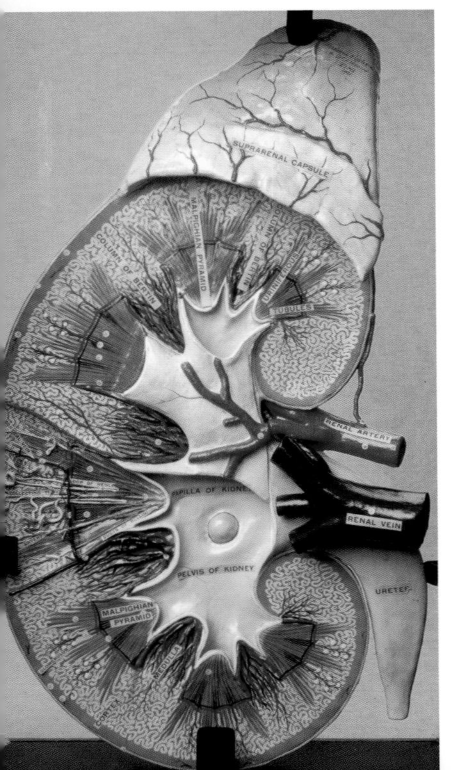

FIGURE 2
Enlarged model of the kidney, comprising several anatomical parts that could be disassembled to show deeper parts, 1921, papier-mâché, by Établissements du Docteur Auzoux, Paris.
University of Aberdeen, Anatomy Museum. Photograph by John McIntosh.

Model-making in the field of medicine is performed not by lone 'inventors' but by many practitioners and participants in particular settings. It engages artists, designers and photographers, as well as medical professionals, educators, museum curators, conservators and students. As a collaborative design process, modelling in anatomy and surgery cuts across distinctions between medical practice and art. Creative and rigorous, inventive and disciplined, this modelling is important in research, teaching and training; it can be crucial in gaining knowledge of the human body and in communicating that knowledge to others.

Designing models is a matter of doing, not just thinking and planning. Through hands-on trial and error, models are fabricated, tested, used and re-designed, with striking results. Visual and tactile exploration of materials is necessary to bring these tangible, 3D objects into being. To produce MARTYN,

Tompsett's corrosion casts and Hicks' limb models, practitioners experimented with many different materials such as wood and plastics. Model design for anatomical and surgical purposes has also involved work with the physical human body, alive and deceased. So parts of bodies donated to medical science and preserved in medical museums have been used as material from which models are developed, as have the living bodies of patients who are observed by surgeons aiming to improve operating methods. In addition to manipulating and shaping materials into models using techniques from casting to sculpting, practitioners have also employed a wide range of media – such as drawings, photographs and printed diagrams – to aid in both model production and use.

From the 1920s onwards, in Britain, substantial shifts in the design of models within anatomical and surgical practices have taken place, changes in which the RCS' models have played a significant part. Medical schools in the early decades of the 20th century continued to purchase anatomical models from established manufacturing firms in continental Europe, especially Auzoux and N Rouppert (successor to Maison Trammond) in Paris and Ziegler in Freiburg. Building strong reputations for high-quality educational models in the 19th century, these firms dealt in anatomical parts rendered in wax [Figure 1] or in a special paper paste, like papier-mâché [Figure 2].[1] The London-based company Adam,Rouilly distributed models in plaster by the Somso® firm founded in Sonneberg, Germany [Figure 3]. By the 1950s, Somso® was producing models in plastics, which were materials that would become predominant in this kind of commercial product owing to malleability during manufacture and durability in use [Figure 4]. Models in plastics could withstand much more handling than their plaster and papier-mâché predecessors, which – although designed for disassembly into a number of anatomical parts – were much more open to wear and tear.

FIGURE 3
Plaster model, 'Trunk with head', with removable half brain, ribs, lungs and intestines, around 1928, by Somso® models from Adam,Rouilly.
Photograph from *Somso®: Anatomical Models*, commercial catalogue, 1928.

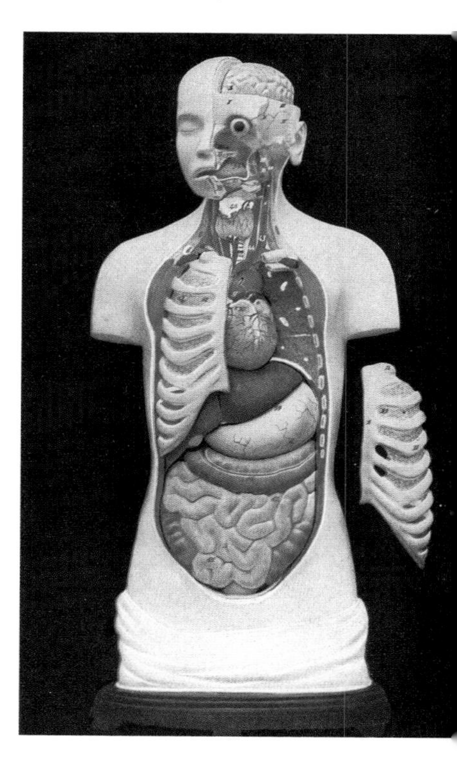

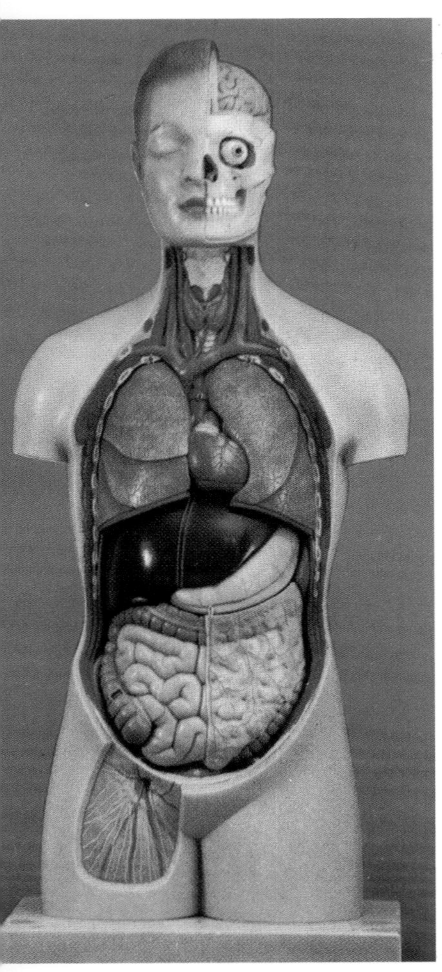

FIGURE 4
Plastic model, 'Trunk of a Young Man with Head', with removable parts, in the 'new design' without imitation loincloth and without 'external sexual organs', 1960s, by Somso® models from Adam,Rouilly. Photograph from *Somso® models: Anatomy*, commercial catalogue, 1970.

Alongside these commercial models, distributed from centres of model manufacture, were those regularly devised and made in-house in medical school workshops by anatomists, technicians and artists throughout Britain. During at least the past 100 years, these models have been constructed in easily accessible and affordable materials such as clay, paper and wool, as well as from parts recycled from other objects. Such models tend to be created for specific purposes, as one-offs or in small numbers for local on-site use rather than in large quantities for international distribution.[2] Mid-20th-century makers interested and involved in model design within medical teaching saw the bespoke nature of in-house models as a distinct advantage compared with commercial models, which were regarded as useful but 'rarely designed' to suit the particular needs of specific medical teaching situations. 'Exploratory', experimental and flexible, on-site modes of model-making was attuned to the everyday requirements of medical educators.[3]

The mid-20th-century and contemporary design of in-house, purpose-made models held at the RCS, then, is the concern of this chapter. This contrasts with recent exhibitions of – and academic research on – anatomical models that tend to focus on the extensive and painstakingly crafted continental European models of the 1700s and 1800s, especially those in compellingly life-like wax. Chapter 2 provides further discussion of these dramatic creations with particular reference to their materials and Chapter 3 moves back to Britain to trace a history of anatomical modelling, especially in wax and plaster from 1750 to 1920. But what follows below is concerned with the to-date far less-celebrated yet significant practices of small-scale model design with 'modern materials', often conducted with a distinctively hands-on, DIY approach.[4] Medical model-making in wax continued into the 1960s and 1970s – for example, in the work of Alice Gretener's prolific moulage production at the St John's Hospital for Diseases of the Skin in London and Richard Neave's wax casting of pathological conditions at the University of

Manchester. However, by then further materials and techniques were already being effectively used in 3D model design geared towards enhancements in medical understanding and treatment of the human body.[5]

DESIGNING VESSELS

Plastics 'opened up completely new possibilities...'

David Hugh Tompsett (*Anatomical Techniques*, 1956, p. 95)

Referring to the ready availability in late-1940s Britain of commercially manufactured cold-setting synthetic polyester resins, Tompsett recognised that these materials made it possible to 'produce beautiful, rigid, coloured casts of any comparatively large anatomical cavity'.[6] Motivated by these possibilities while working as RCS prosector, Tompsett devoted much time and attention to the production of corrosion casts that were designed to expose the anatomy of often-complex vessels, and to exhibit the many bodily tubes, channels and cavities [see Cat. 1–42]. It was difficult, if not impossible, to make these vessels visible through other methods of display, such as the dissection of deceased bodies. And, unlike parts of bodies preserved as specimens for medical study, resin casts would 'last indefinitely without deterioration'.[7]

Corrosion casting of vessels necessarily began with a human body part – an organ or a limb – to which Tompsett had access in the anatomy department of the RCS. Many of these were from people who donated their bodies after death to medical science. Amputated limbs from surgical operations and organs from post-mortem examinations of the dead (probably in one or more of the London hospitals) were also used to produce casts.[8]

Although the bulk of Tompsett's work was on human anatomy, it also encompassed casting from organs of animals, including brains, hearts and lungs – of dogs, cats and horses, for example – to enable the study of comparative anatomy [Figure 5].

FIGURE 5
David Hugh Tompsett
Corrosion cast of the bronchial tree in the lungs of a dog, 1949, resin.
Royal College of Surgeons of England.
Photograph by John Carr.

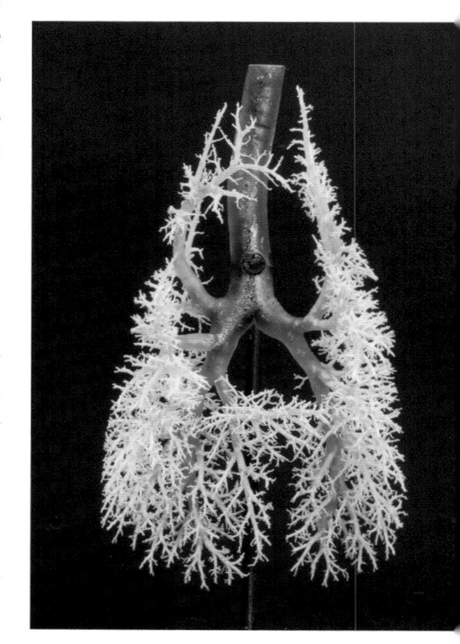

Tompsett injected vessels in prepared human body parts (or entire bodies in the case of deceased newborn infants) with fluid resin that filled the vessels and then quickly solidified. Next, the flesh of body parts was corroded or dissolved away with hydrochloric acid to reveal the cast vessels inside. Lungs, livers, kidneys, brains, hearts, arms and legs were processed in this way, creating casts that were seen as intimately related to the bodies that gave them shape. These were a type of model with particular claims to being almost identical to their original body moulds. Yet these powerfully convincing models were designed; they were created, sculpted and displayed.

Making and accumulating educationally valuable casts at the RCS from 1945 onwards, Tompsett worked in a context of reconstruction following the Second World War, a setting in which the College and its museum displays were substantially rebuilt following extensive bomb damage [Figure 6]. His casts were to feature in the newly built Hunterian Museum, which opened in May 1963 on the 150th anniversary of its first opening [Figure 7].

During the period in which the museum's interior was redesigned, Tompsett experimented with resins and developed techniques for effectively displaying the human body's anatomical interior. Debates regarding medical museums were critical of 'obsolete' holdings, especially aging wax models and specimens without a 'vestige of colour', for these could not be easily pressed into service when teaching the 'new anatomy', with its emphasis on the form and function of living bodies and processes of bodily 'growth, repair and adaptation', not simply the dissected dead.[9] Models, including Tompsett's casts, would help students to understand the anatomy of the living body. Indeed, these casts of the dead were made to seem (in some sense) alive, especially in their form – composed as though in a living body – and in their vibrant colour. Furthermore, through his modelling work, Tompsett approached these resin vessels as trees that took form or grew with a life of their own in the process of their making.

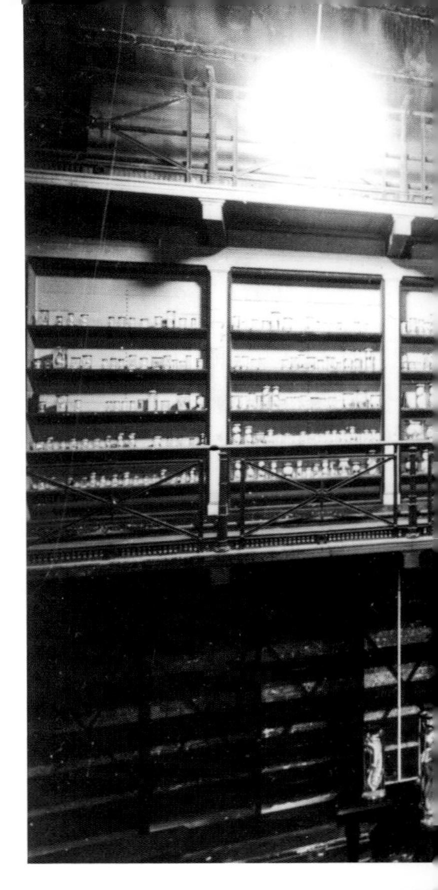

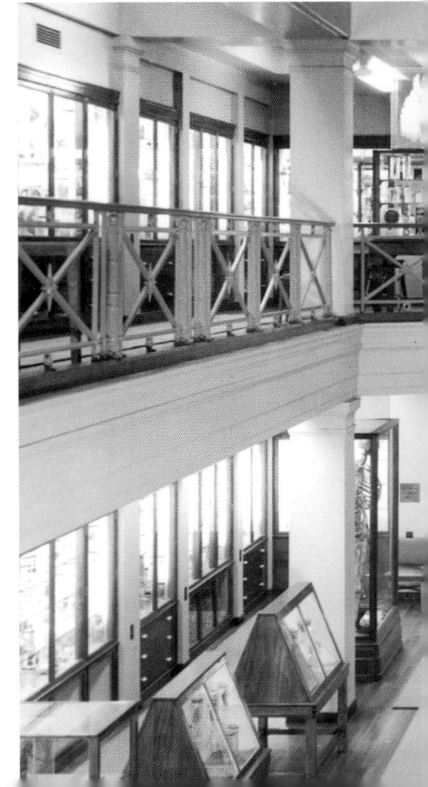

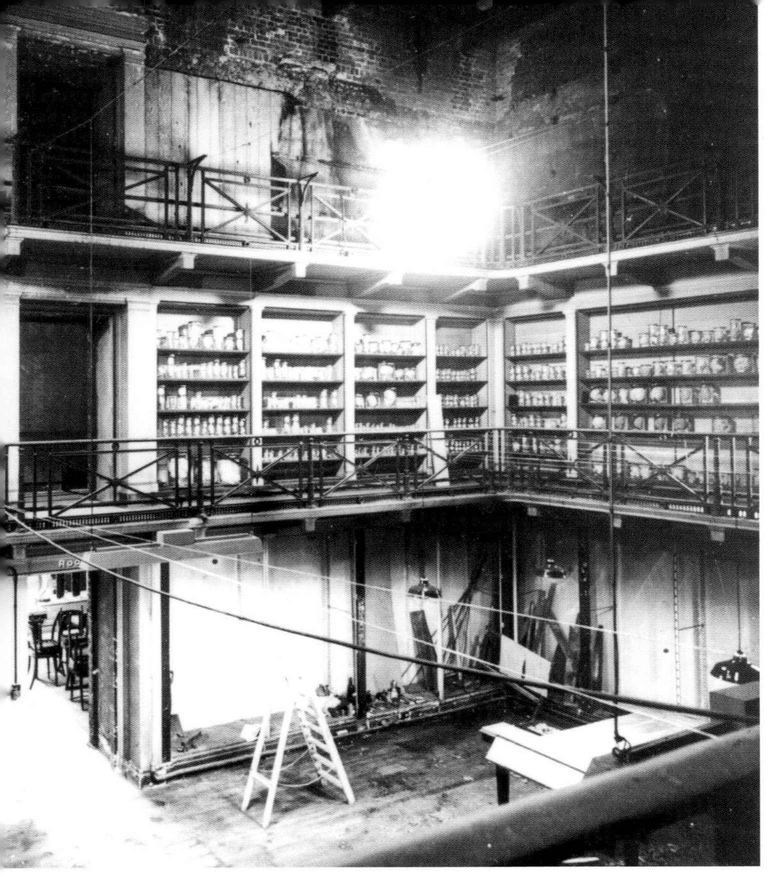

FIGURE 6
Hunterian Museum after bomb damage during the Second World War, around 1945.
Royal College of Surgeons of England.

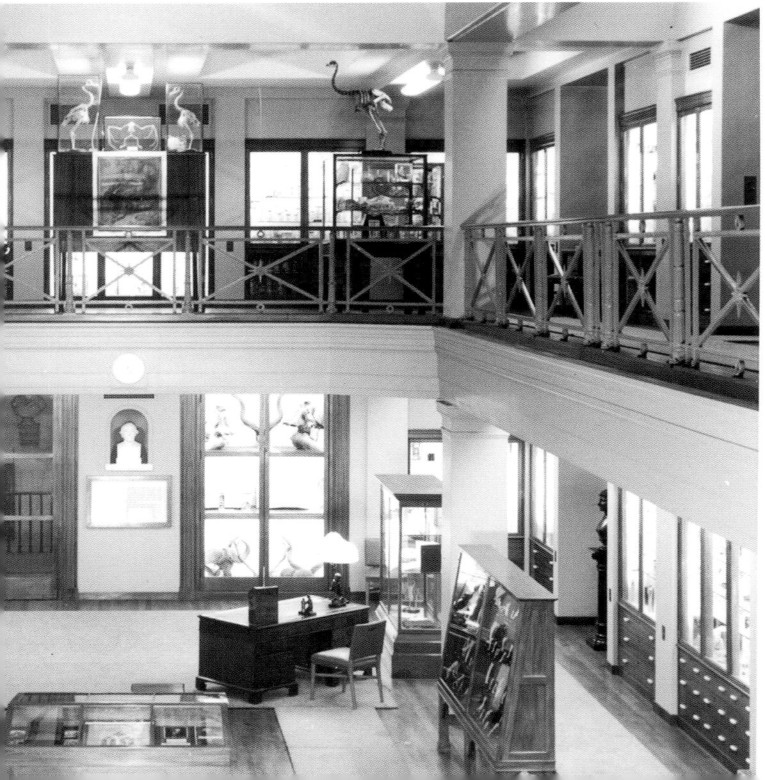

FIGURE 7
The new Hunterian Museum at the RCS, shortly after opening in 1963, with David Tompsett's cast of horse lungs on display (white cast, top left).
Royal College of Surgeons of England.

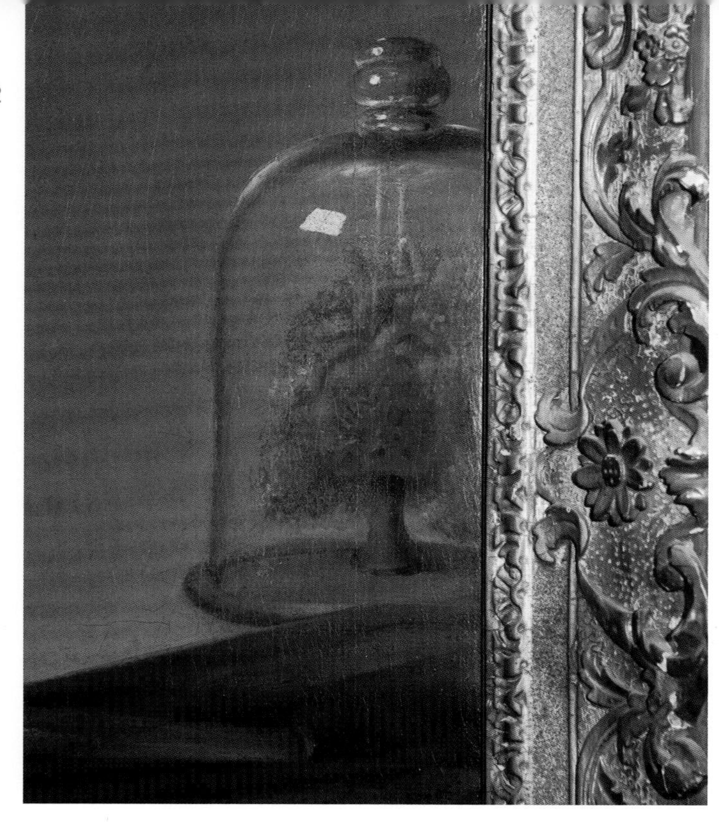

FIGURE 8
Robert Edge Pine
Wax corrosion cast of the heart and lungs, in a portrait of William Hunter, probably 1760s.
Royal College of Surgeons of England. Photograph by John Carr.

Respected as an important pioneer in corrosion casting with plastics, Tompsett selected his working materials carefully as these substances imbued casts with vitality. He was familiar with previous methods used in this type of casting, including William Hunter's 18th-century wax compositions [Figure 8] and early-20th-century uses of metals [Figure 9]. Wax, for Tompsett's purposes, was too fragile and metals so heavy that they distorted the vessels they were meant to cast. For the 'modern' anatomy museum, the material properties of resins produced much more effective results when used to compose casts according to Tompsett's tried and tested techniques.[10] Resins' initial fluidity and capacity to readily impress with detail along the course of very fine vessels before hardening was especially valued.

Tompsett's technical manual, *Anatomical Techniques*, published in 1956 and revised in 1970, provided detailed instructions for workers in medical schools who made specimens and models of anatomy. In these, he aimed to 'reveal as completely as possible all the tricks of his trade' with

FIGURE 9 (OPPOSITE)
JL Livingstone
Painted corrosion cast (in Wood's metal) of the trachea and bronchi in the lungs of an adult male, prepared by Dr Livingstone when a physician at King's College Hospital, London, 1920s.
Royal College of Surgeons of England.

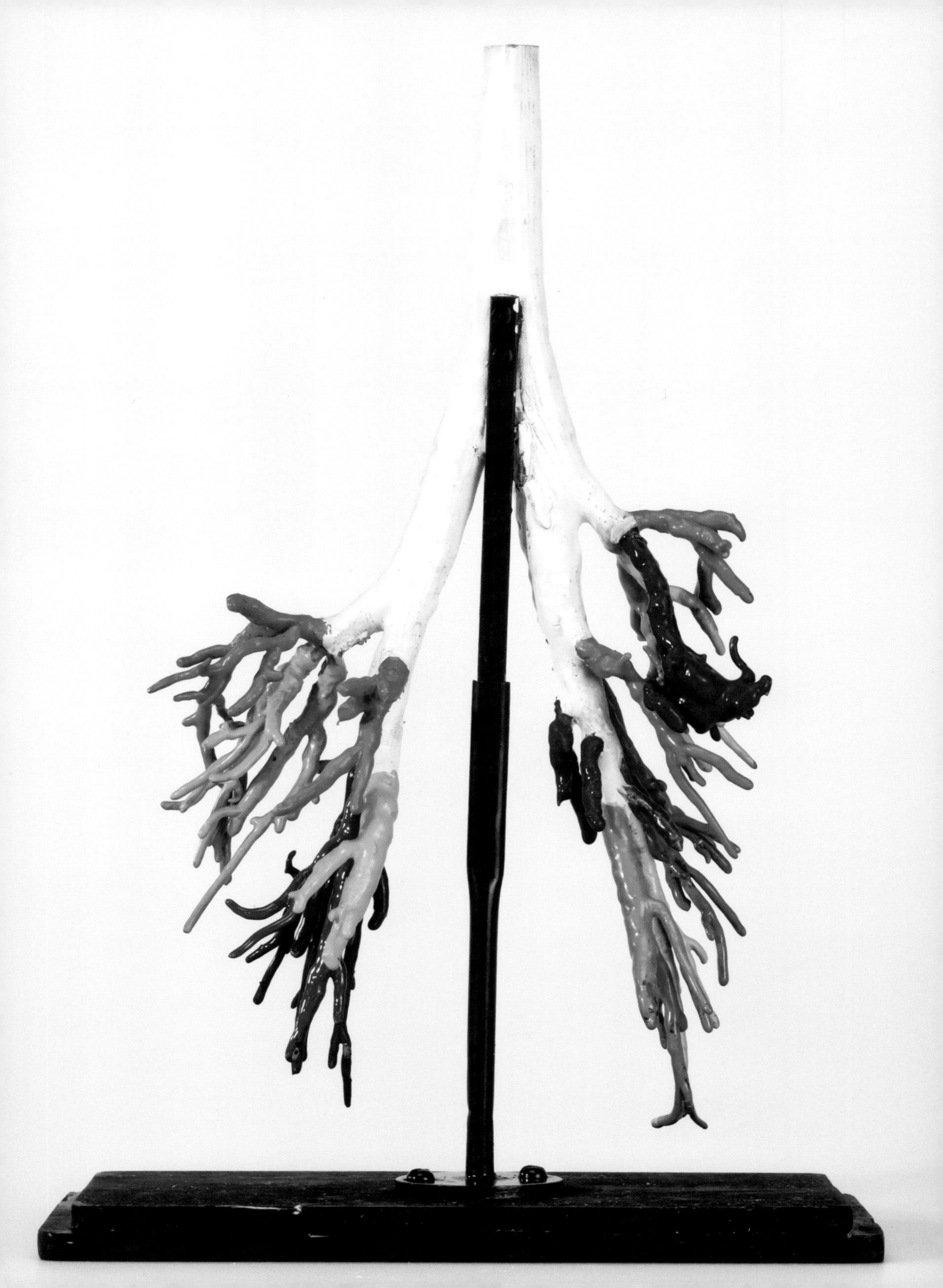

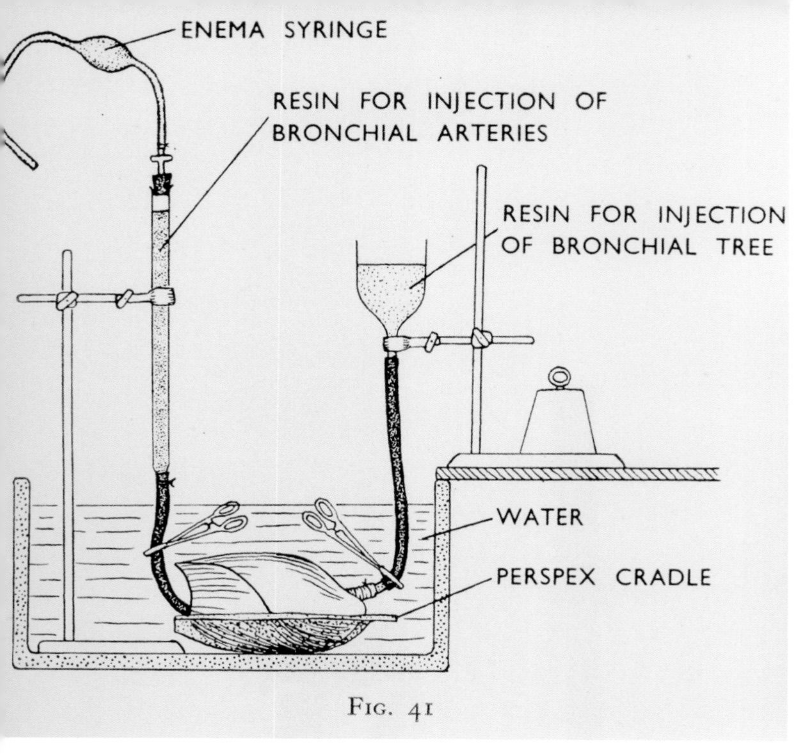

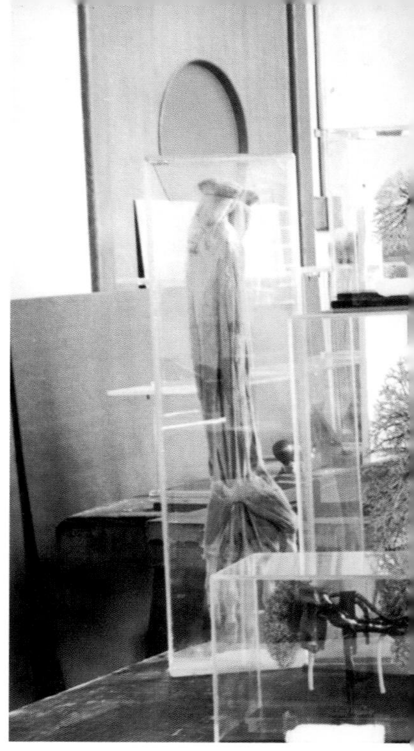

FIGURE 10 (ABOVE)
Diagram of apparatus for the injection of the bronchial tree and bronchial arteries.
From DH Tompsett, *Anatomical Techniques*, 1st Edition (Edinburgh: E&S Livingstone Ltd., 1956).
Photograph by John Carr.

FIGURE 11 (BELOW)
Apparatus used by David Hugh Tompsett to make corrosion casts: enema syringe, customised tubing and two cannulas.
Royal College of Surgeons of England.
Photograph by John Carr.

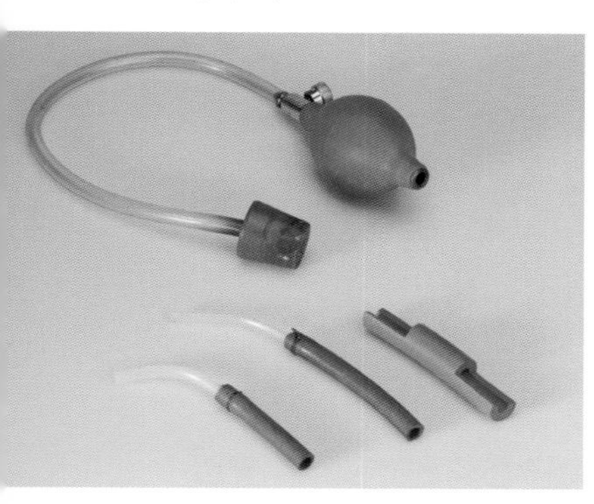

descriptions and illustrations. Diagrams showed workers how to inject vessels with resin using apparatus, including tubing and an enema syringe for applying the pressure needed to inject the resin [Figures 10 and 11]. Medical equipment was thus in his toolkit, as were dissecting instruments and paraphernalia from the home such as button thread and linen carpet thread. Tompsett appreciated this 'homemade' equipment for its 'simplicity', affordability and adaptability to the task in hand.[11] He was praised for his craft, for developing his tools and for his techniques inspired by the 'cult of "Do it yourself"'.[12]

After casting vessels, Tompsett carefully 'pruned' these resin 'trees' to expose deeper areas, which would otherwise be hidden, to tidy the cast and to create contours [Figure 12]. Casts then required mounts and cases to display and protect them. This model-making may have been influenced by DIY but it was not carried out by Tompsett alone; he was supported and assisted at the RCS within a community of practitioners. Sydney Bartlett, for example, who became chief museum technician, helped Tompsett with the construction of Perspex containers and other devices for exhibiting casts [Figure 13]. Bartlett also learnt

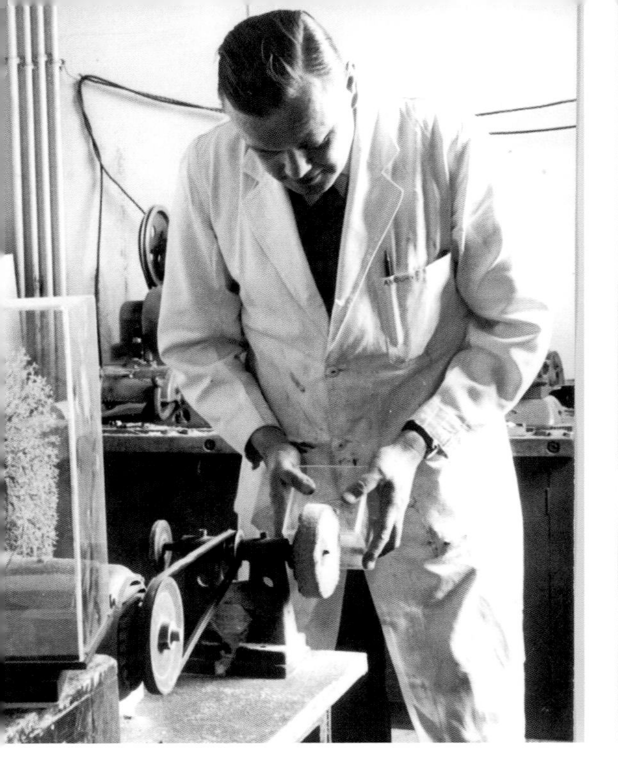

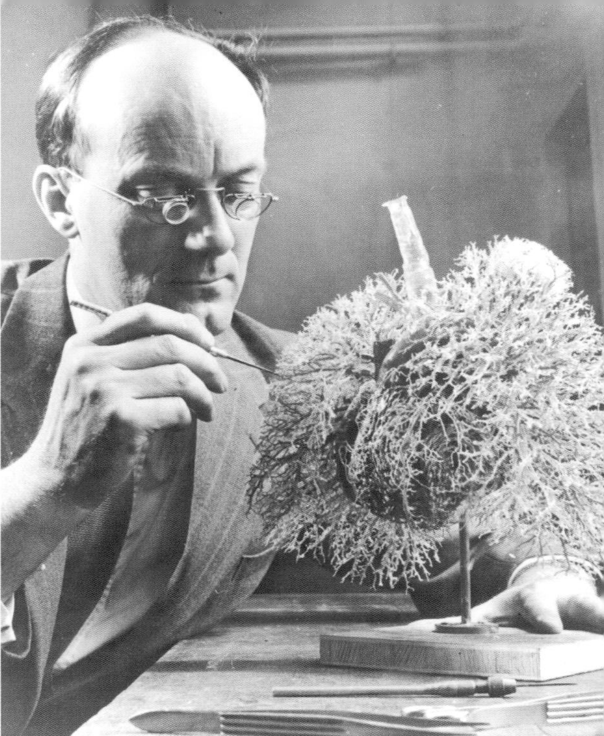

FIGURE 12 (ABOVE RIGHT)
David Hugh Tompsett working with his tools, pruning a corrosion cast of the heart and lungs, 1950s.
Royal College of Surgeons of England.

FIGURE 13 (ABOVE LEFT)
Museum technician Sydney Bartlett making Perspex cases for corrosion casts and specimens at the RCS, 1958.
© Keystone Press Agency.

corrosion casting techniques [Figure 14]. Tompsett's techniques were, furthermore, taken up more widely among anatomists and medical educators, promoted through his manual and in live demonstrations that he held at the RCS. His published work was read in medical schools from the north of Scotland to the south of Australia. Casts of the liver, for instance, were made, following Tompsett's methods, by Daryl H Nye and Kenneth J Hardy in the University of Melbourne's departments of surgery and anatomy, where they carried out research on veins to help improve surgical procedures in these areas of the body [Figure 15].

DISPLAYING FORM

Central to Tompsett's work was the drive to create effective ways of displaying the form (shape or structure) of vessels in organs and bodily parts. Casts were designed to demonstrate anatomical parts in three dimensions. These models could be viewed up close and in the round, to encourage observation from different angles and positions. The depth, position and relations between vessels, such as those in the lungs, were made clearly visible [Figure 16; see Cat. 18 for front view].

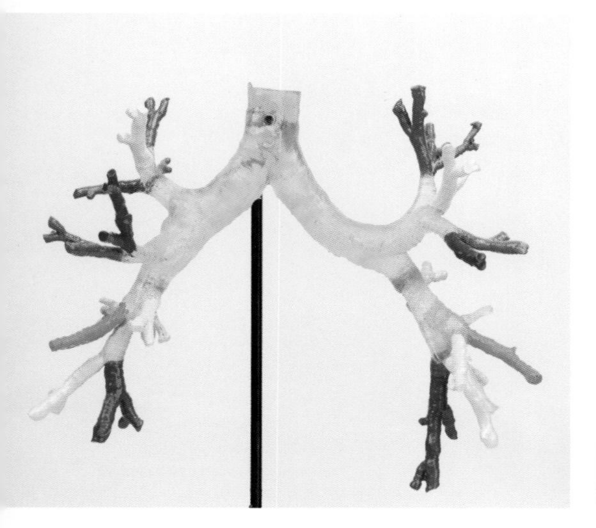

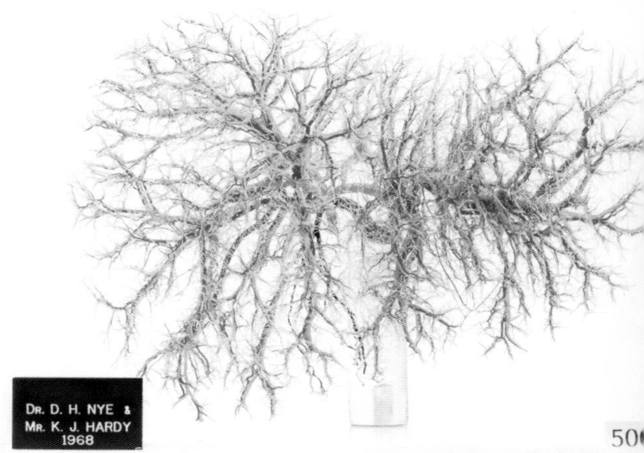

Because Tompsett cast body parts derived from the young and the old, these models could be compared to see how vessels grow during the life course, always varying in different people. The finest blood vessels in stillborns were carefully injected with resin to create delicate models of anatomy at both the beginning and end of life. Casts made inside organs from women and men exhibited these vessels in adulthood.

Careful, skilled casting highlighted anatomical detail, as when vessels in the kidney – the finest it was possible to show with this injecting method – were displayed [Figure 17; see Cat. 27 for full view]. Colour was also strategically employed, often to dramatic effect. Red and blue were widely recognised as colours for indicating arteries and veins but Tompsett went further with his anatomical palette of turquoise, orange, pink, green, grey and yellow. This use of colour enabled viewers to visually distinguish and trace the course of many different vessels in the same organ while showing the relations between them. Pigments were either mixed into the resin before injection or sometimes coloured paint was applied after the cast

FIGURE 14 (ABOVE LEFT)
Sydney Bartlett
Corrosion cast of the trachea and bronchial tree in the lungs, 1975, resin and paint.
Royal College of Surgeons of England. Photograph by John Carr.

FIGURE 15 (ABOVE RIGHT)
DH Nye and KJ Hardy
Corrosion cast of the liver, 1968, resin.
Harry Brookes Allen Museum of Anatomy and Pathology, Melbourne. Photograph by Gavan Mitchell.

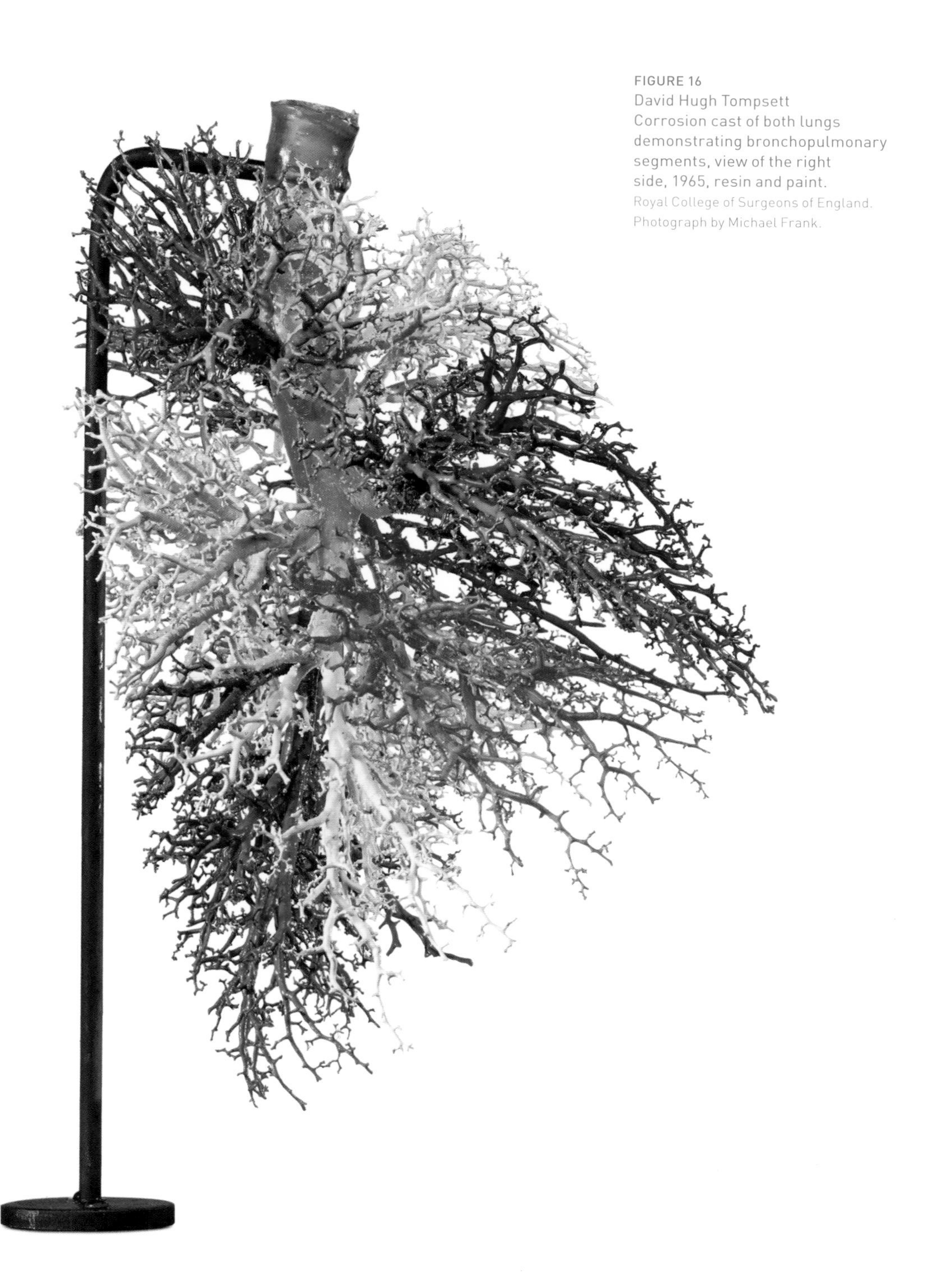

FIGURE 16
David Hugh Tompsett
Corrosion cast of both lungs demonstrating bronchopulmonary segments, view of the right side, 1965, resin and paint.
Royal College of Surgeons of England.
Photograph by Michael Frank.

had hardened [see Cat. 18]. Use of the former method can be seen in many of Tompsett's casts: for example, vessels in the placenta of triplets were made clearly visible [Figure 18], as were those in the organs of the thorax and abdomen of a male aged 14 – one of Tompsett's most complex and accomplished casts [see Cat. 36].

These resin compositions were exhibited in the Hunterian Museum [see Figure 7] and in the Wellcome Museum of Anatomy at the RCS from the 1950s onwards. In the latter, medical students could view multiple casts in relation to preserved specimens of human anatomy and diagrams of the same [Figure 19].

Cases for casts were, like the models themselves, designed for purpose. Transparent tailor-made boxes would ensure that casts were not only protected from dust but also from the hands of museum visitors. Although these models were certainly hands-on projects for their dexterous makers, for users they were presented for eyes only. Tompsett designed museum apparatus that would present casts to maximum visual effect, such as rotating mounts to facilitate 360° views. Cases were often crafted in Perspex but Tompsett also devised a mould for

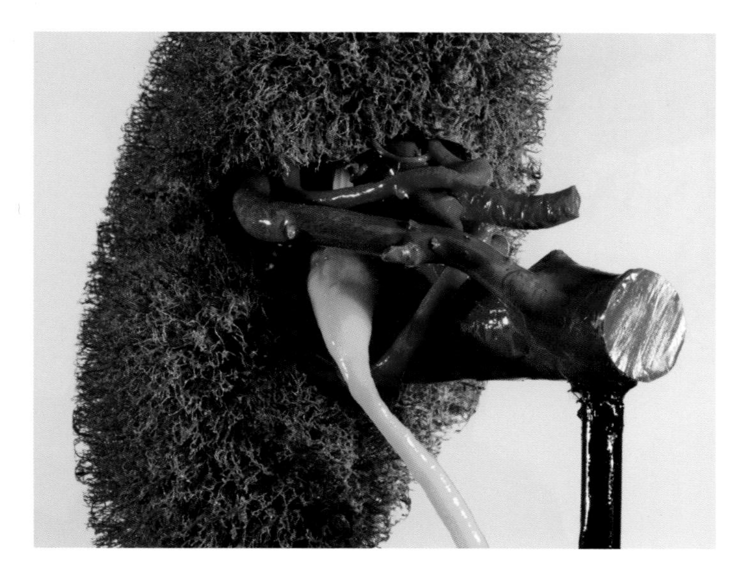

FIGURE 17
David Hugh Tompsett
Corrosion cast of vessels in the kidney, close up, 1950s–60s, resin.
Royal College of Surgeons of England.
Photograph by Michael Frank.

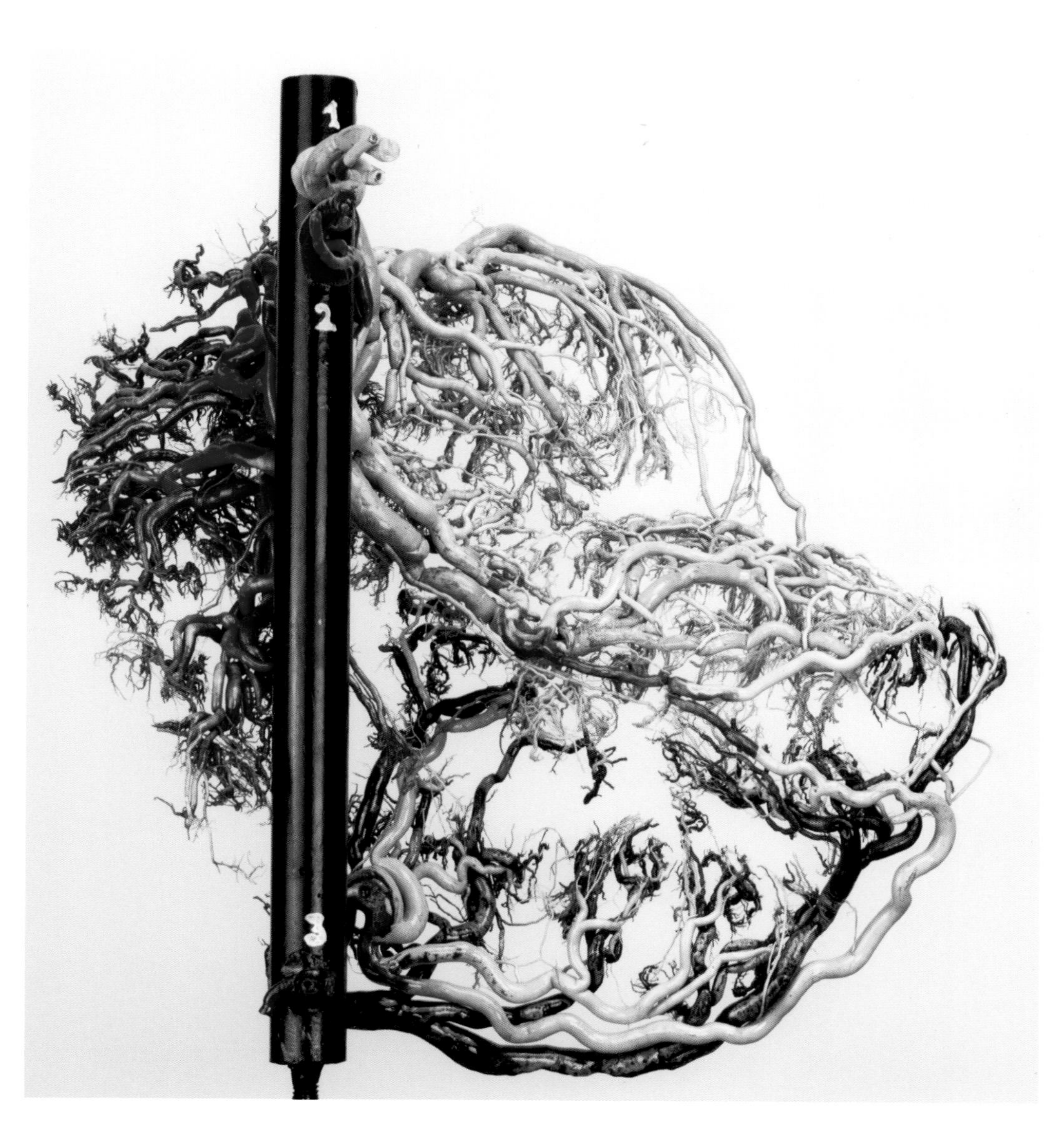

FIGURE 18
David Hugh Tompsett
Corrosion cast of vessels in the placenta of triplets, view from the back, with the supporting metal post labelled 1, 2, 3.
Royal College of Surgeons of England. Photograph by John Carr.

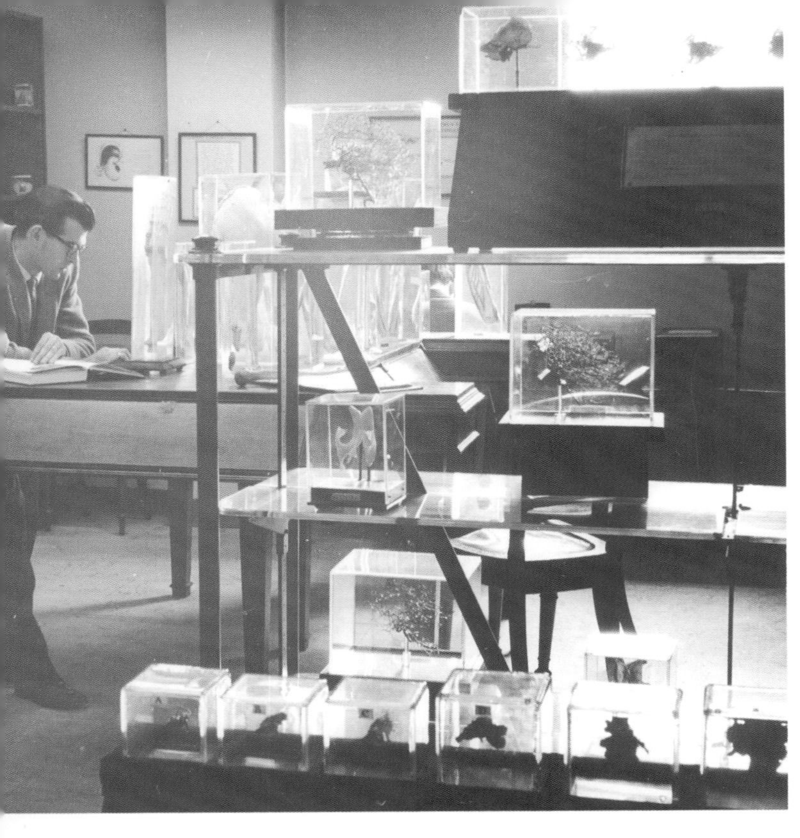

FIGURE 19
Display of corrosion casts in the Wellcome Museum of Anatomy at the RCS, 1958.

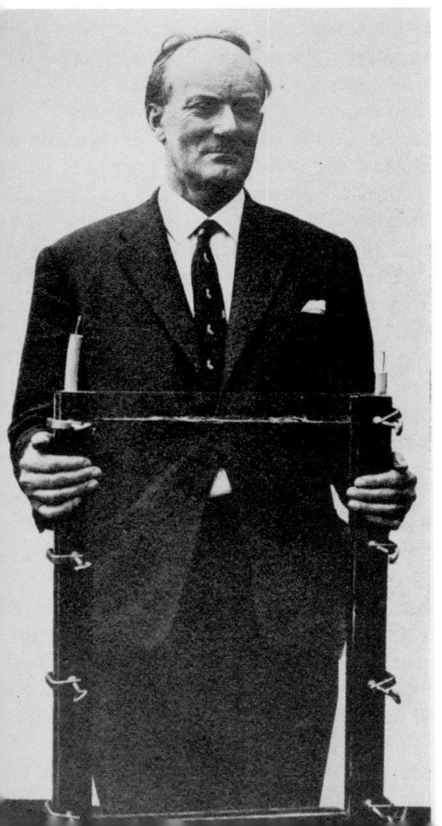

FIGURE 20
David Tompsett holding a mould for casting sheets of transparent resin, from which museum boxes were made.
From DH Tompsett, *Anatomical Techniques*, 2nd Edition (Edinburgh: E&S Livingstone Ltd., 1970). Photograph of original by John Carr.

casting sheets of clear resin with which to build them [Figure 20]. Although these boxes were intended to be robust constructions, 30 years later at the RCS some of them were apt to explode. By contrast, the large majority of Tompsett's casts have endured, with their intricate form and intense colour. Displayed in the 1990s with diagrams and photographs [Figure 21], they continue to be exhibited and interpreted in anatomy and surgical teaching at the RCS today.

DESIGNING LIMBS

> *'It is difficult to visualize... but the model... will help'*
>
> John Hicks ('The Mechanics of the Foot. I. The Joints', 1953, p. 355)

A different mode of modelling was developed by John Hicks at the Birmingham Accident Hospital, established in 1941 to improve injury treatment for patients. In this context, through the mid-20th century (from 1951), Hicks made and used models as means to research and demonstrate the workings of the lower leg and foot – models credited as 'ingenious' (see Cat. 43–60).

FIGURE 21
Display of corrosion casts in the Wellcome Museum of Anatomy at the RCS, mid-1990s.
Royal College of Surgeons of England.

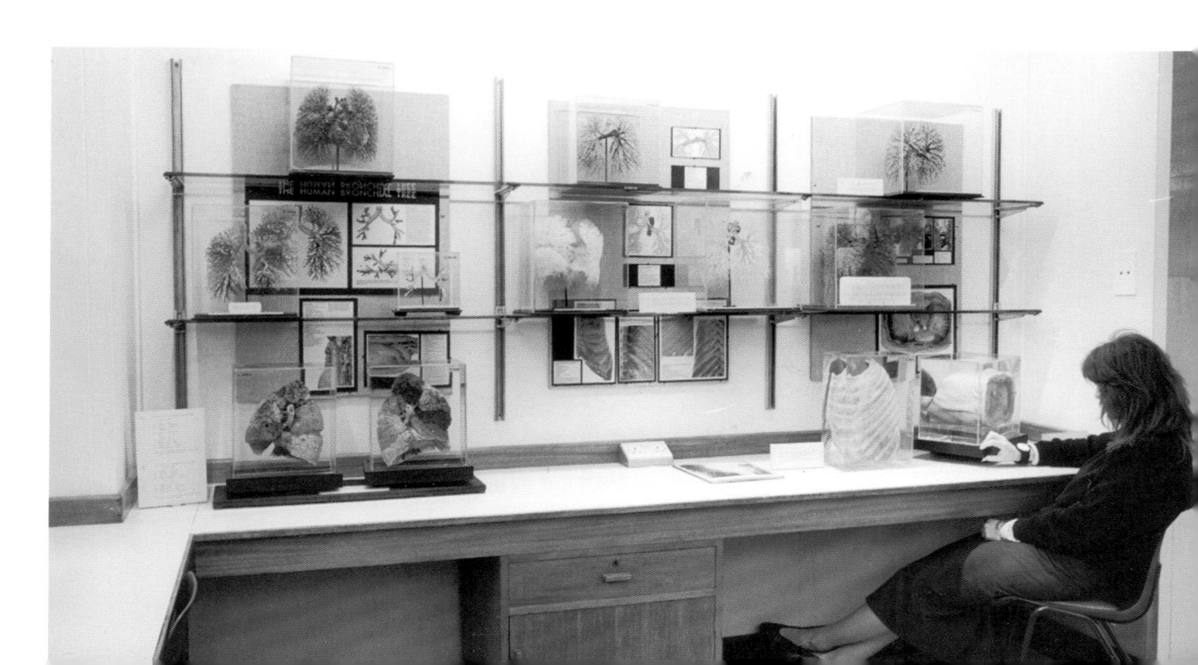

FIGURE 22 (OPPOSITE)
Photograph of John Hicks' investigations and experiments with a human foot, 1950s.
Royal College of Surgeons of England. Print by John Carr from original negative.

Fascinated by the 'mechanics' of these anatomical parts, Hicks' work in the designing of models was driven by his attempts to better describe and display movement, and to improve medical treatment of injuries, especially fractured bones. Like Tompsett's, his modelling practice contributed to the understanding of living anatomy, yet the materials and techniques that he used – and consequently the anatomical forms that he produced – were very different. Contrasting with Tompsett's fluid, colourful vessels, Hicks' limbs were geometric and angular. And if the former's model design captured intricate curving detail, the latter's design tended to simplify into cube-like shapes, almost to the point of abstraction.

Like Tompsett, however, Hicks dissected amputated limbs and observed anatomical specimens preserved from deceased bodies; this anatomical work formed the basis of his model design.[13] Working as a surgeon in a hospital setting, Hicks had access to amputated limbs, which he examined in his research [Figure 22]. He dissected feet to investigate and experiment with bones and tendons so that their form and function in the living body could be better interpreted.

One of Hicks' main working materials was wood, fitted with metal components and wire. These suited his purpose well; they could be assembled into model limbs that sought not a close resemblance to anatomical parts of the body but rather to provide a clarified demonstration of motion.

Again like Tompsett, Hicks also recycled household or domestic items, building models with, for example, a wooden sewing-thread bobbin, ribbon, a drawing pin and part of a broom handle [see Cat. 56, 60]. Using materials from everyday life in anatomical modelling was consistent with Hicks' approach to anatomical descriptions, in which he compared parts of the human body (such as the foot) with household items (such as, a stool) to help readers to grasp his points more fully.[14] In the same

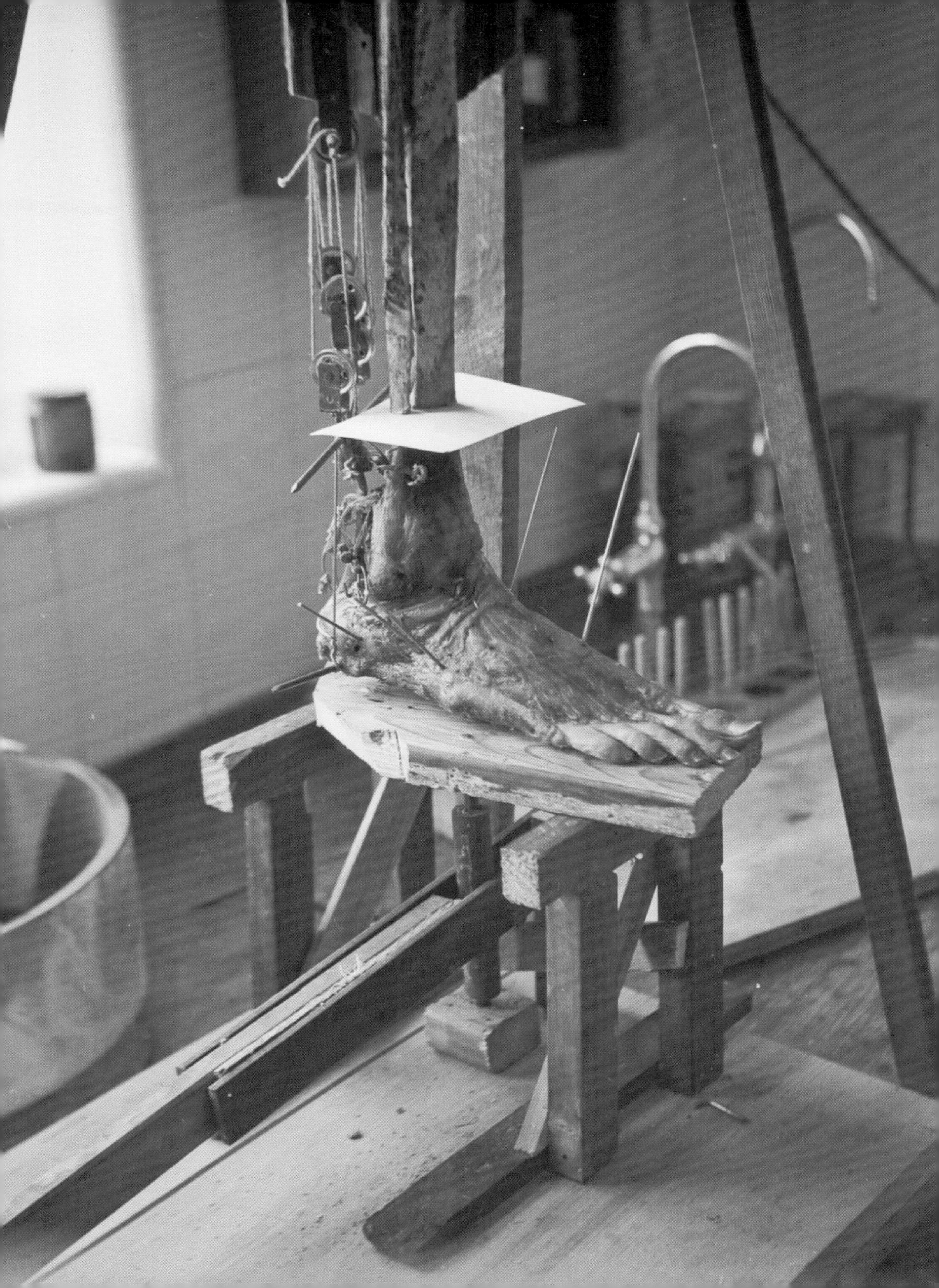

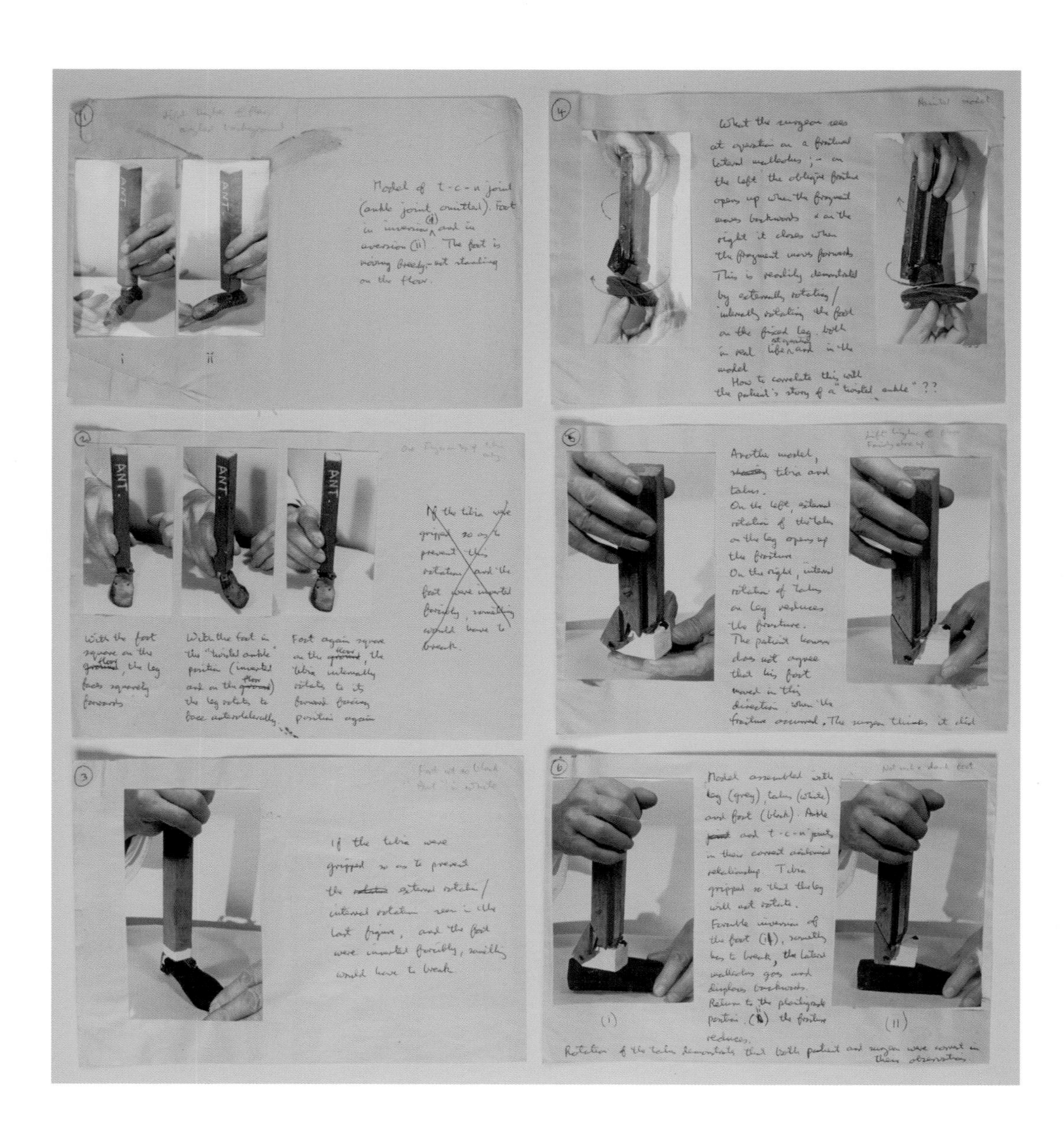

FIGURE 23
Photographs of John Hicks' models in action, with notes by Hicks, 1950s.
Royal College of Surgeons of England. Photograph of original documents by John Carr.

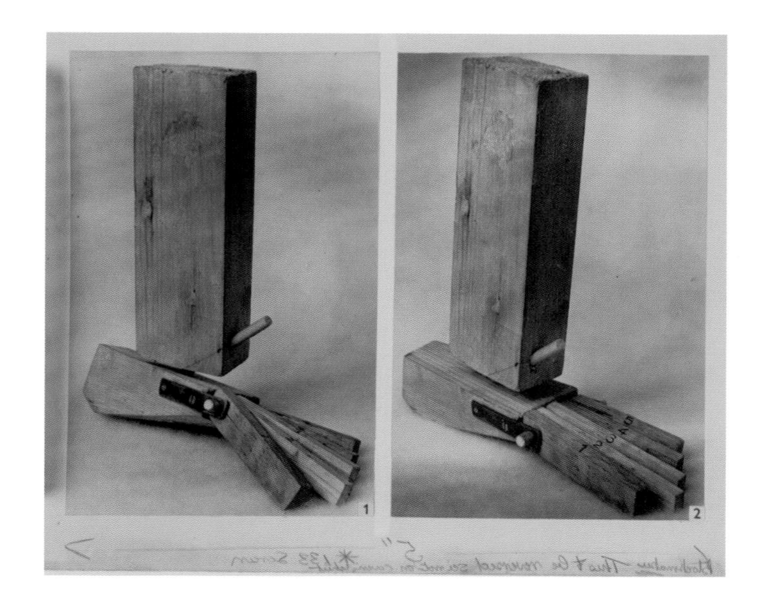

FIGURE 24
Photographs of John Hicks' models in action, demonstrating movement in the leg and the foot, including tarsal and metatarsal bones, 1953.
Royal College of Surgeons of England. Photograph of original documents by John Carr.

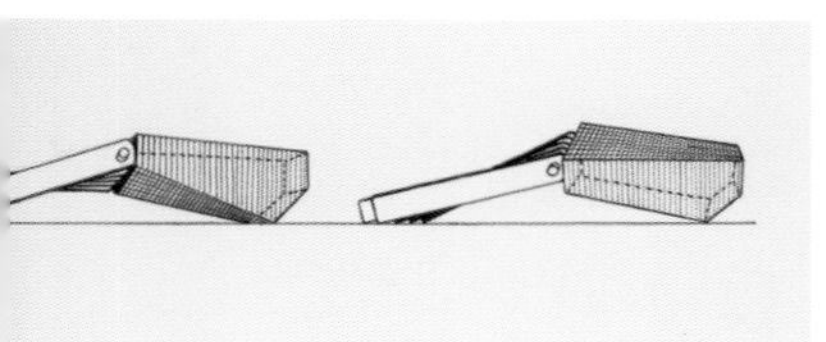

FIGURE 25 (ABOVE)
John Herbert Hicks
Drawings of Hicks' foot model, including tarsal and metatarsal bones, 1950s.
Royal College of Surgeons of England. Photograph by John Carr.

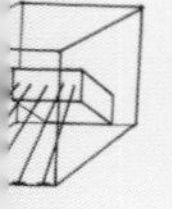

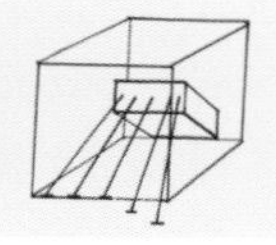

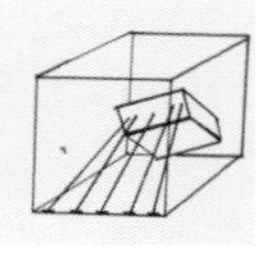

FIGURE 26 (ABOVE)
John Herbert Hicks
Diagrams of Hicks' foot model, showing bone movement and raising of the arch, as viewed from the front, 1950s.
Royal College of Surgeons of England. Photograph by John Carr.

vein, he also used analogies that linked joints in the leg/foot with the hinges of wooden fixtures in houses.[15]

Hicks drew upon various media to communicate through his models as effectively as possible. He made films of models in action, and produced a series of photographs showing models demonstrating particular movements and potential injuries [Figure 23]. To show the workings of a 'simple hinge movement', he would use photographs of a model shifting from one position to another [Figure 24].[16] Cleanly executed drawings of models further demonstrated movement in the foot [Figure 25], helping viewers to visualise – to imagine and grasp – dynamic form and function. And with diagrams Hicks distilled his models of foot movement even further, honing them (and therefore the moving body part that they represented) into clear, sharply visible lines [Figure 26].

MODELLING MOVEMENT

Much of Hicks' model design was put into practice on and with paper. Finding ways to display how limbs twist, shift, rotate and maintain balance, Hicks sculpted, assembled and made visual

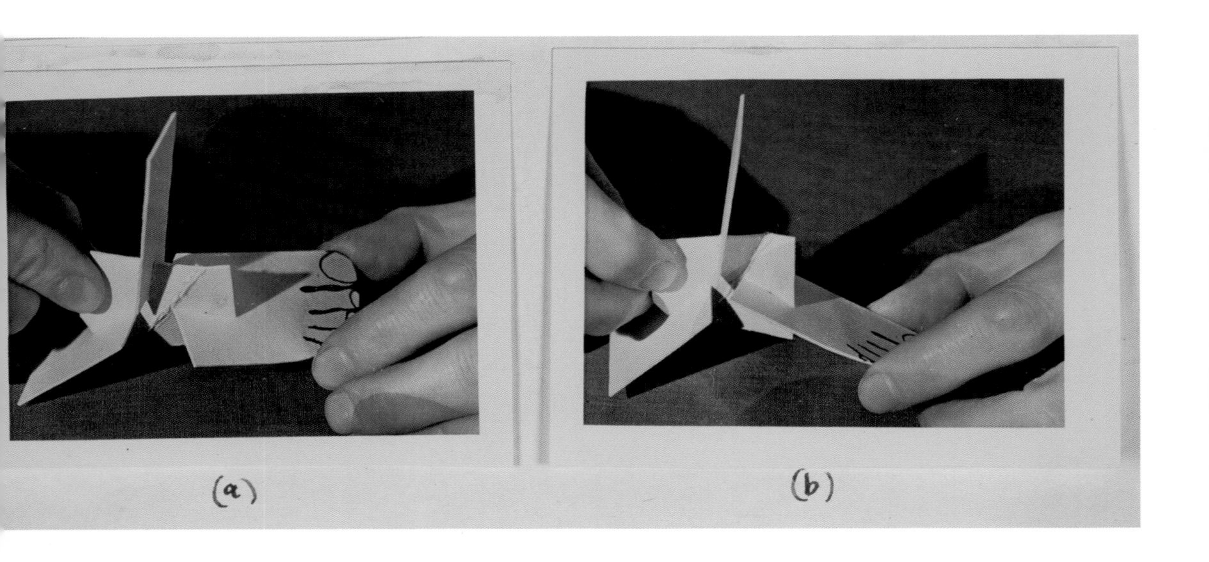

FIGURE 27
Photographs of John Hicks' cardboard model of the foot, made to demonstrate oblique (diagonal) hinge movement, 1950s.
Royal College of Surgeons of England. Photograph of original documents by John Carr.

images of models. With a range of visual media he brought his models to life – animated them – with assistance from hospital nurses and technicians.

Hicks modelled motion in the foot with cardboard, taking photographs to display how a model worked in 'demonstrating oblique (diagonal) hinge movement' [Figure 27; see Cat. 51].[17] Surviving negatives of these photographs in Hicks' archive at the RCS reveal how they were cropped for publication in his articles; the nurse operating the cardboard foot model was cut out of the frame, isolating and thereby focusing attention upon the model in action on the page [Figure 28]. A further negative shows another nurse demonstrating this model [Figure 29], indicating the collective nature of work associated with model-making and use.

Investigating limbs of the living as well as the dead, Hicks translated his observations into models [Figure 30]. He mapped the same structures, such as the arch of the foot, across 3D models [see Cat. 52–56], x-rays [Figure 31], outline tracings

FIGURE 28
An assistant operating John Hicks' model of the foot. This is a print from a photographic negative that was masked to frame the foot model for publication in a journal, 1950s.
Royal College of Surgeons of England.
Print by John Carr from original negative.

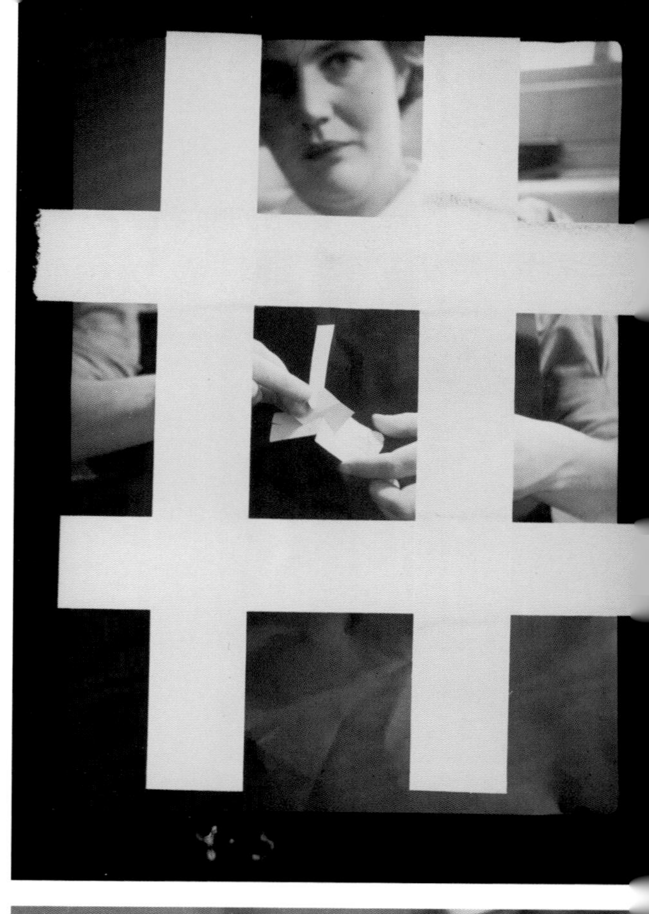

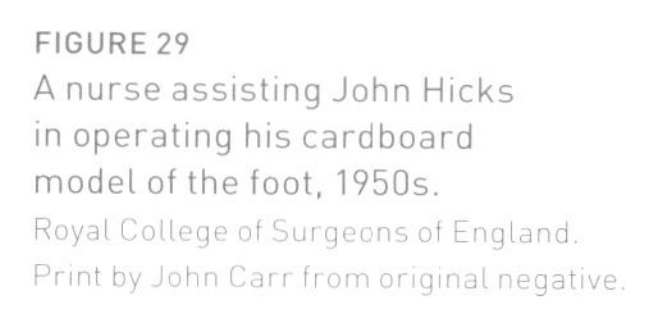

FIGURE 29
A nurse assisting John Hicks in operating his cardboard model of the foot, 1950s.
Royal College of Surgeons of England.
Print by John Carr from original negative.

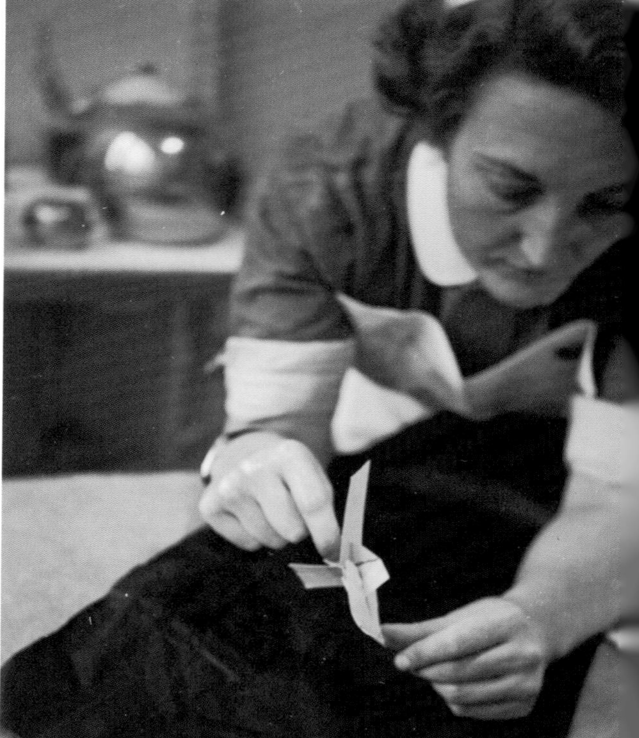

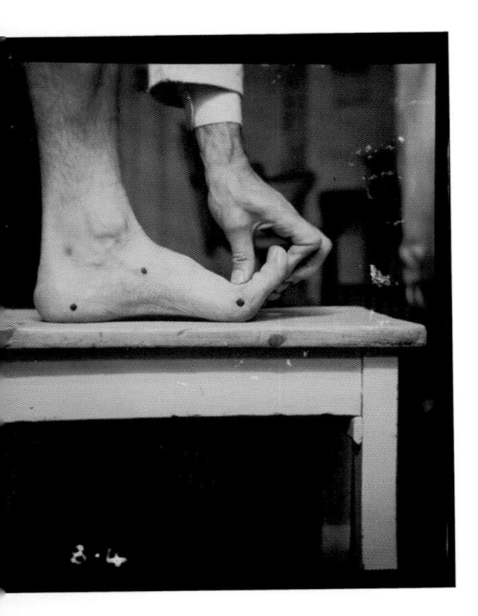

FIGURE 30
Photograph of John Hicks' investigations of the living foot, including the extension of the toe and rising of the arch, 1950s.
Royal College of Surgeons of England. Print by John Carr from original negative.

of those x-rays and sequences of minimal diagrams to develop and reinforce his anatomical descriptions of them. While Hicks modelled the arch of the foot as a rounded form, he also claimed the simplest way to depict it was as a triangle [Figure 32]. The triangle was central to his model for demonstrating what he described as the windlass mechanism, which happens when the big toe extends, the tissue underneath the foot shortens and the arch of the foot rises [see Cat. 54–56]. In describing this, Hicks used the image of the windlass, an apparatus with a winch mechanism often used to lift weights.

Just as Hicks' models helped him to study, understand and display movement in the foot and ankle, so did his sketches on paper. Outlines of foot anatomy and explorations of balance were worked out in this way [Figure 33], and repeated, rapidly drawn stick figures were for Hicks a means to analyse a wide range of everyday human movements, from rising off a chair to walking upstairs and standing on one leg [Figure 34].

Hicks' modelling of movement was directed towards improving medical provision and design work included that with fixation plates for helping bone fractures to heal. He produced models of fractures in arms and legs, displaying effective and ineffective fixation with metal plates [see Cat. 57–59]. Carrying

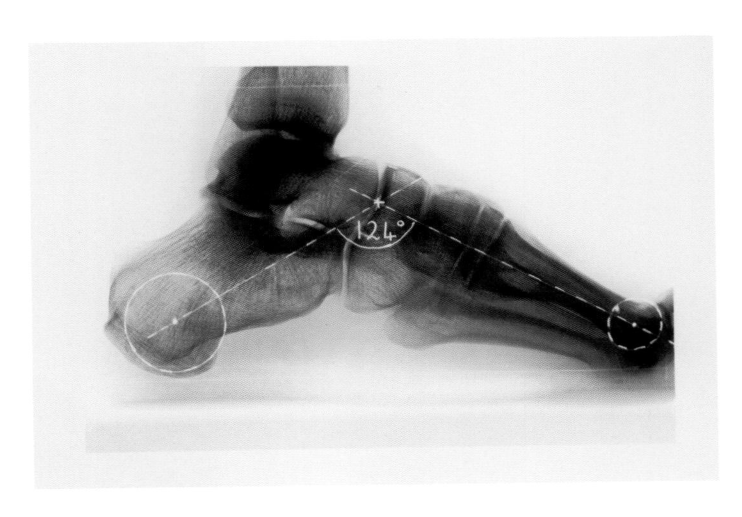

FIGURE 31
Photograph of an x-ray of the foot, used by John Hicks to investigate the arch of the foot when rising, 1953.
Royal College of Surgeons of England. Photograph by John Carr from original document.

FIGURE 32 (RIGHT)
John Herbert Hicks
Diagrams of bones and joints in the foot to illustrate the arch rising, the foot as a triangle (long/flat and short/high) and the windlass mechanism (unwound and wound up), 1950s.
Royal College of Surgeons of England. Photograph by John Carr.

FIGURE 33 (BELOW LEFT)
John Herbert Hicks
Diagram of the bones in the foot (tarsal and metatarsal) on tracing paper, drawn to investigate movements that maintain balance when standing (reverse of drawing shown here), 1950s.
Royal College of Surgeons of England. Photograph by John Carr.

FIGURE 34 (BELOW RIGHT)
John Herbert Hicks
Quick sketches of stick figures to investigate everyday movements such as rising from a chair, walking up stairs and standing on one leg, 1950s.
Royal College of Surgeons of England. Photograph by John Carr.

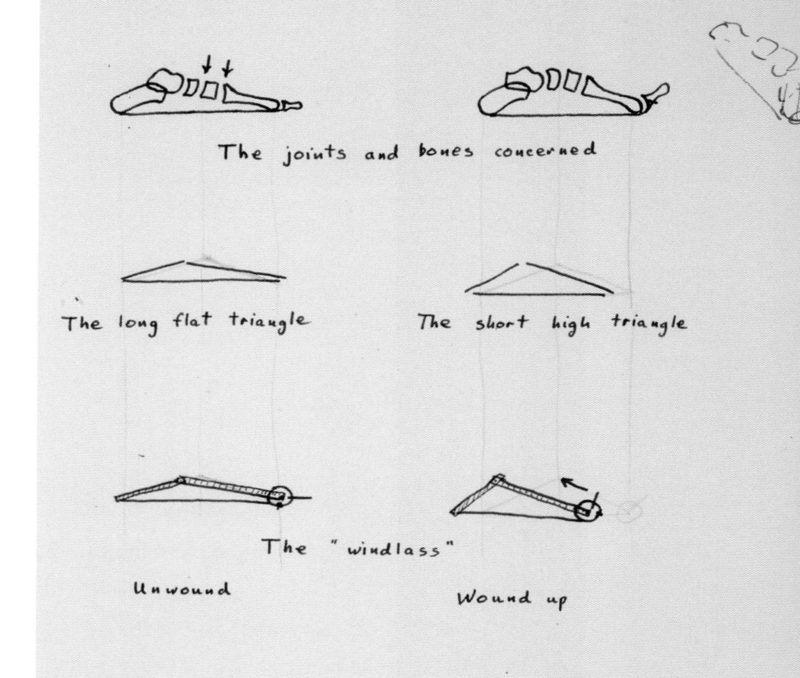

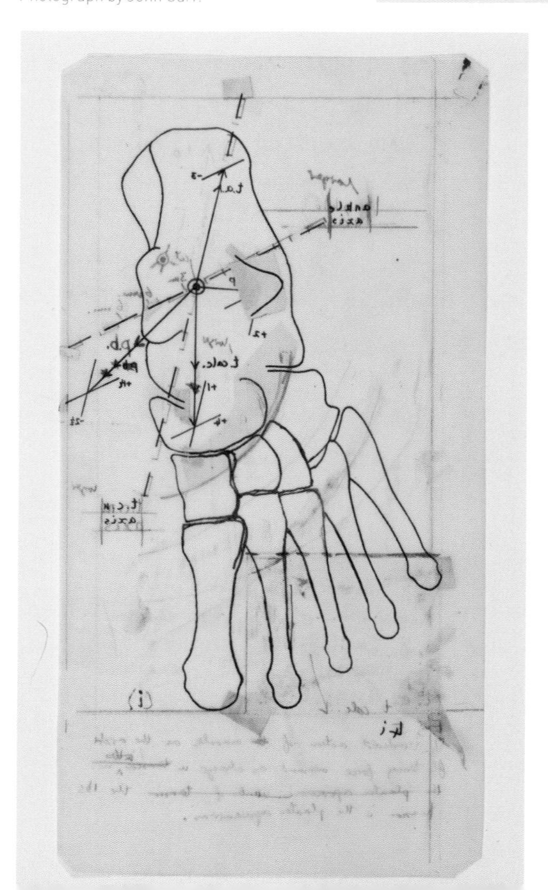

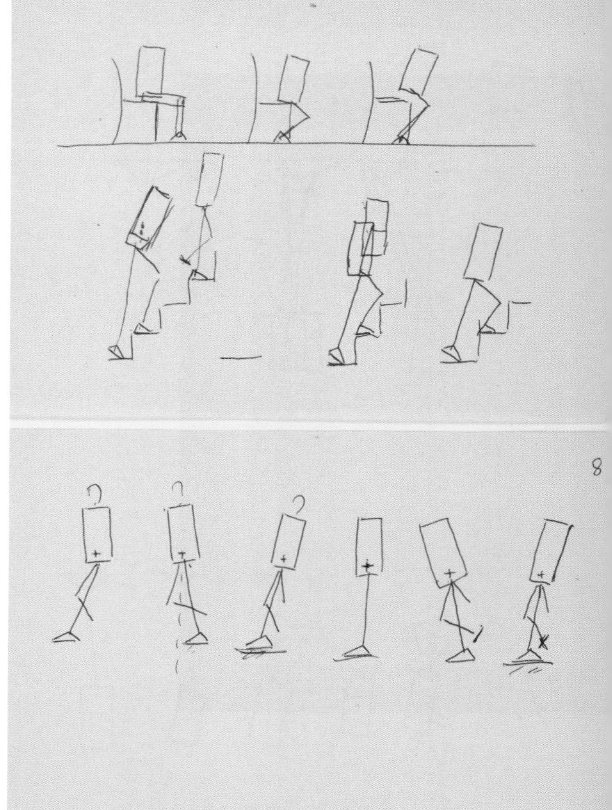

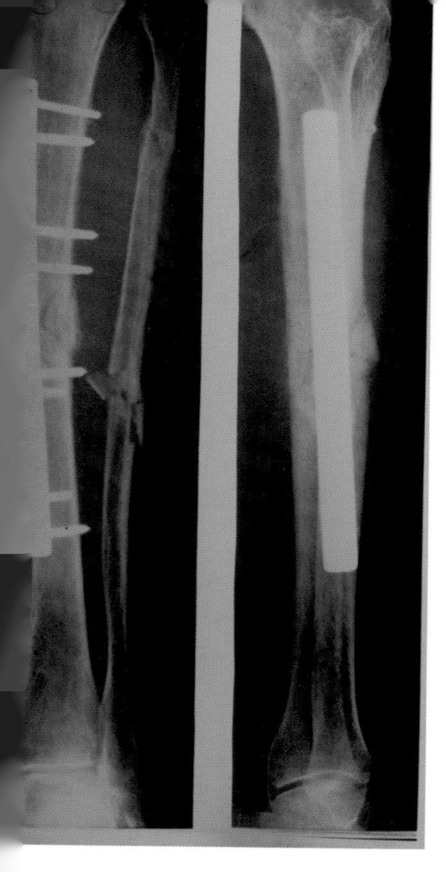

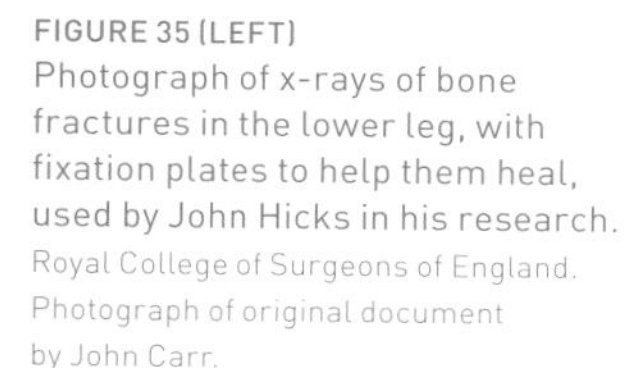

FIGURE 35 (LEFT)
Photograph of x-rays of bone fractures in the lower leg, with fixation plates to help them heal, used by John Hicks in his research.
Royal College of Surgeons of England. Photograph of original document by John Carr.

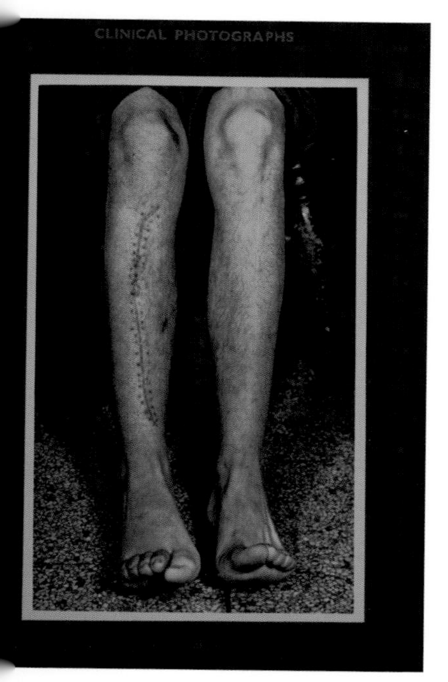

FIGURE 36 (BELOW LEFT)
Clinical photograph of a patient's legs following surgery for a fracture, used by John Hicks in his research.
Royal College of Surgeons of England. Photograph of original document by John Carr.

out investigations of these plates, Hicks made extensive, documented observations of patients' cases [Figures 35 and 36].

To encourage readers of his research articles to more fully understand his work, he suggested that readers themselves participate by making – and even becoming – anatomical models of feet. Thus Hicks suggested to readers:

> To overcome the difficulties of a description confined to the two dimensions of this page the reader if he wishes to be convinced of the essential simplicity of all this he must make for himself the cardboard model illustrated [see Figure 27].
>
> The essential part of the model is a piece of cardboard with an oblique (diagonal) fold across it.
>
> If the model is held [...] and moved about the hinge, foot movement will be simulated with surprising faithfulness.[18]

Hicks went on to instruct:

> If the reader has not done the experiment before perhaps he will now stand on one foot and observe the movements he makes to preserve his balance. He will see that his leg is constantly moving, rotating alternately a little one way and then the other.[19]

The reader became their own living anatomical model, just as – in medical schools – students were encouraged to act as models by observing the surface anatomy of their own bodies and those of fellow students, all while appropriately dressed.[20] By making and becoming models, readers of Hicks' work engaged with his descriptions of motion through the responsive movement of their own bodies.

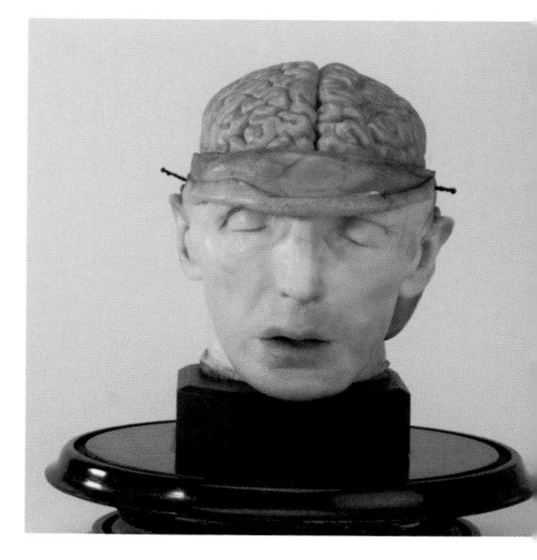

FIGURE 37
Joseph Towne
Wax model of the brain, mid to late 19th century.
Royal College of Surgeons of England. Photograph by John Carr.

DESIGNING BRAINS

> *'"Can you make a brain?" That was the key question.'*
> Martyn Cooke, 2015

Models that engage not only the eyes but also the hands of medical students have become important teaching resources in Britain, especially from the mid-20th century onwards. Wax models from the 1800s, such as those of Joseph Towne [Figure 37, see Chapter 3] tended to be redefined as 'historical' artefacts rather than models with which to learn current anatomy; this shift into the category of valuable artefact from the past reinforced their status as 'hands-off' exhibits. Just as there was growth in commercial plastic models for teaching anatomy, so too the interest rose in models for simulating the bodily – especially tactile – experience of medical and surgical procedures. Adam,Rouilly in London, for example, while marketing and distributing models of anatomy made by Somso®, began to develop and manufacture models for demonstrating and practising skills in patient care and surgery from the 1930s. In the past 30 years, surgical simulation in medical training has accelerated, along with developments in medical imaging and digital technologies.

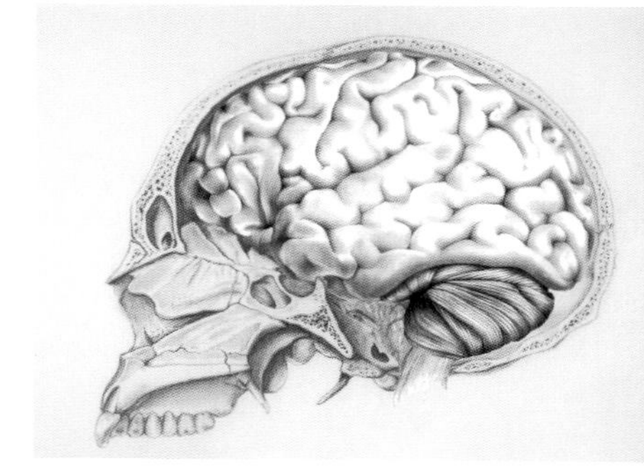

FIGURE 38
Lydia Carline
Drawing produced during the development of MARTYN at the RCS, 2013.
Courtesy of Lydia Carline.

Designing models to train in advanced surgical procedures often involves teams of people who have many different contributing skills.[21] At the RCS in 2011, when Major David Baxter, a neurosurgeon in the Royal Army Medical Corps, asked if a brain and skull could be made for training in head-trauma surgery, a collaborative and ongoing design process began, led by Martyn Cooke, Head of Conservation in the Museums Department.[22] The team also drew in medical artist Lydia Carline and Imperial College London medical student Claudia Craven.

The agreed aim was to make a model that allowed trainee surgeons to practise surgery in preparation for cases of emergency head injury. MARTYN had to be makeable within the museum laboratory facilities at the RCS and it had to be useable by junior trainees, who would gain practical experience of several procedures with the model, including cutting into the skull and draining fluid from the brain. Such practice is intended to increase the skill of surgeons and therefore the safety of patients undergoing operations. These requirements established a framework for the process of model design, and informed the choice of key modelling materials and methods. Central to the latter was casting, a method that Cooke was already familiar with from previous projects.

Research and development for MARTYN required sketching, drawing [Figure 38] and, crucially, exploration of materials for creating the 3D model. Cooke carried out a series of tests with materials for making the model in several parts. For casting the brain, gelatine variants mixed with other substances were trialled [Figure 39], as were methods for adding colour to the model brain. Acrylic paint would not properly mix with the gelatine brain material [Figure 40] but watercolour paint was found to mix well, and a blend of white, yellow and grey was used to produce a uniform approximation of living brain colour [see Cat. 67]. Failed and rejected materials were recorded for future reference. For casting the skull, Cooke explored Cascamite® wood glue (powder) mixed with water [Figure 41] and variations of silicone rubber with different densities for making muscle [Figure 42]. The modelled *dura mater* (a membrane lining the inside of the skull) was tested in rice paper, which had a convincing feel when wet but was far too crispy when dry.

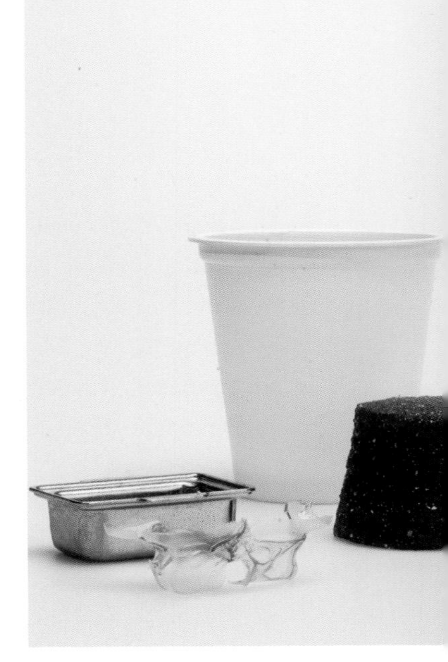

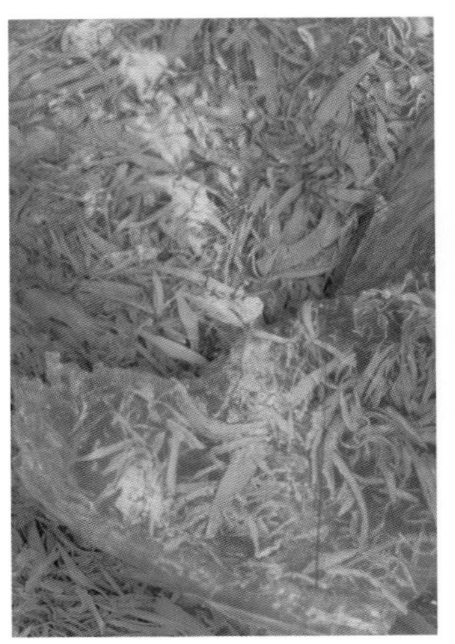

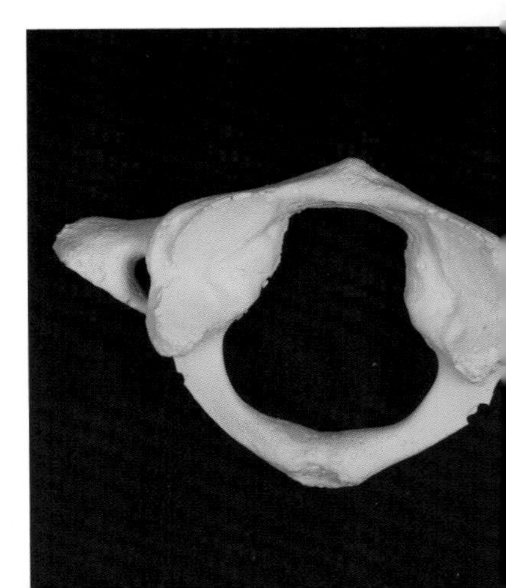

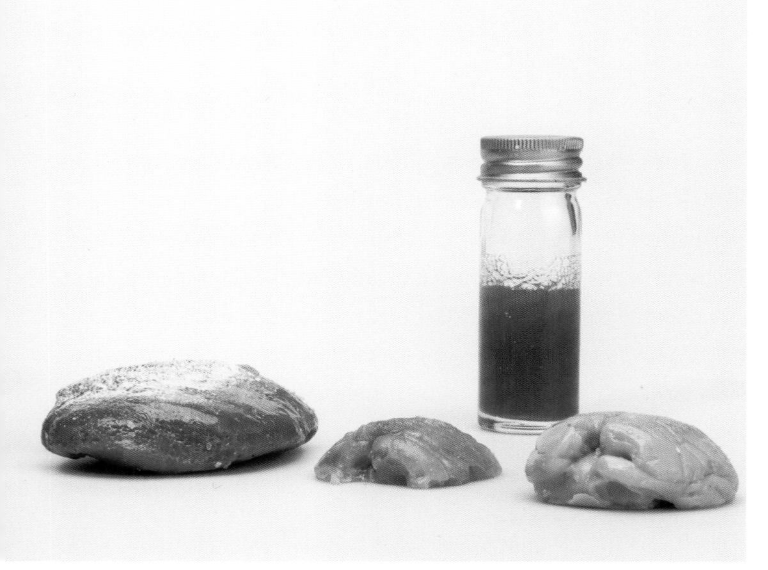

FIGURE 39
Six tests of materials – gelatine variants mixed with other substances – for casting the brain in MARTYN, with two containers used as moulds (left).
Photograph by John Carr.

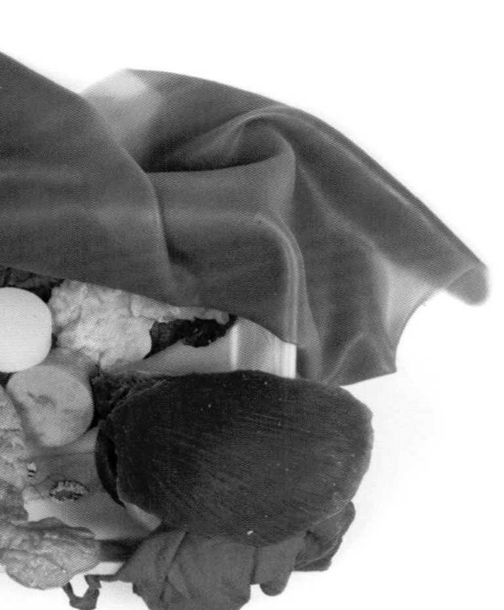

FIGURE 40 (LEFT)
Tests with gelatine and acrylic paint to find a colour for the brain in MARTYN. The paint was rejected as it would not mix properly.
Photograph by John Carr.

FIGURE 42 (RIGHT)
Exploring materials: variations of silicone rubber. One was selected for the muscle in MARTYN (muscle shown at bottom right of box).
Photograph by John Carr.

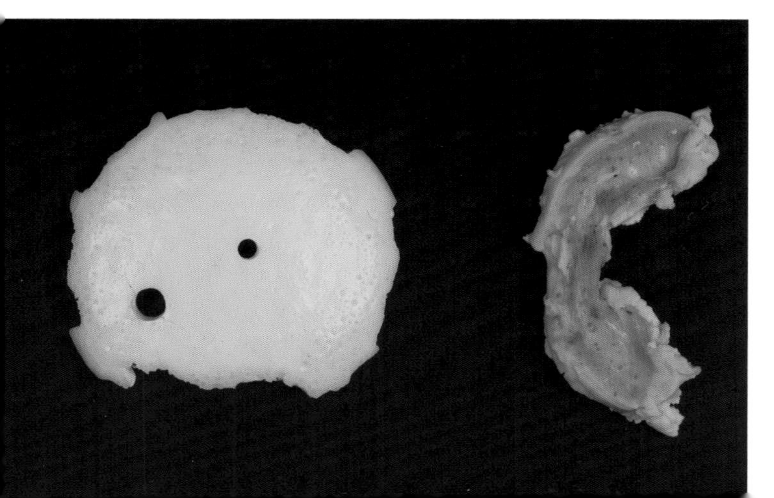

FIGURE 41
Three tests of materials – Cascamite®, powdered wood glue mixed with water – for casting the skull in MARTYN. This material was rejected as it took too long to set.
Photograph by John Carr.

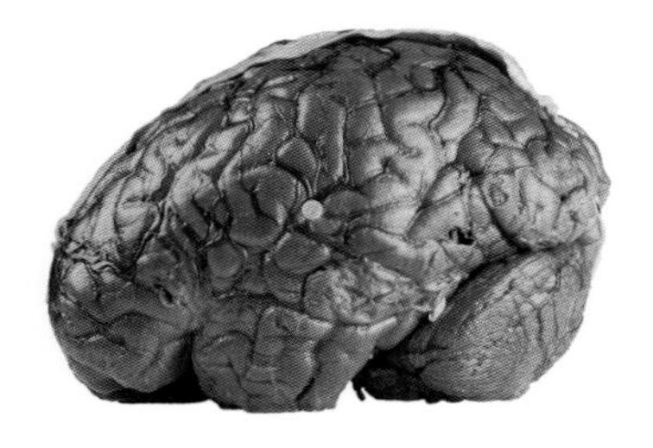

FIGURE 43 (ABOVE)
The preserved human brain that was studied to produce a model of a brain. The model was then cast to create a mould in which the brain in MARTYN could be repeatedly cast.
Royal College of Surgeons of England. Photograph by Michael Frank.

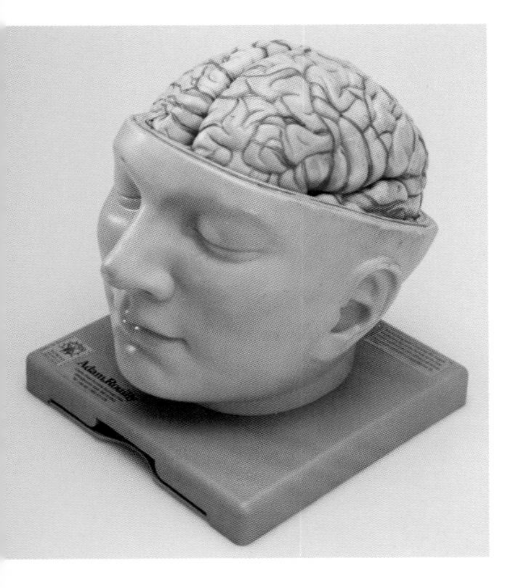

FIGURE 44 (ABOVE)
Plastic model of the head and brain, by Somso® models from Adam,Rouilly.
Wellcome Museum of Anatomy, RCS. Photograph by John Carr.

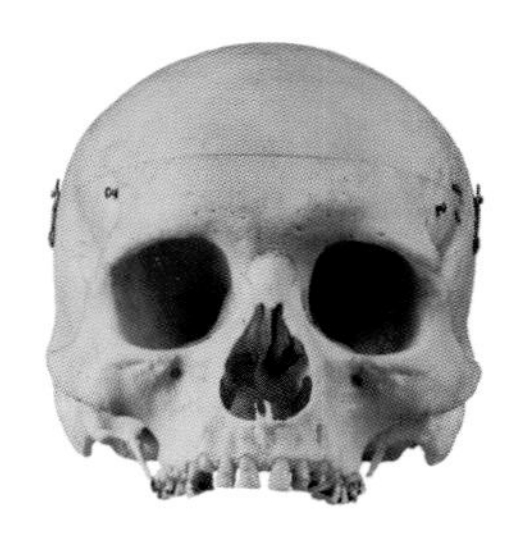

FIGURE 46 (ABOVE)
Human adult skull (without mandible). A skull similar to this was cast to produce a mould from which the skull in MARTYN could be repeatedly cast.
Royal College of Surgeons of England. Photograph by Michael Frank.

The selection of materials for MARTYN was guided as much by their expense, and the ease with which they could be obtained and worked with, as by their resemblance to the relevant parts of the living human head in both look and feel. Visual resemblance was deemed important but the feel of it was crucial, given that MARTYN was to be a hands-on training device. Cooke consulted with surgeons on the feel of test materials to ensure the most appropriate choice was made based on their experience of operating procedures.

To create a flexible silicone mould for casting the model brain in MARTYN, an initial model brain was crafted using modelling wax. Making this modelled brain with the appropriate shape and surface structures involved close visual study of a preserved human brain specimen from the Wellcome Museum of Anatomy [Figure 43]. Further models of the brain, especially a Somso® model [Figure 44], were also studied to guide this modelling. The brain made in modelling wax was then cast in silicone – bound with retaining walls assembled with LEGO® bricks – to form a mould [Figure 45]. Using this mould, the brain model in MARTYN could be repeatedly cast in a gelatin mixture. To create spaces for the model brain's ventricles [fluid-filled cavities; see Cat. 5], clay ventricles were positioned in the mould before the gelatin mixture was poured around them to cast the brain (each clay ventricle was later removed to create a cavity).

Just as a human brain specimen was used to create a mould, so a human skull [Figure 46] was cast to make a silicone mould from which the skull in MARTYN could be repeatedly cast. The MARTYN skull, like the MARTYN brain, was cast in two halves using polyurethane resin [Figure 47]. The *dura mater* was painted on in latex [Figure 48], and the two halves of the skull containing the modelled brain (with ventricles filled with paraffin to represent cerebrospinal fluid) were then assembled together and fixed with resin (Figure 49). Muscles (temporalis) cast in silicone were attached to the fully assembled MARTYN [see Cat. 61].

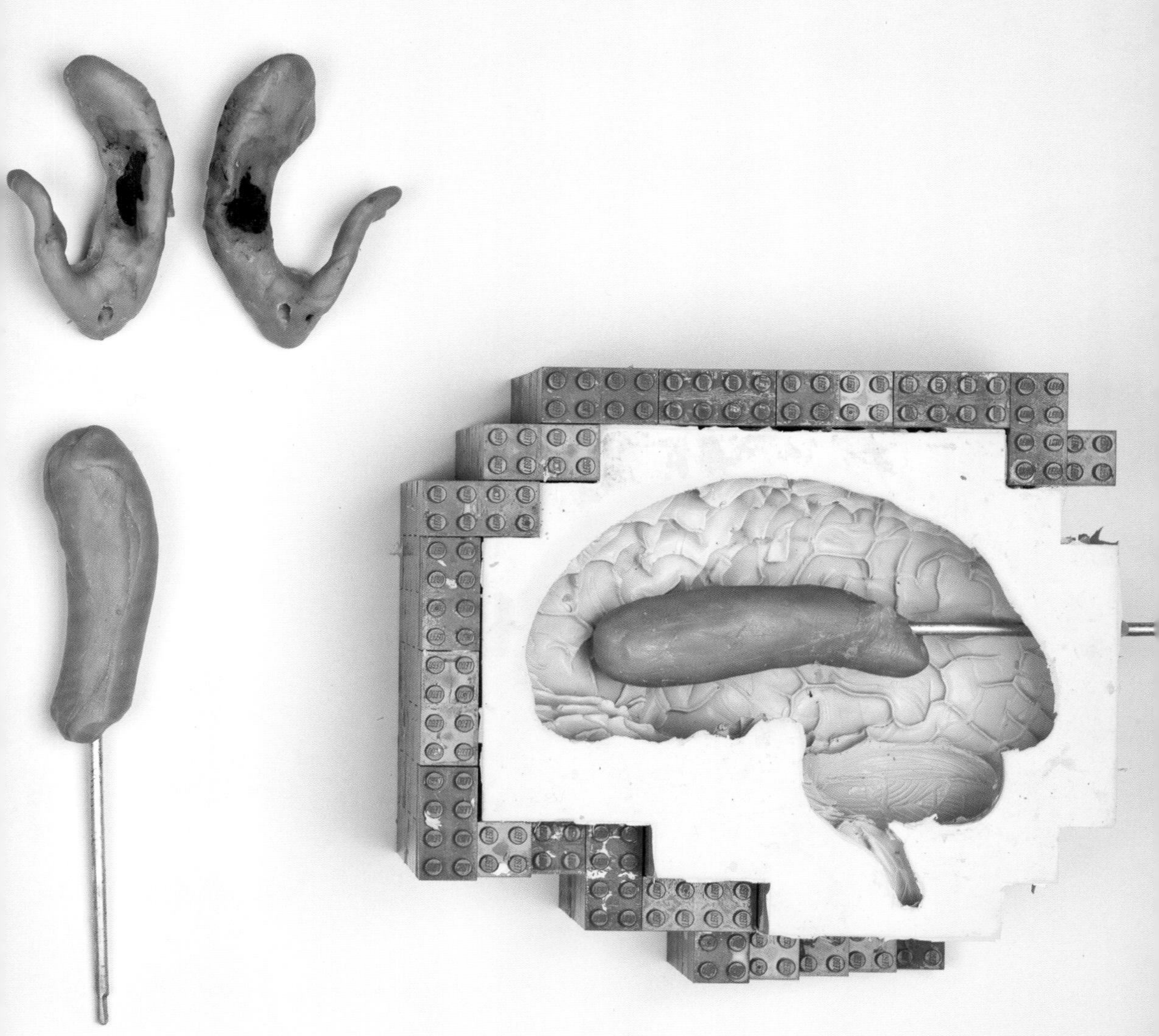

FIGURE 45
Silicone brain mould (one half of a pair) with LEGO® retaining walls, and a second-generation modelled ventricle inserted, for casting the brain in MARTYN (right). First-generation modelled ventricles (top, left) and second-generation model ventricle (bottom, left).
Photograph by John Carr.

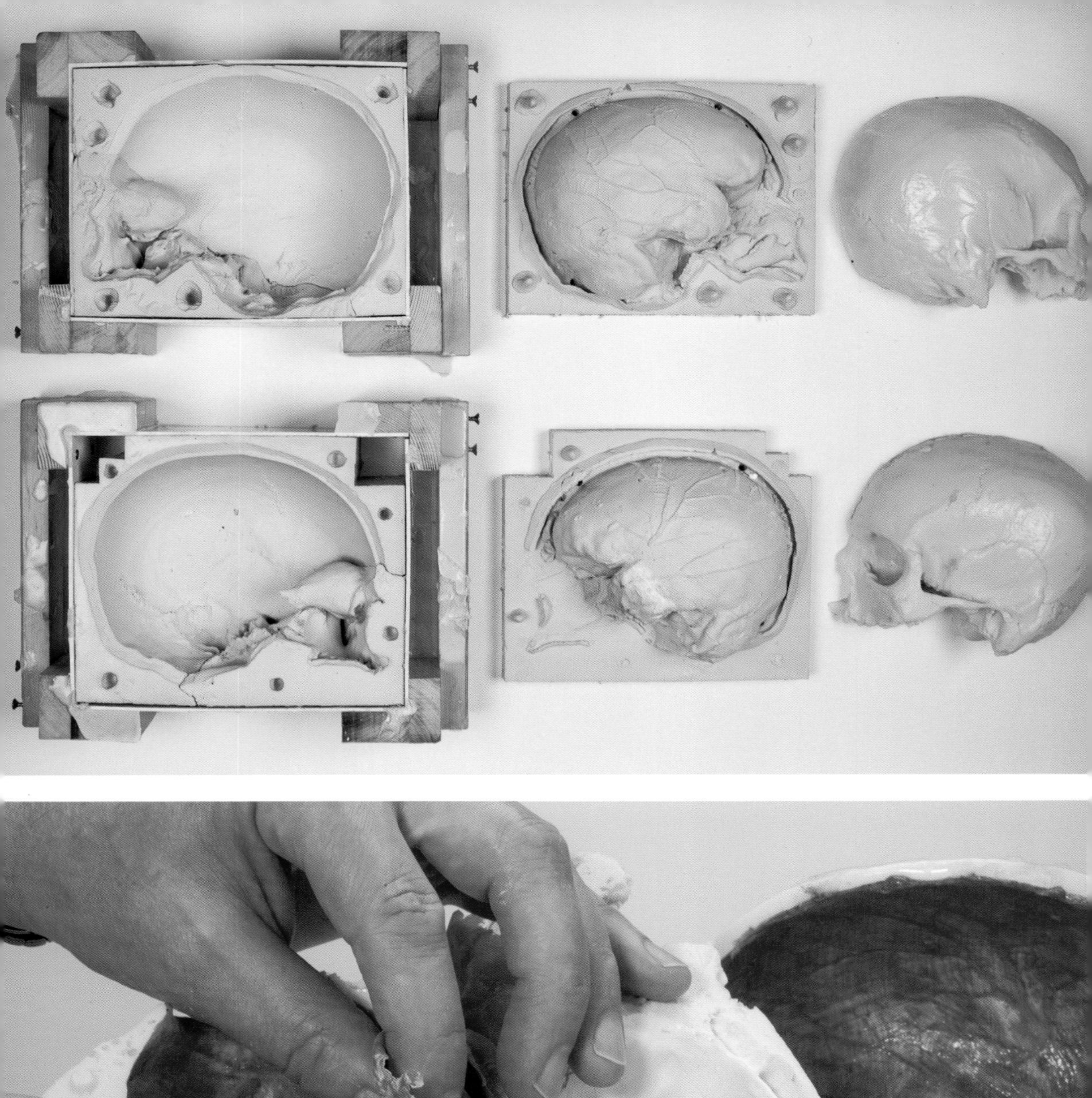

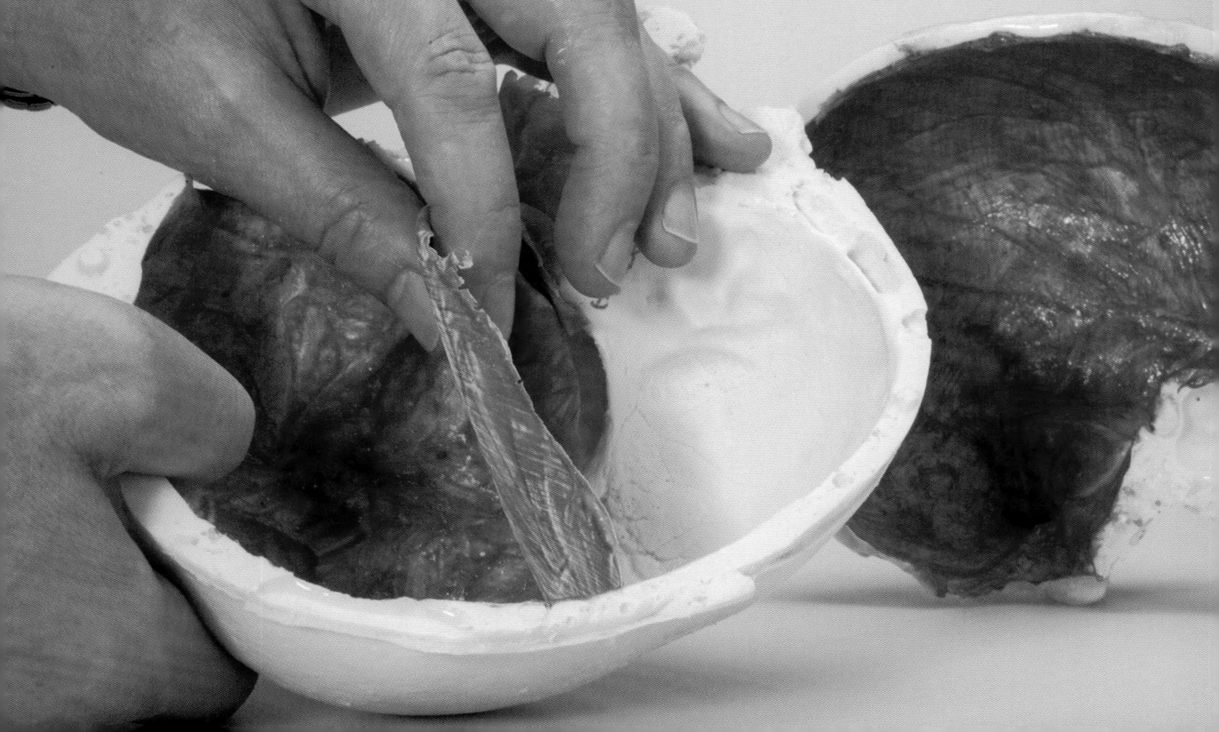

FIGURE 47 (LEFT)
Two pairs of silicone moulds (left and centre) for casting two halves of the skull in MARTYN (right).
Photograph by John Carr.

FIGURE 48 (LEFT)
Making the latex *dura mater* in MARTYN.
Photograph by John Carr.

Further experiments undertaken as part of MARTYN's design included attempts to work out how best to create the ventricle cavities inside the model brain. The first step had been to work up free-hand clay models of the ventricles based on Tompsett's casts of this part of the brain [see Cat. 5]. These initial ventricle models for MARTYN were carefully shaped and the aim was to place these in the brain cast so that they could be removed later, thereby creating the ventricle cavities [see Figure 45, top left]. These proved too difficult to remove from the cast brain. A further step was to model the ventricles in ice and then use these ice models to create the cavity, as the ice would melt away to leave a cavity inside the brain. Again, the plan failed. The solution so far has been to place very simplified clay ventricles inside the cast brain [see Figure 45, bottom left and inside brain mould], which can be easily removed.

Designing MARTYN to date has involved sequences of improvised solutions to problems occurring as plans are put into action and modified in practice.

SIMULATING SURGERY

MARTYN is designed to simulate the look, feel, texture and weight of a human skull and brain for purposes of surgical training. Although it simplifies the head, reducing it to six main model

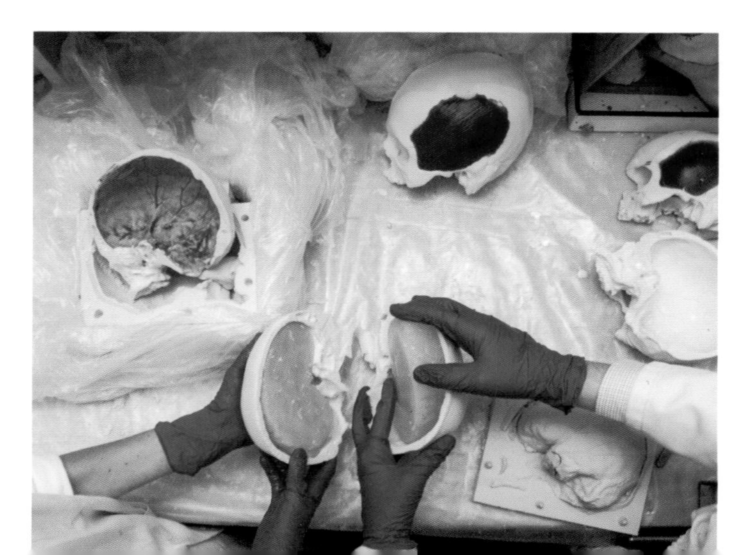

FIGURE 49 (RIGHT)
Assembling two halves of the cast brain and skull of MARTYN in the laboratory, Museums Conservation Unit, RCS, 2013.
Photograph by John Carr.

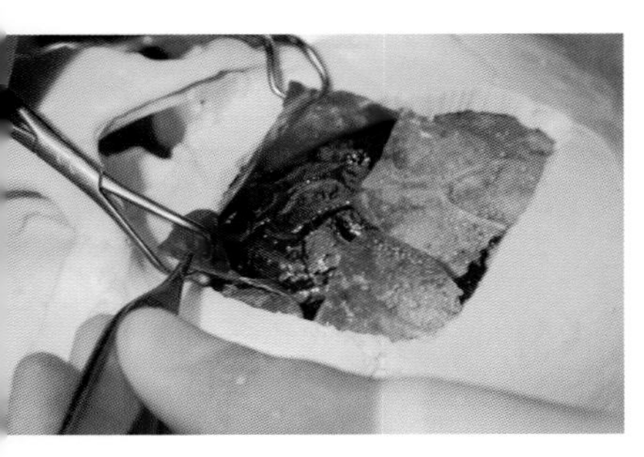

FIGURE 50
Testing the MARTYN prototype: a hole was cut in the skull and the ***dura mater*** peeled back to reveal the brain, 2012.
Photograph by John Carr.

components – brain, ventricles, cerebrospinal fluid, *dura mater*, skull and muscle – the model aims for 'visual and tactile' realism.[23] MARTYN is made to seem like a real, live head to facilitate learning. This life-like quality is seen as advantageous when compared with surgical training with the use of deceased, preserved bodies.

To mobilise MARTYN as an effective 'training tool', it has been used in specially designed workshops at the RCS since 2011.[24] Prior to use by students, the first MARTYN prototype [see Cat. 63] was trialled [Figure 50] so that students' potential experiences of the model could be anticipated. Trainees performed the recommended surgical procedures with the model at the RCS [Figure 51] and provided feedback on the experience. Cooke and further participants in the making of MARTYN take note of such responses to the model in action so that improvements can be implemented. One issue under consideration is the dust that is created when the modelled skull is drilled [Figure 52]. The model's design thus continues to evolve as it is put to work, evaluated and improved through dialogues between makers and users. Used models that have been taken apart in learning workshops have been retained so that they can be used to devise improved versions [see Cat. 64–66].

Recent developments of MARTYN have involved the design of further generations of the model, some fitted with pathologies

FIGURE 51 (BELOW)
Trainees learning surgical procedures using MARTYN, head injury course, RCS, 2012.
Photograph by John Carr.

FIGURE 52 (BELOW RIGHT)
Hands-on training with MARTYN, 2012.
Photograph by John Carr.

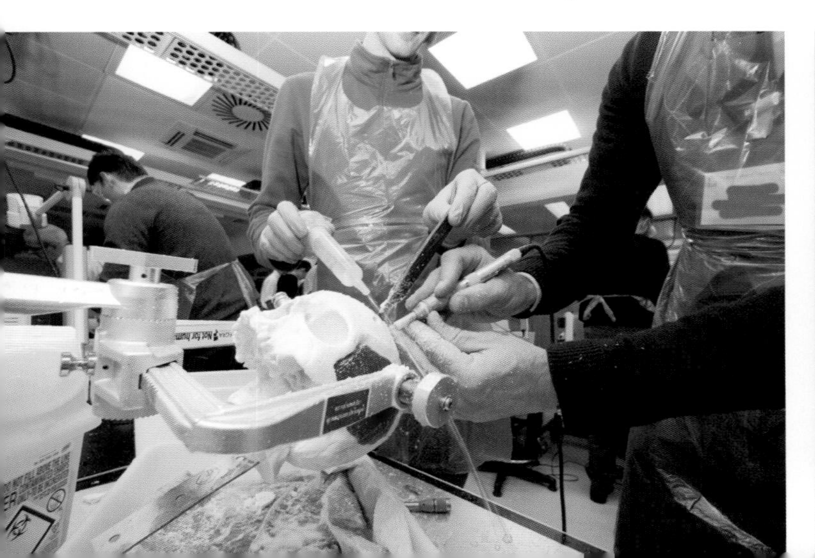

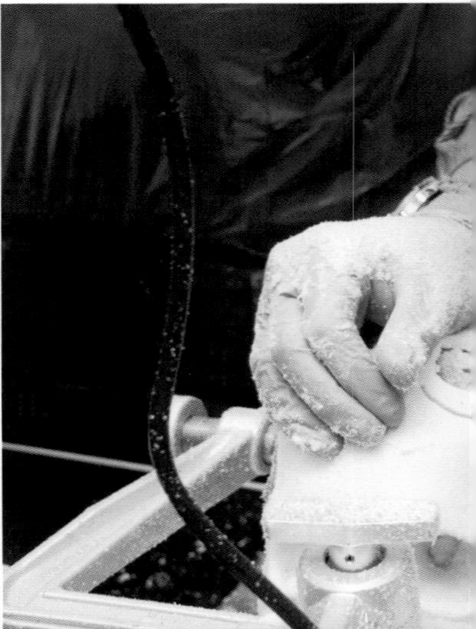

such as blood clots and aneurysms (a bulge in a blood vessel due to weakness in it) [see Cat. 68–70], for training in a wider range of procedures. A Paediatric MARTYN is also currently in its early stages, as Martyn Cooke collaborates with professional medical model-maker Clare Rangeley [see Cat. 71–76]. Modelling methods developed in the making of MARTYN are being adapted in the making of this version for training in surgery performed on infants. Again, the model was initially derived from a human skull in the Wellcome Museum of Anatomy [Figure 53]. Drawing on recent technological innovations, the infant skull was printed in 3D (initially at the wrong size by mistake) [Figure 54] and the (correctly sized) print was then cast to create the skull in Paediatric MARTYN. The design of this latest version of MARTYN – MARTYN's next of kin – thus combines a range of techniques and technologies in its collaborative design.

To date, about 53 MARTYN models have been produced at the RCS and put to work in hands-on surgical training at the RCS, Imperial College London and in Edinburgh.

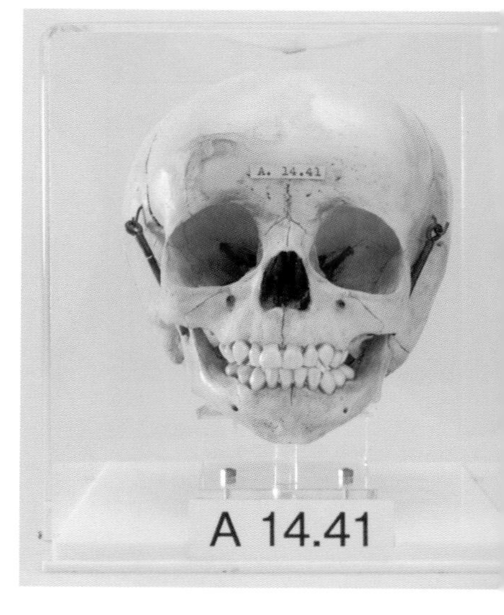

FIGURE 53 (ABOVE)
Skull of an infant, around 1900, from which a 3D print was made, for casting the skull in Paediatric MARTYN.
Wellcome Museum of Anatomy, RCS.
Photograph by John Carr.

FIGURE 54 (BELOW)
3D printing of the infant skull: first print at the wrong size (left), second print at the correct size (right); the second print was used to cast Paediatric MARTYN.
Photograph by John Carr.

MATERIAL DESIGN IN PRACTICE

These three striking sets of models at the RCS have been designed for different purposes in a variety of materials, each set building up within particular working environments and giving

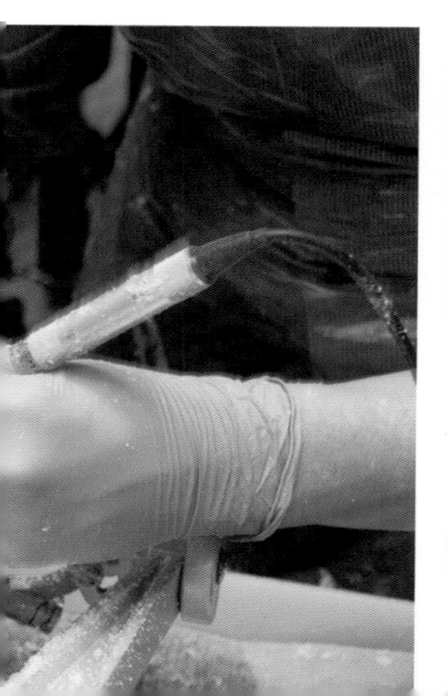

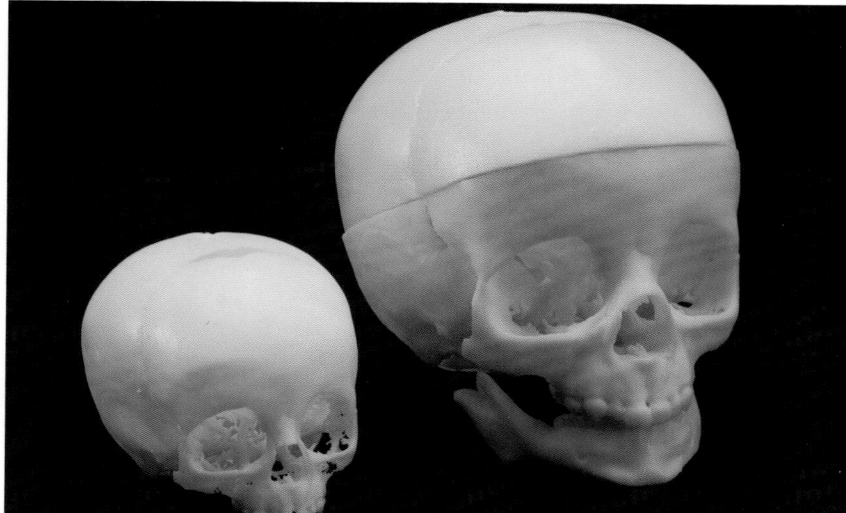

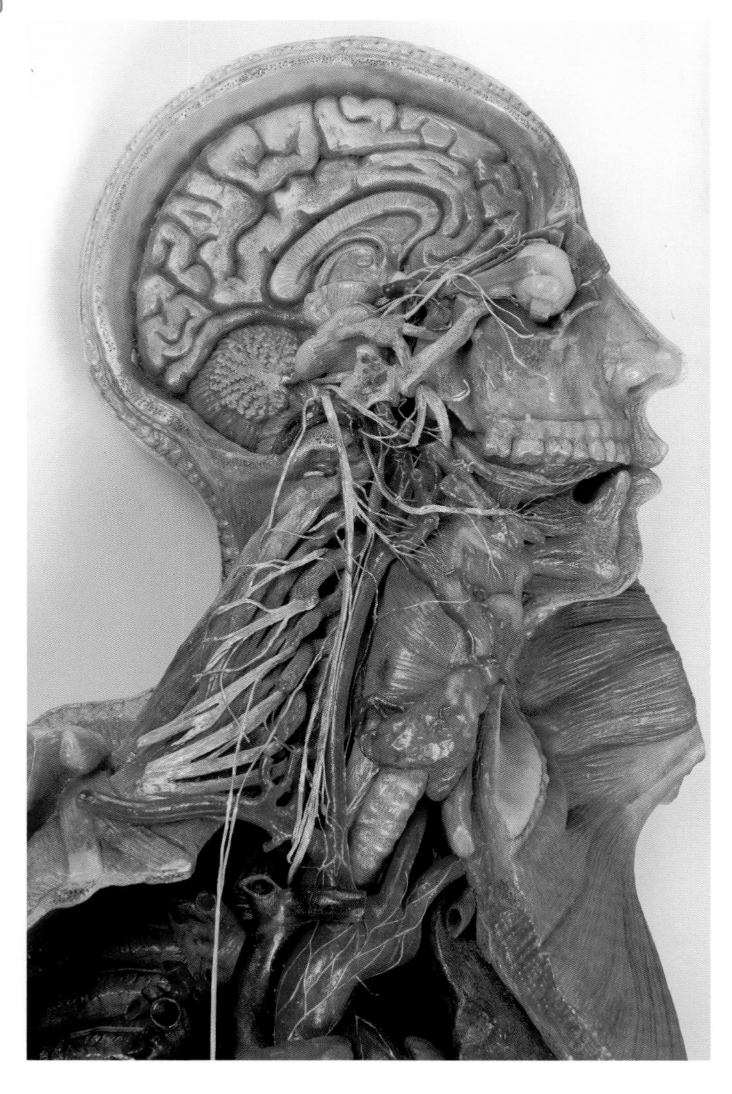

FIGURE 55
Rudolf Weisker
Wax anatomical model,
around 1877, Leipzig.
University of Aberdeen, Anatomy Museum.
Photograph by John McIntosh.

form to the human body in distinctive ways. These sets of models are related in terms of their emphasis on the utility of mundane, everyday materials for modelling the body, with techniques that are accessible or can be learnt in a hands-on or DIY way. This 3D improvised in-house modelling is designed to investigate and communicate in specific settings for anatomical and surgical learning. Such careful design – attuned to particular medical issues and requirements – is what makes them so effective and compelling.

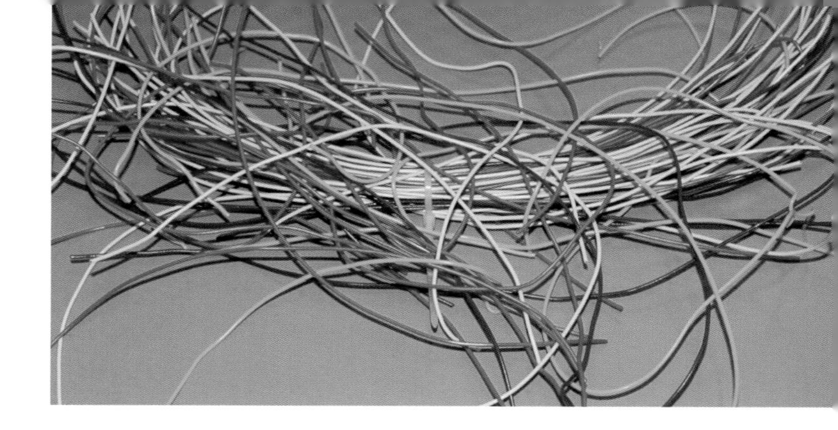

FIGURE 57
Plastic-coated wire used to model nerves, at the University of Aberdeen, Anatomy Facility, School of Medicine and Dentistry, 2010.
Photograph by Elizabeth Hallam.

The RCS' models explored in this book and related exhibition can be interpreted within a broad trajectory that shifts from 19th-century wax models designed predominantly for the eyes [Figure 55], through plastic models for handling [Figure 56], to models that require more active making and engaged participation on the part of the learner [Figure 57]. Yet in practice, each of these phases of material model design has not fully displaced their predecessors. Many bodies modelled in three dimensions persist over time, are reinterpreted and used in previously unanticipated ways, just as existing materials for anatomical and surgical design can be rejuvenated and infused with new meanings alongside new materials that offer up further possibilities for modelling the human body.

NOTES

1. Nick Hopwood, *Embryos in Wax: Models from the Ziegler Studio* (Cambridge and Bern: Whipple Museum of the History of Science, University of Cambridge; Institute of the History of Medicine, University of Bern, 2002, reprinted 2013); Anna Maerker, 'Anatomizing the trade: designing and marketing anatomical models as medical technologies, ca. 1700–1900', *Technology and Culture*, 54 (2013), 531–62.
2. Elizabeth Hallam, 'Anatomical Design: Making and Using Three-Dimensional Models of the Human Body', in Wendy Gunn, Ton Otto and Rachel Charlotte Smith, eds, *Design Anthropology: Theory and Practice* (London: Bloomsbury, 2013), 100–16.
3. LH Hamlyn and Patricia Thilesen, 'Models in medical teaching, with a note on the use of a new plastic', *The Lancet*, 5 September 1953, 472–75, p. 472; George Blaine, 'Biological teaching models and specimens', *The Lancet*, 25 August 1951, 337–40, p. 339.
4. Blaine, 'Biological teaching models and specimens', p. 339.
5. AJ Barson and RAH Neave, 'Teaching models of abnormal infants', *Medical Education*, 11 (1977), 136–38; Richard Neave, 'Pictures in the

round: moulage and models in medicine', *Journal of Audiovisual Media in Medicine*, 12 (1989), 80–84.

6. DH Tompsett, *Anatomical Techniques*, 1st Edition (Edinburgh: E&S Livingstone Ltd., 1956).
7. Tompsett, *Anatomical Techniques*, p. 95.
8. Elizabeth Hallam, 'Anatomopoeia', in Elizabeth Hallam and Tim Ingold, eds, *Making and Growing: Anthropological Studies of Organisms and Artefacts* (Farnham: Ashgate, 2014), 65–88.
9. Anon. 'Future of the medical museum', *The Lancet*, 24 March 1945, 376–77, p. 376; Royal College of Physicians of London, *Planning Committee Report on Medical Education* (London: Harrison and Sons Ltd., 1944), p. 13.
10. DH Tompsett, 'The bronchopulmonary segments', *Medical History*, 9 (1965), 177–81.
11. Tompsett, *Anatomical Techniques,* p. 3, p. 95; DH Tompsett, *Anatomical Techniques*, 2nd Edition (Edinburgh: E&S Livingstone Ltd., 1970), p. 74.
12. D Brown, 'Review of Anatomical Techniques, by DH Tompsett', *British Medical Journal*, 1 (1957), 689.
13. JH Hicks, 'The mechanics of the foot. I. The joints', *Journal of Anatomy*, 87 (1953), 345–57; JH Hicks, 'The mechanics of the foot. II. The plantar aponeurosis and the arch', *Journal of Anatomy*, 88 (1954), 25–30, plate I; JH Hicks, archival materials, 1949–1993 (53 boxes), MS0186, RCS Archive.
14. JH Hicks, 'The mechanics of the foot. I. The joints', p. 354.
15. JH Hicks, 'Mechanics of the Foot: The Posterior Hinge Movement', p. 13, typescript, around 1955, MS0186/3/2, RCS Archive.
16. Hicks, 'The mechanics of the foot. I. the joints p. 356.
17. JH Hicks, 'Mechanics of the foot: the joints', p. 24, typescript, around 1953, MS0186/3/5, RCS Archive.
18. Hicks, 'Mechanics of the foot: the posterior hinge movement', p. 15.
19. JH Hicks, 'Mechanics of the foot III: the 'windlass', p. 12, manuscript, early 1950s, MS0186/3/3, RCS Archive.
20. RD Lockhart, *Living Anatomy: A photographic atlas of muscles in action and surface colours* (London: Faber and Faber, 1948).
21. Rachel Prentice, *Bodies in Formation: An Ethnography of Anatomy and Surgery Education* (Durham, NC: Duke University Press, 2013).
22. Martyn Cooke, 'Surgical simulation: the way ahead', *Bulletin of The Royal College of Surgeons of England*, 95 (2013), 158.
23. Claudia Craven, David Baxter, Martyn Cooke, Lydia Carline, Samuel JMM Alberti, Jonathan Beard and Mary Murphy, 'Development of a modelled anatomical replica for training young neurosurgeons', *British Journal of Neurosurgery*, 28 (2014), 707–12, p. 707.
24. Craven et al., 'Development of a modelled anatomical replica for training young neurosurgeons'.

FIGURE 56 (OPPOSITE)
Plastic model of the hand, 2005, by Somso® from Adam,Rouilly.
University of Aberdeen, Anatomy Museum. Photograph by John McIntosh.

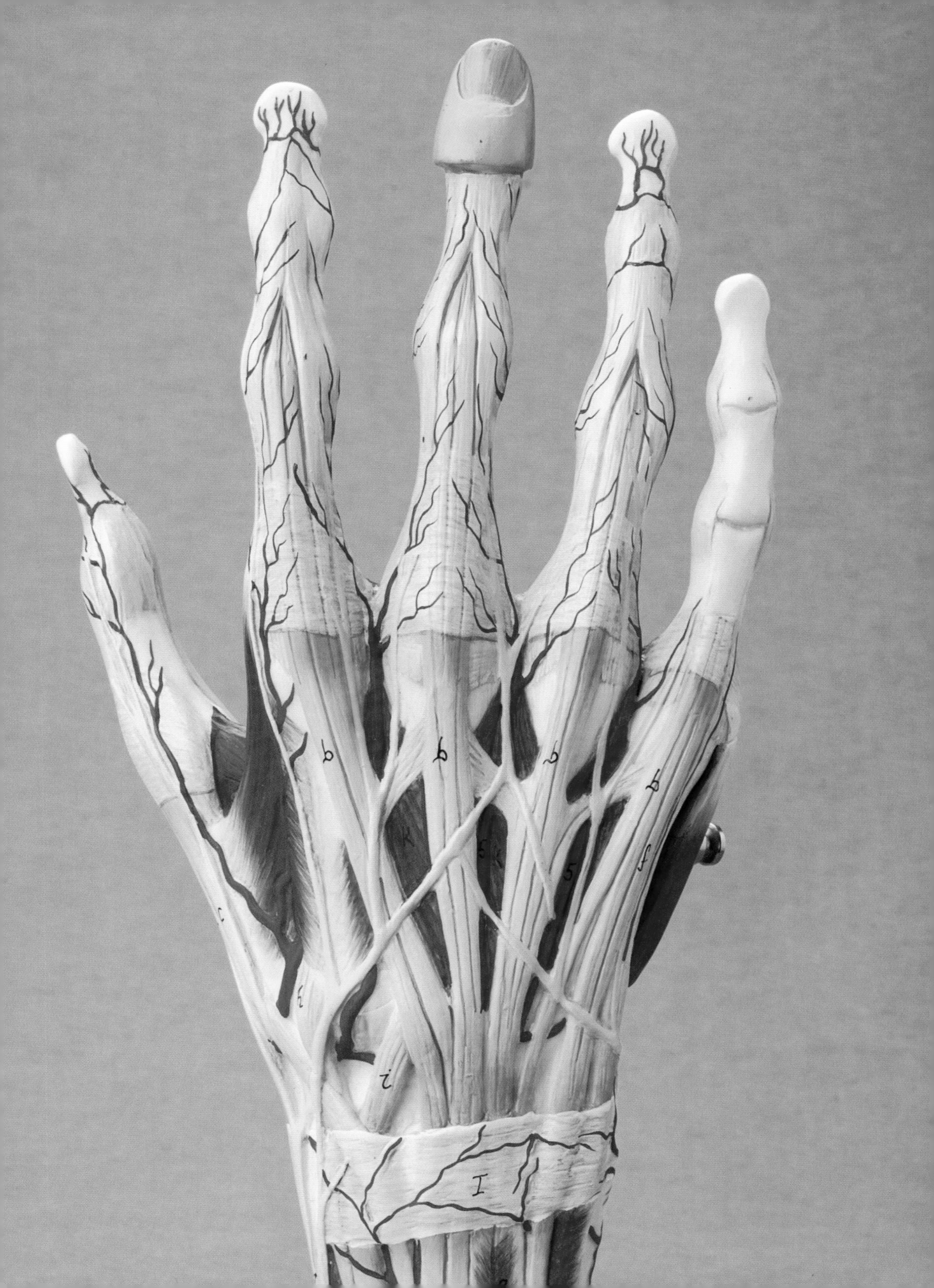
b
b
b
b
k
f
h
i
I

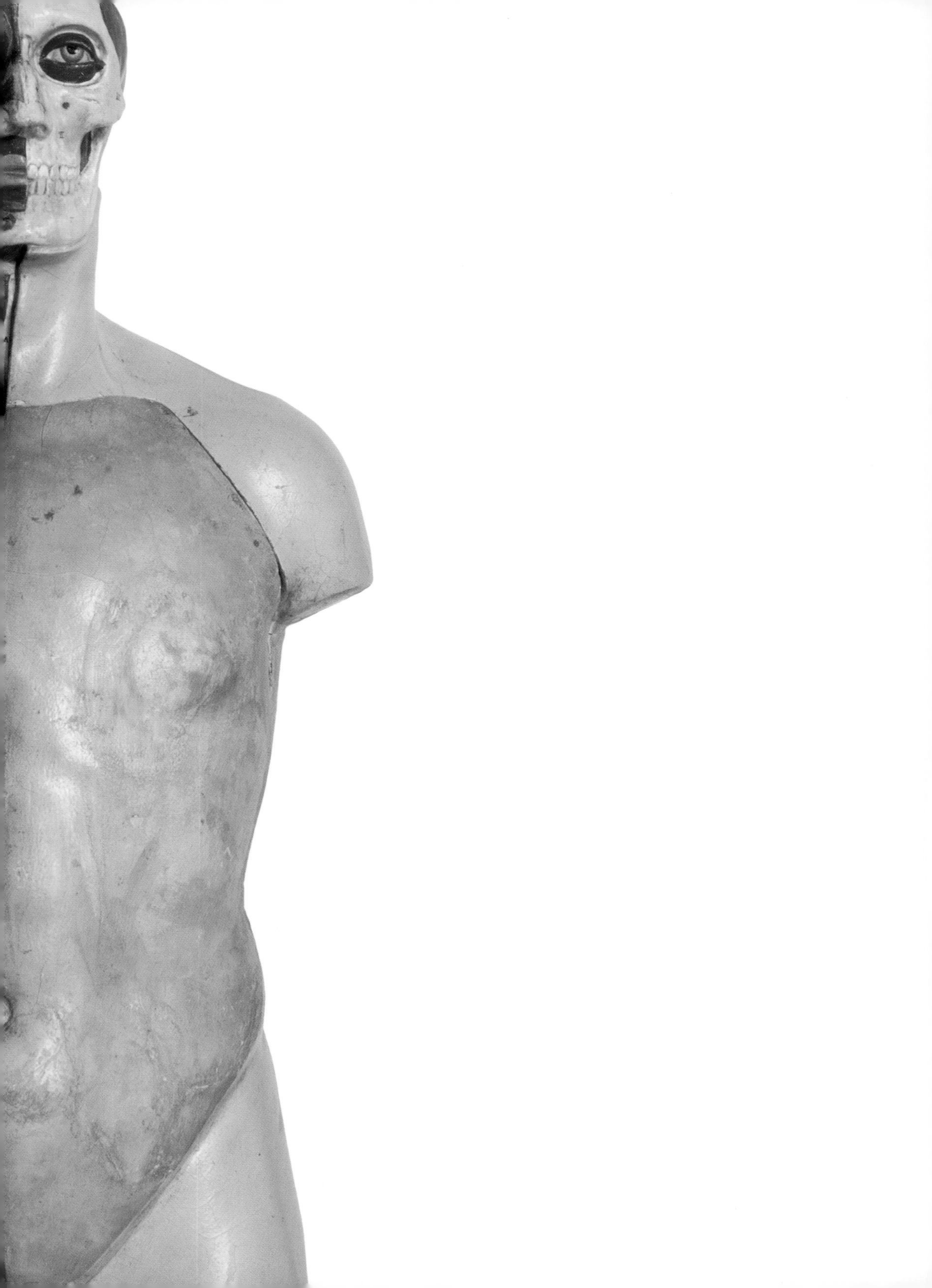

HISTORICAL CONTEXT

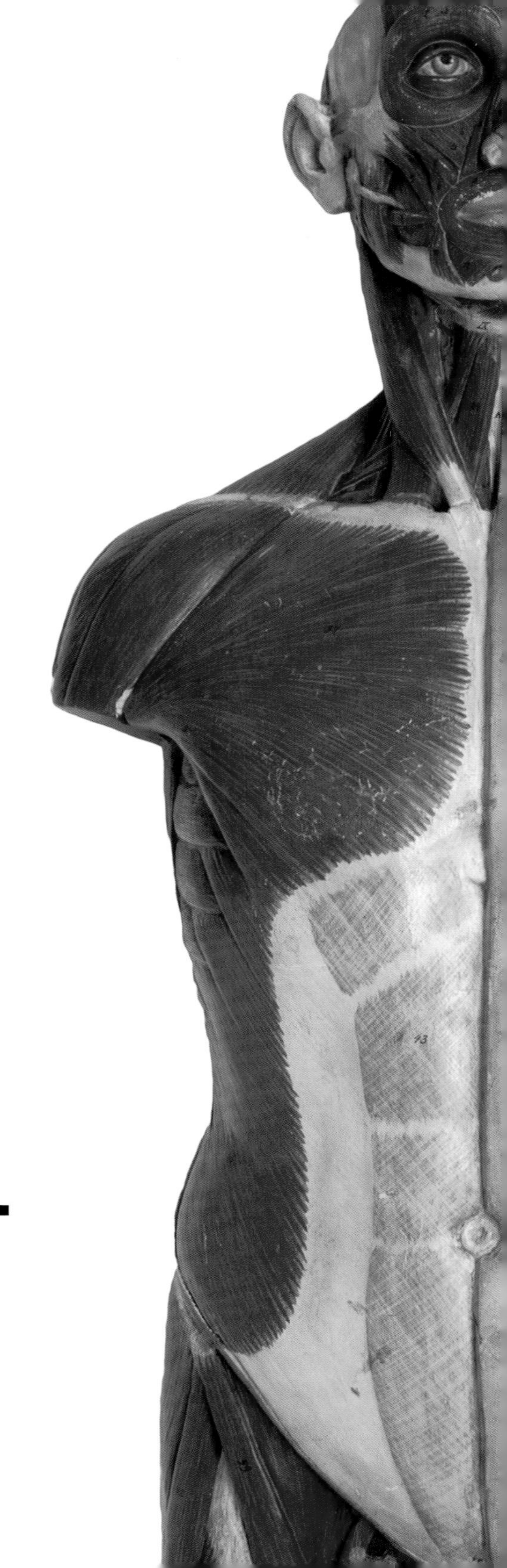

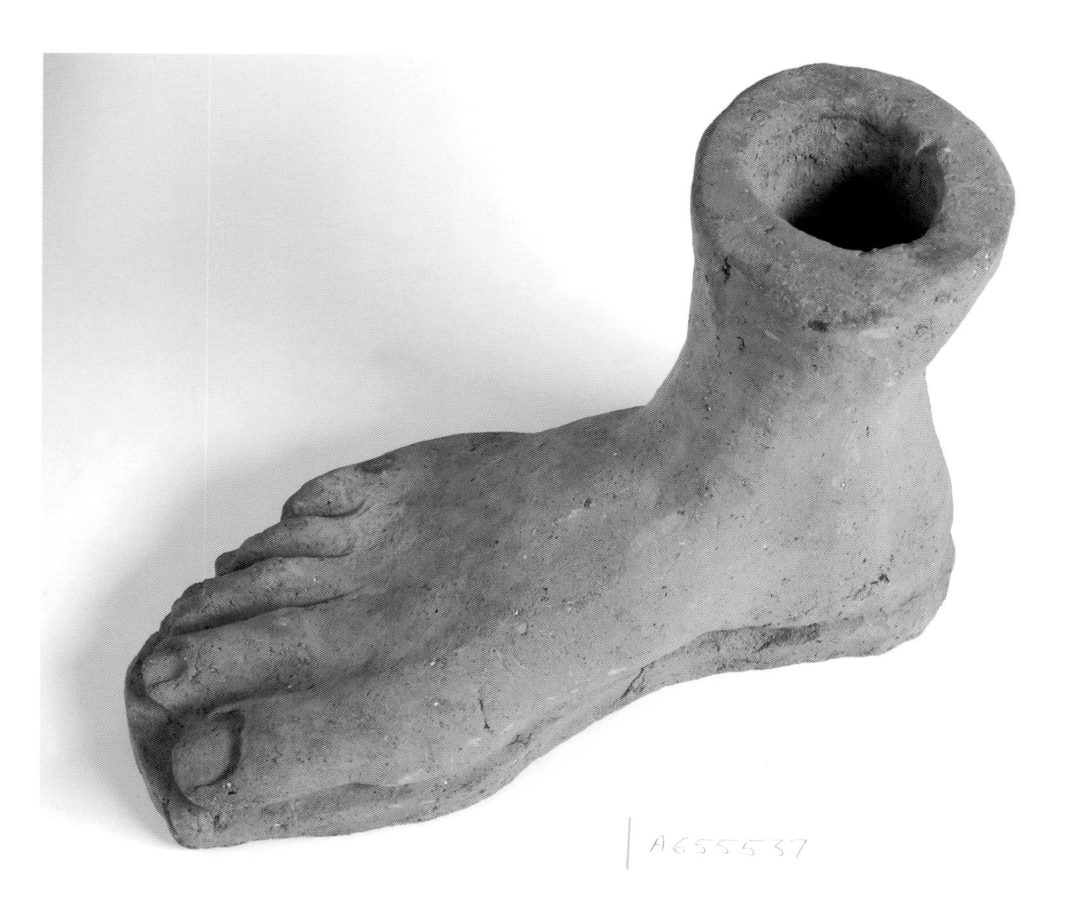

FIGURE 1
Roman votive offering of a foot, clay, 200 BC to AD 200.
Wellcome Library, London.

Models and materials in Europe 1650–1890

Anna Maerker

Europe has a rich and diverse tradition of representing the human body in three dimensions, for purposes ranging from portraiture and religious practices to public entertainment and royal spectacle. Dating back as far as antiquity, these traditions have influenced the evolution of modern anatomical models. The diversity of uses of these representations was matched by a diversity of materials, from wax and wood to plaster and papier-mâché. Throughout the evolution of anatomical models there was a reciprocal relationship between uses and materials: to match an intended use, modellers would select certain materials whose properties best suited their needs. At the same time, artisans and artists experimented with new materials and combinations of materials, which in turn enabled new uses.

One of the most important roots of anatomical representations was in religious practice. In ancient Greece and Rome, supplicants gave thanks for divine intervention by displaying 3D representations of the relevant body part at temples [Figure 1]. These so-called votive offerings were simplified models in materials suited to the supplicant's purse – for instance, in cheap clay or more expensive waxes. The practice of votive offerings was continued in Christian Europe. Artisans fashioned more or less elaborate miniature sculptures of arms and legs, breasts and eyes, in materials ranging from wax to precious metals.

Although verisimilitude was not important for the simplified votives, modellers working in wax also explored the material's suitability for the highly naturalistic representation of human bodies and body parts. Like skin, wax possesses a slight translucency and lustre. Wax can be coloured any shade by mixing it with pigments; other additions change its pliability. It can be freely sculpted, or melted and cast in moulds. It even allows for the easy application of natural hair, teeth and nails. In early modern Europe, these properties made wax a material that was prized in magical practices, as well as in the creation of highly naturalistic portraits of the living and effigies of the dead.

The waxiness of flesh – or perhaps the fleshiness of wax – made this an ideal material through which to understand and to imitate the human body. For the physician and polymath Walter Charleton, an early member of the Royal Society, wax and flesh were the two substances that most exemplified the quality of softness.[1] The properties of wax also provided a way to understand the formation of embryos in early modern Europe. Just as malleable wax received its shape at the hands of the sculptor, early modern philosophers argued, so the child was shaped in the womb through the impressions the mother received during pregnancy:

> the Embryo being like soft wax, is capable of every impression never so little proportionate to its subject; yea, sometimes it is so extravagant, that the effect cannot be attributed to any other cause. Such was that young Girl... which, besides that she was all hairy like this, had the feet of a Camel; her Mother having too wistly consider'd the Image of Saint John Baptist clothed in Camel's hair: And this consideration satisfi'd the Father, who at first disown'd her. The same was the Opinion of Hippocrates, when he sav'd the Honour and Life of a Princess who had brought forth an Aethiopian, through the too attentive minding

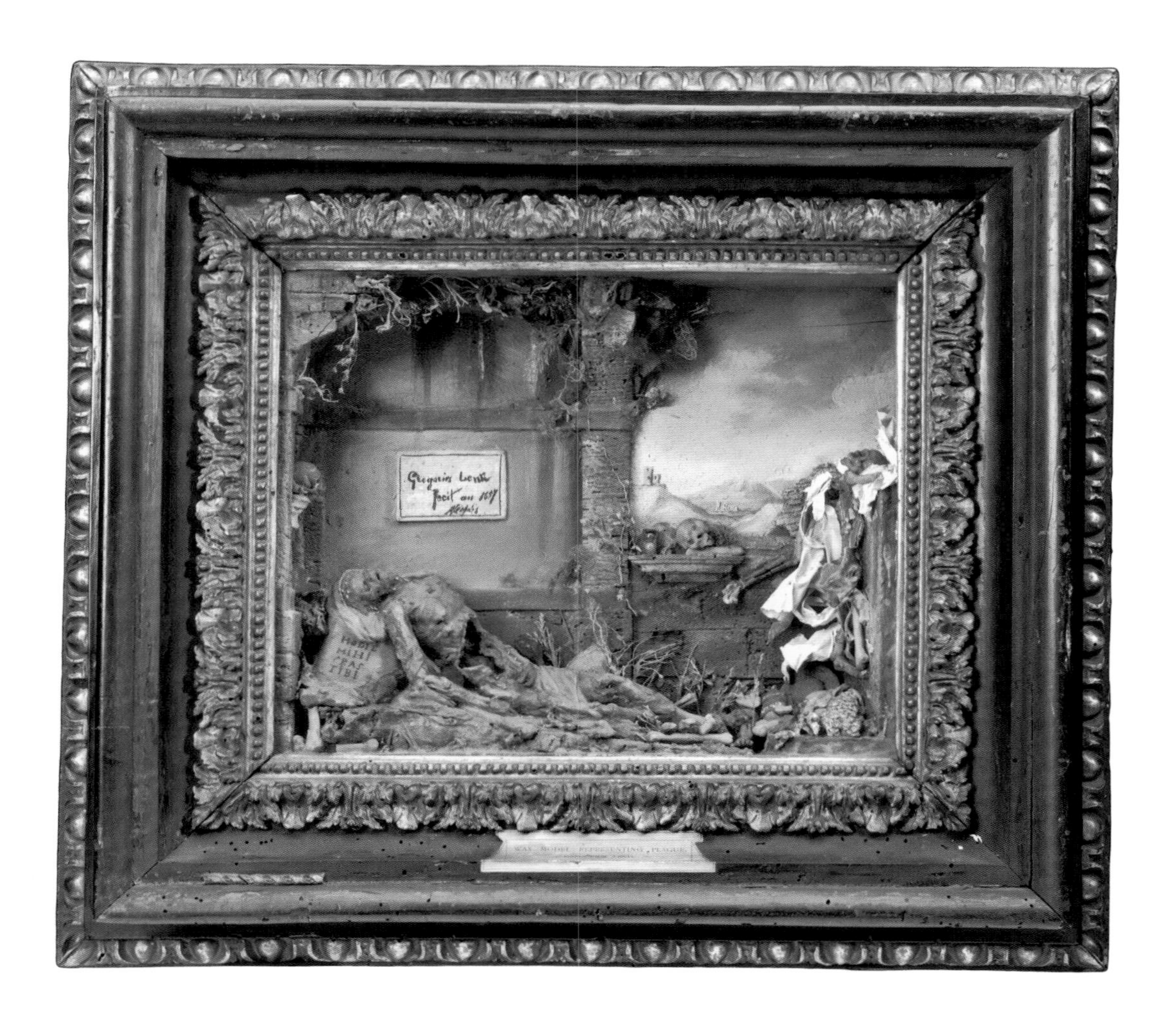

of the picture of a Moor hanging at her beds-feet. Which mov'd Galen to advise such Ladies as would have fair Children, to behold those that are such frequently, at least in picture.[2]

The close association of wax and flesh took on a more sinister aspect in magical practices. In ancient Egypt and Greece, wax effigies were damaged or destroyed in attempts to injure or kill enemies; this practice remained widespread in many different cultures and epochs.

FIGURE 2
Gregorius Lenti
The Plague, 1657, Italy, wax, cork, dried plants.
Wellcome Library, London.

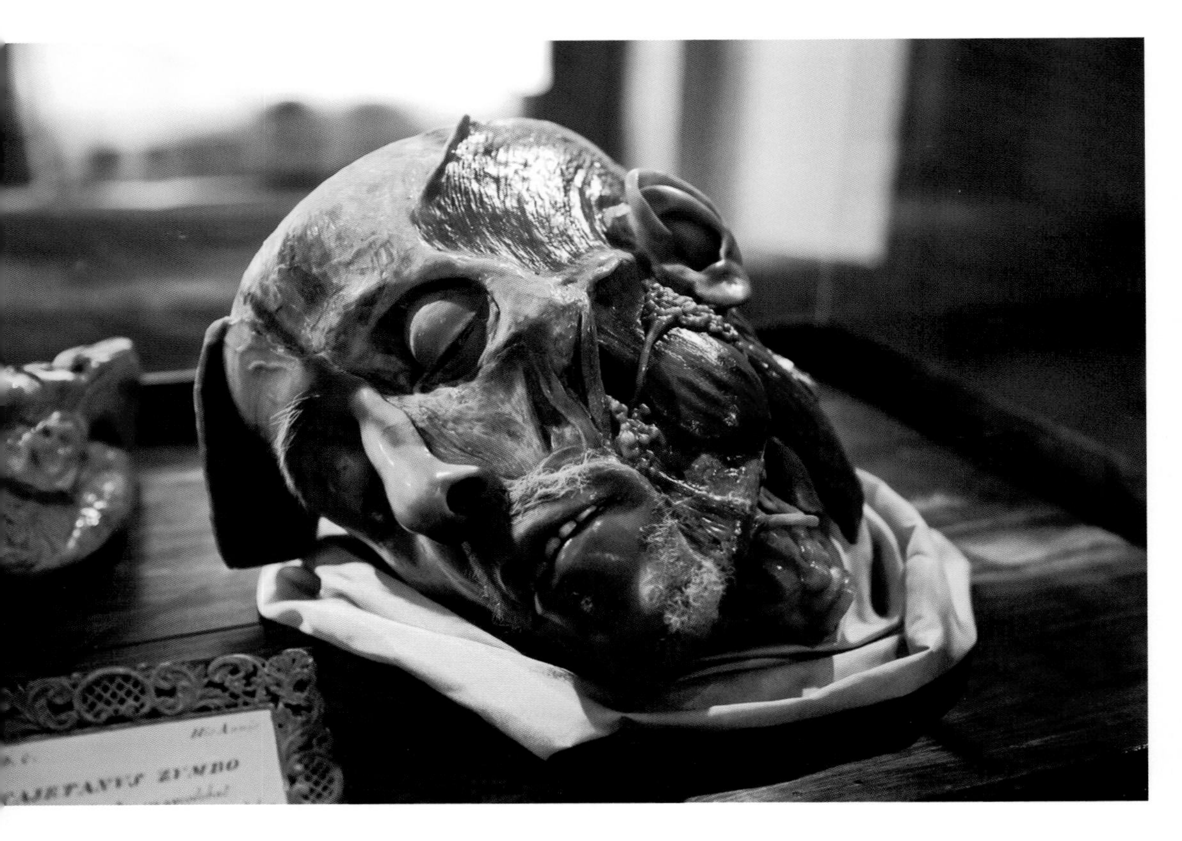

FIGURE 3
Gaetano Zumbo
Study of a dead man's head, late 17th century, Italy, wax.
Photograph by Joanna Ebenstein.

The translucency, malleability and colouration of wax, coupled with its uncanny resemblance to human flesh and skin, also enabled the creation of highly naturalistic 3D portraits. This led to its use in the production of effigies and portraits for public and personal use. Wax effigies of European kings and queens were used in processions and public celebrations; examples are still on display in places such as the museum of Westminster Abbey in London. Affluent noblemen and burghers had their portraits done in wax, adorned with real hair and clothing, glass eyes and even the stubble of a growing beard.

The artists who developed wax-modelling skills in early modern Europe began to put them to use for more gruesome representations as well. Wax was frequently used in the tradition of the memento mori: depictions of bodies and body parts in states of decay that served to remind spectators of their mortality, and to prompt them to lead appropriately blameless lives [Figure 2]. This intense preoccupation with the human body enabled early modern artists in wax to use their skills for explicitly anatomical works. Anatomists teamed up with artists to create representations of the human body in three dimensions. In particular, the Italian sculptor Gaetano Zumbo – who had undertaken religious training before turning to art – was widely praised in the late 17th century for his works, which included miniaturised scenes of death and decay in the memento mori tradition, as well as life-sized, naturalistic studies of dead bodies and body parts [Figure 3]. Zumbo collaborated with the Paris surgeon and anatomist Desnoues to create wax models of human bodies in various stages of dissection that took 18th-century Europe by storm when they went on travelling display. One of the viewers was the Marquis de Sade, who memorialised Zumbo's art in his novel *Juliette*:

> So powerful is the impression produced by this masterpiece that even as you gaze at it your other senses are played upon, moans audible, you wrinkle your nose as if you could detect the evil odours of mortality... These scenes of the plague appealed to my cruel imagination: and I mused, how many persons had undergone these awful metamorphoses thanks to my wickedness?[3]

Beyond prompting spectators to moral contemplation, however, wax models were increasingly explored for their potential to contribute to anatomical research and training in the age of enlightenment, and especially to public education. Unlike real corpses, wax models did not decay and thus they enabled users to study anatomy at leisure, without being offended by the smells and health hazards of a real dissection. In Bologna, the learned Cardinal Prospero Lambertini (who became Pope Benedict XIV in 1740) commissioned a large set of anatomical wax figures from

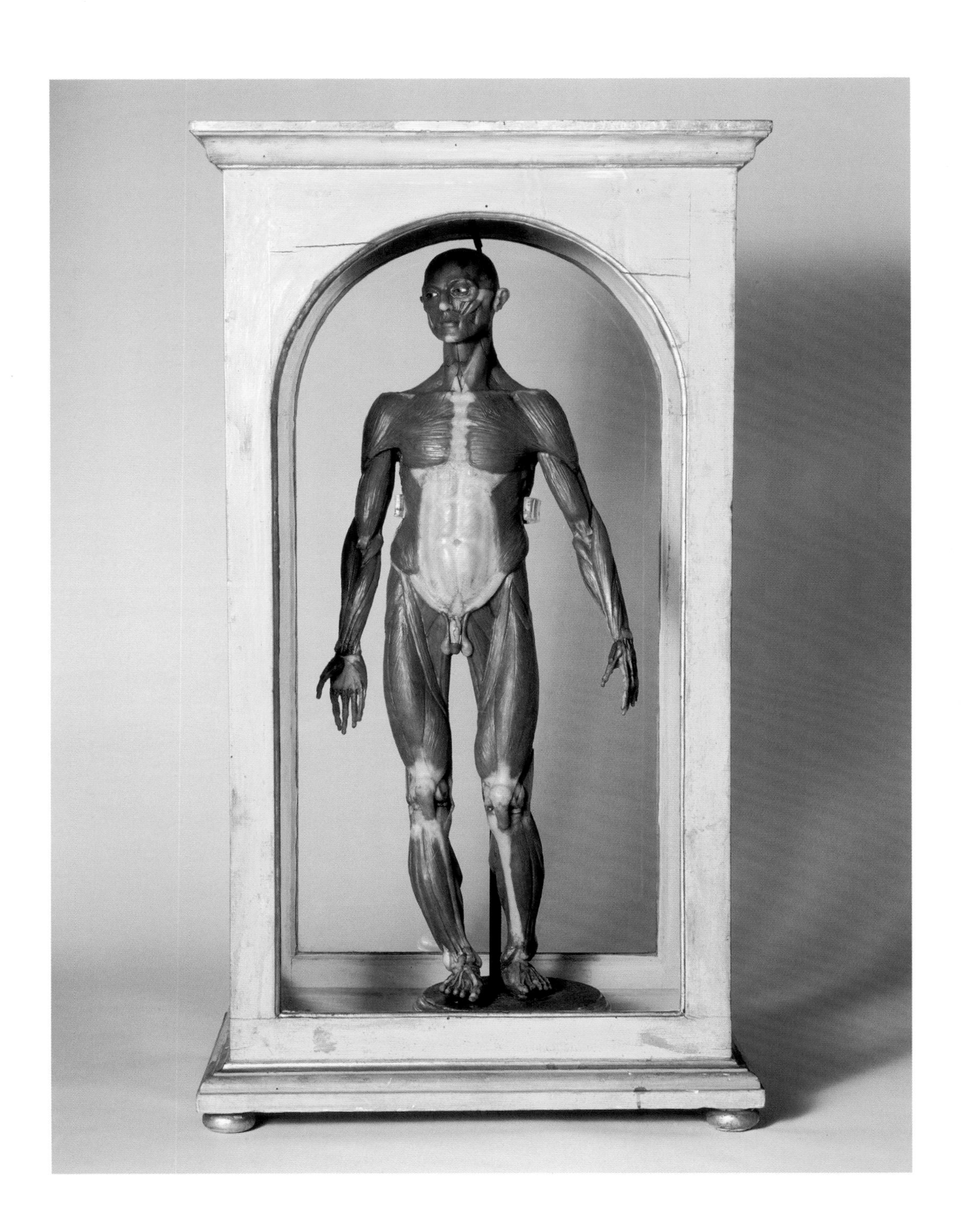

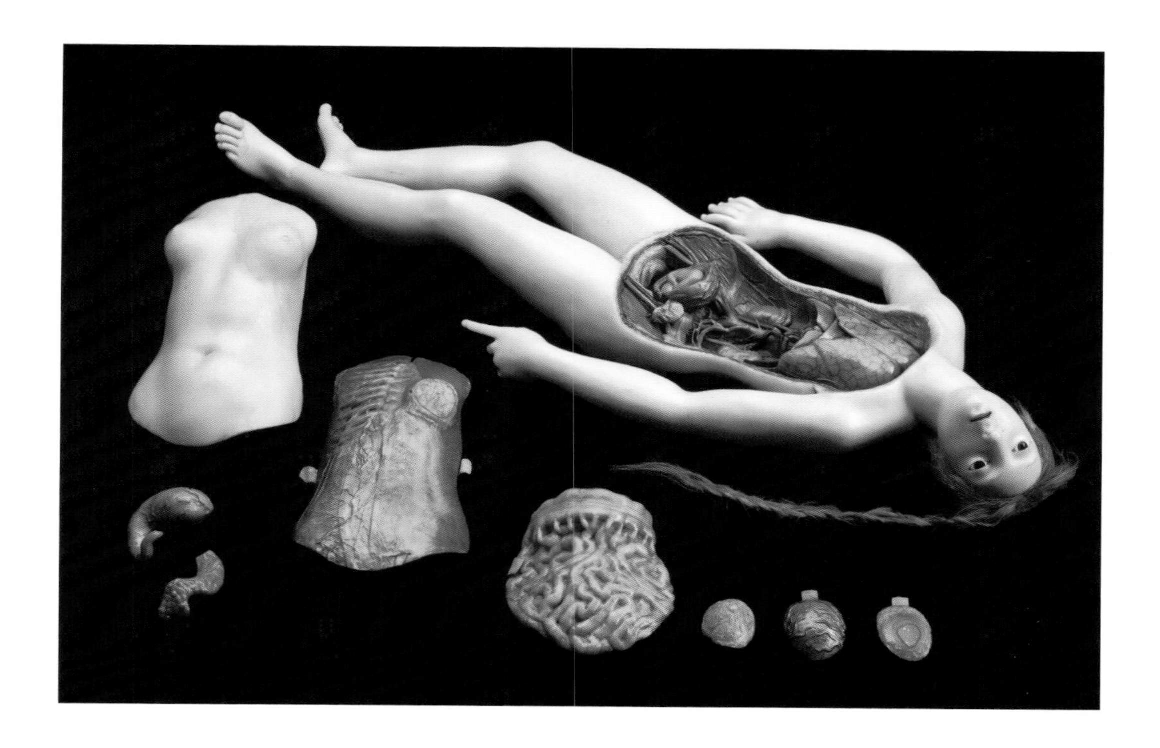

the sculptor Ercole Lelli to be put on display at the local Academy of Sciences.[4]

Wax models similarly contributed to a project of public enlightenment in Florence, where the Tuscan Grand Duke Pietro Leopoldo founded one of the first public museums of science. A large collection of anatomical wax models, produced in-house under the supervision of the renowned court scientist Felice Fontana by modellers such as the classically trained sculptor Clemente Susini, was praised both for the models' accuracy and their beauty, echoing classical works of art [Figure 4]. Visitors from all over Europe, grand tourists and locals alike, admired these depictions of (what was defined as) normal human anatomy. These were based on an amalgamation of numerous actual dissections of bodies and body parts from the local general hospital, which the Grand Duke had permitted the museum's

FIGURE 4 (OPPOSITE)
Clemente Susini (attributed)
Half-sized study of the superficial muscles, 1776–1780, Italy, wax.
Wellcome Library, London.

FIGURE 5 (ABOVE)
Clemente Susini (attributed)
Female model with detachable parts ('Anatomical Venus'), 18th century, Italy, wax.
Wellcome Library, London.

anatomists to use for their studies. Unlike modellers such as Joseph Towne, whose depictions of bodies did not hide the fact that they were based on studies of the dead [see Chapter 3], the Florentine models seemed to represent the living. They were posed in an upright position or relaxed repose and sometimes partly covered with rosy skin.

The museum's visitor books of the time attest to the Tuscan collection's popularity. As many visitors observed, the models lacked nothing but the stench of real corpses. Unlike those, the waxen replicas presented serene beauties, languidly reclining on cushions or posing on pedestals. Stripped of the horrors of dissection, the collection was educational entertainment for families as well as for adult visitors. Family groups who visited included mothers and their daughters, and the collection became a popular means to teach young men and women something of pregnancy and childbirth. Spectators paid particular attention to the museum's life-sized reclining female models – some opening up to reveal a fetus inside – one of which came to be known as the 'Anatomical Venus' [Figure 5]. Eighteenth-century grand tourists admired the skill of the artists, and the anatomists' learning, but also the spectacle of uncovering the figure's pregnancy:

> Under a glass cover, which is removable, in the first chamber, there is a beautiful female figure, in wax, of the size of life. Surprised as we were, at the workmanship of the external parts, how much more fearfully were we astonished, and how was our curiosity excited, when, after removing successively the outward membranes of the body, which are in different divisions, the entire internal structure of a pregnant woman was exhibited![5]

Soon, the fame of the Florentine collection inspired imitations across Europe, and some artists made a living travelling with and exhibiting copies of models – the Anatomical Venus foremost among them. The Italian Sarti, for instance, brought his 'celebrated Florentine Venus' to mid-19th-century England, where he advertised its 'public utility' and announced that the

FIGURE 6
Advertisement for Signor Sarti's celebrated 'Anatomical Venus', around 1850.
Wellcome Library, London.

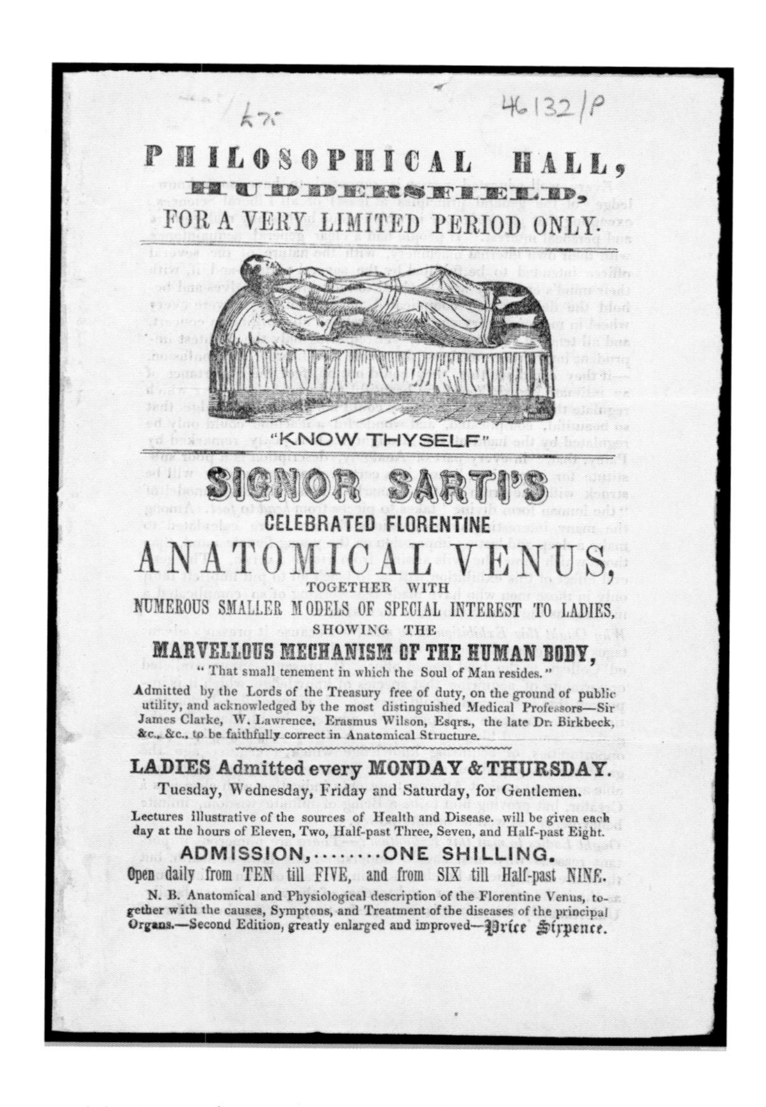

model might be 'of special interest to ladies' – presumably for its ability to illustrate matters of reproduction and pregnancy in a socially acceptable manner [Figure 6].

However, despite their celebrated ability to look just like the real thing (that is, the human body), wax models did not feel real at all. They were hard and dry, and too fragile to be handled frequently. Naturalists such as the Florentine Felice Fontana ultimately found this fragility an obstacle to the models' use for teaching purposes. To enable dissectible representations (figures that could be disassembled), modellers drew on materials other than wax to create very different kinds of artificial bodies. Fontana experimented with wood to enable students to take models apart with their own hands. Detachable wooden models were already known from earlier periods but these were coarse and lacking in anatomical detail [Figure 7]. Fontana tried to improve on wooden models by adding details with the help of skilled carpenters but after several years he had to concede that this project had failed. The wood had a tendency to warp under changing climactic conditions to the point where the model was no longer detachable.

FIGURE 7
Detachable anatomical figure of the female body, 1650–1750, Germany, wood.
Wellcome Library, London.

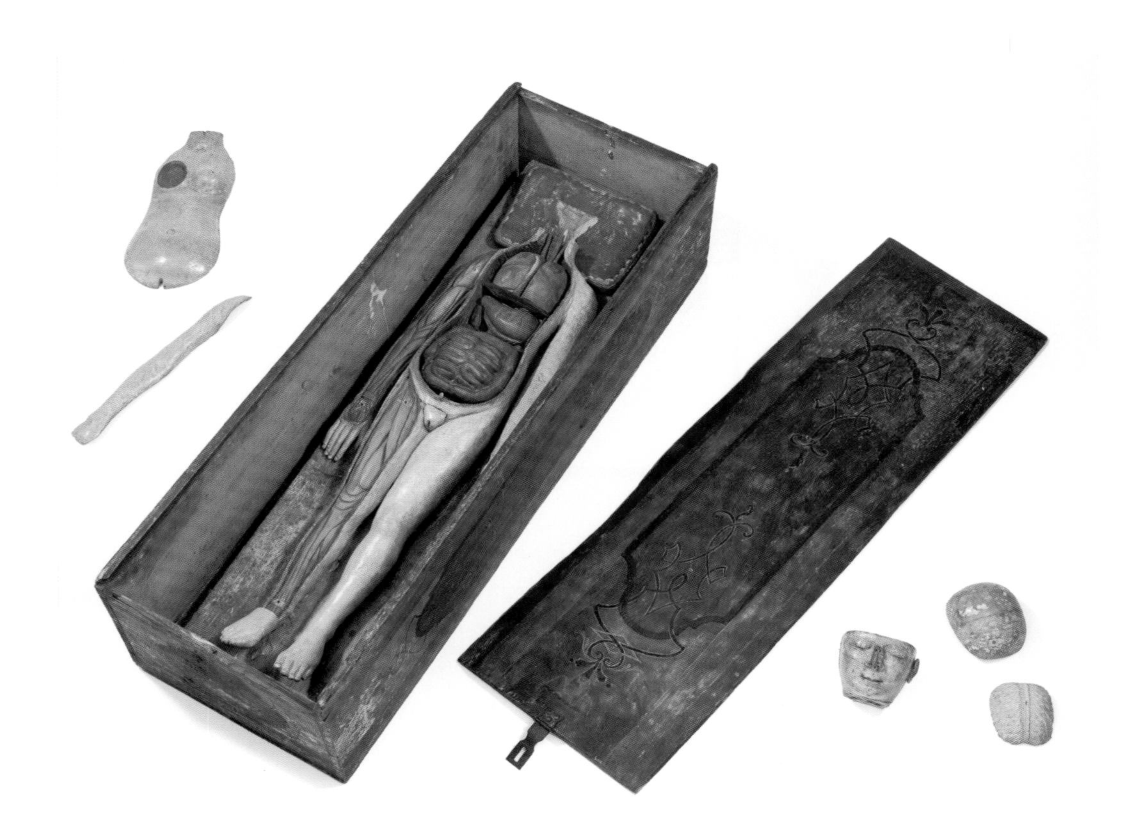

The use of wood was more successful in the production of other, less-detailed anatomical models. Unlike the anatomical waxes that aimed to represent minute structures with accuracy and naturalism, the so-called 'obstetric phantoms' or 'birthing machines' were designed to facilitate practical training [Figure 8]. They were robust dummies that came into use in the 18th century, designed to enable students of obstetrics and apprentice midwives to grasp – quite literally – the basics of midwifery. These 'phantoms' were much less detailed and visually attractive than the coloured waxes. Instead, they reproduced the haptic or tactile properties of the birthing body in a mix of materials such as leather, wood, fabric and, in some cases, a real pelvic bone. Although this material composition opened up anatomical models

FIGURE 8
Obstetric phantom or birthing machine, 18th century, wood and leather.
Wellcome Library, London.

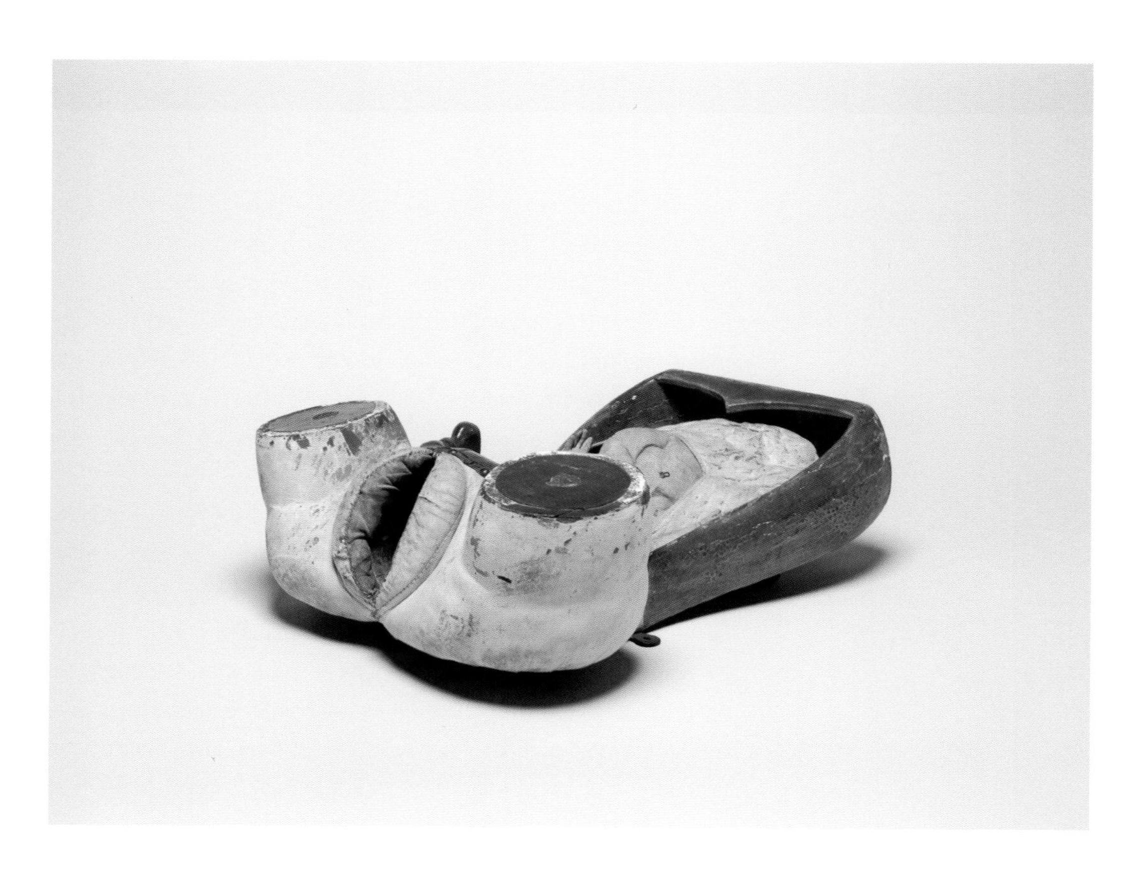

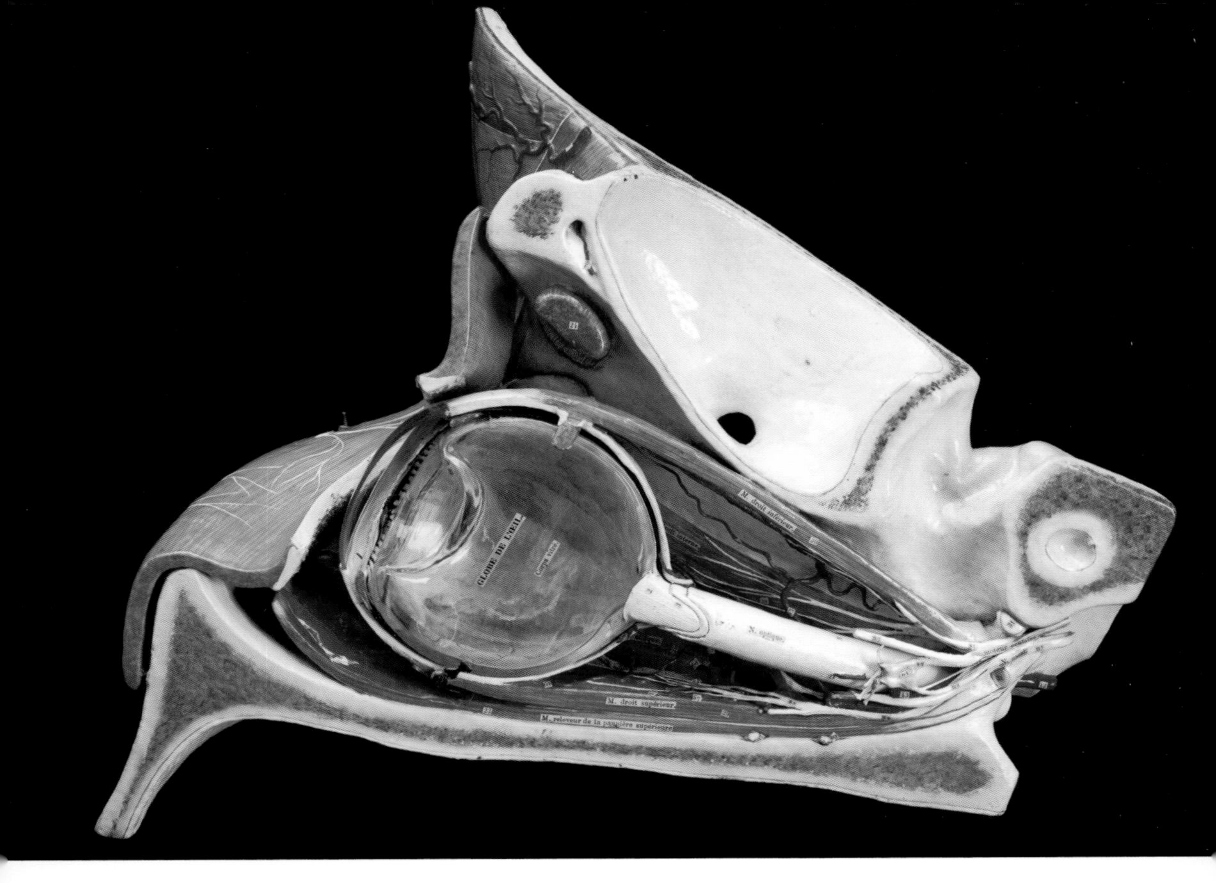

FIGURE 9
Model of the eye, 1884, papier-mâché, by Établissements du Docteur Auzoux, Paris.
Wellcome Library, London.

to a wholly different area of use, the materiality of these 'birthing machines' also raised concerns among practitioners. Some male obstetricians and female midwives rejected these novelties for fear that training with coarse, unresponsive dummies might make practitioners insensible to the experience – and the potential suffering – of the living patient.[6] Not all technological innovations, they suggested, were necessarily an improvement on established practices of training.

Felice Fontana's dream of fully 'dissectible' models was finally realised in the 19th century. Thirty years after Fontana's frustrated attempts to model in wood, the French surgeon-physician Ameline created robust anatomical models by sculpting papier-mâché onto real skeletons. Although his prototypes never evolved into an established modelling business, Ameline's introduction of a new material may have inspired the French doctor Louis Auzoux, who, around 1820, developed a new kind of paper paste for the purpose of anatomical modelling. This paper paste enabled not only the creation of more robust, detachable models but also crucially the development of a production process using moulds and the foundation of a factory for serial production. Production in series by workers rather than trained artists lowered model prices considerably. Unlike the unique, individually sculpted wax models, Auzoux's papier-mâché products were affordable not only to grand dukes and cardinals but also to universities and schools. With the introduction of a monthly rental scheme, they became available to ambitious bourgeoisie such as the novelist Gustave Flaubert, who hired an Auzoux model for a spot of home dissection and drew on this experience in his satirical novel *Bouvard and Pécuchet* (1881).

Auzoux's models of normal human and animal anatomy were brightly painted and extensively labelled to help in the identification of anatomical details [Figure 9].[9] This didactic design, together with the models' robust constitution and comparative affordability, made the artificial anatomies a global success. The French products were exported around the world, and found their way into classrooms in Sudan, Australia and the United States. The Emperor of Brazil and the Pope praised Auzoux's models, and the Japanese started a franchise in the late 19th century. In Egypt, the models served to accustom students of medicine and of midwifery to studying dead bodies, and in China they facilitated the translation of Western works of anatomy.

Methods for casting models generated particular interest among 19th-century anatomists, who responded to new developments in science, especially the rise of pathological anatomy (see Chapter 3). In the 1830s, the French anatomist Félix Thibert developed a method of taking plaster casts of lesions directly from the bodies of the dead. Thibert used this method to create what he advertised as an *encyclopédie vivante*, a 'living encyclopaedia' of pathological cases. Casts of lesions

FIGURE 10
Félix Thibert's 'encyclopédie vivante'. From Thibert, *Musée d'anatomie pathologique* (Paris: Lambert, 1844).

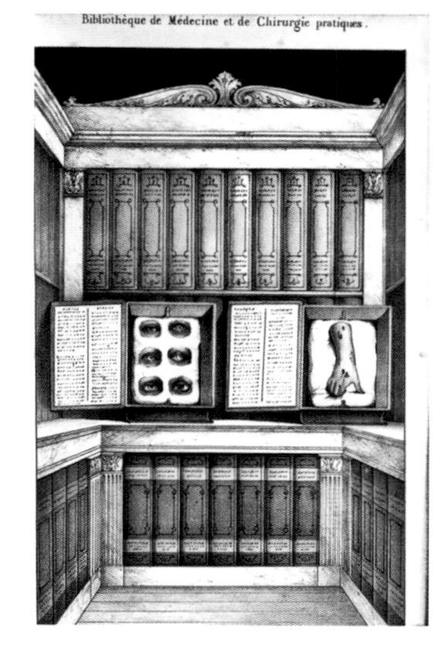

derived from individual patients were painted and then stored in boxes accompanied by brief descriptions of the patient's case; the boxes were shaped like books and could be stored similarly on shelves [Figure 10]. Thibert's encyclopaedia, he suggested, should become a national project of pathological knowledge production that could support not just the work of researchers but also of practitioners. Although medical professionals in Paris had frequent opportunities to observe patients' serious conditions in the many hospitals, practitioners in the provinces might never see a rare case. Conversely, if an interesting case appeared far from the capital, it was difficult for it to be observed by many researchers. Thibert's plaster casts offered a solution to these dilemmas: they allowed for the production of a faithful record of cases that could be multiplied infinitely, shared among researchers and teachers, and consulted by practitioners in the provinces and the colonies. Although Thibert's own casts were based on cases he encountered in Paris, he encouraged his colleagues to turn the encyclopaedia into a collaborative project, and to contribute rare and intriguing cases from across the country.

Throughout the evolution of a continental European tradition of modelling, the diversity of materials enabled the introduction of new uses for anatomical models. Beautiful coloured waxes turned anatomy into a suitable subject for public education during the age of enlightenment, robust 'birthing machines' in wood, leather and textiles enabled hands-on training, while Auzoux's papier-mâché models travelled globally and Thibert's plaster casts offered the prospect of a collaborative project of pathological anatomy. However, during these developments artificial anatomies continued to resonate with other meanings, established through the use of models in religious and magical practices, public entertainment and spectacle.

NOTES

1. Walter Charleton, *Physiologia Epicuro-Gassendo-Charletoniana: or a Fabrick of Science Natural, upon the Hypothesis of Atoms* (London: Newcomb, 1654), p. 326.
2. T Rénaudot, *A General Collection of Discourses of the Virtuosi of France, upon Questions of All Sorts of Philosophy, and Other Natural Knowledge Made in the Assembly of the Beaux Esprits at Paris, by the Most Ingenious Persons of that Nation* [G Havers, transl.] (London: Thomas Dring and John Starkey, 1664), p. 64.
3. Marquis de Sade, *Juliette or Vice Amply Rewarded*, abridged from the translation by Pieralessandro Casavini (Goldstar Publications: London, 1966), pp. 238–39, quoted in Jane Eade, 'The theatre of death', *Oxford Art Journal*, 36 (2013), 109–25 (p. 109).
4. Lucia Dacome, 'Women, wax and anatomy in the "century of things"', *Renaissance Studies*, 21 (2007), 522–50.
5. Tobias Smollett, review of Stolberg's Travels Through Germany, Switzerland, Italy, and Sicily, in *The Critical Review; Or, Annals of Literature* (London: Hamilton, 1797), p. 364.
6. Anna Maerker, 'Florentine anatomical models and the challenge of medical authority in late-eighteenth-century Vienna', *Studies in History and Philosophy of Science Part C: Studies in History and Philosophy of Biological and Biomedical Sciences*, 43 (2012), 730–40.
7. Anna Maerker, 'Anatomizing the trade: designing and marketing anatomical models as medical technologies, ca. 1700–1900', *Technology and Culture*, 54 (2013), 531–62.

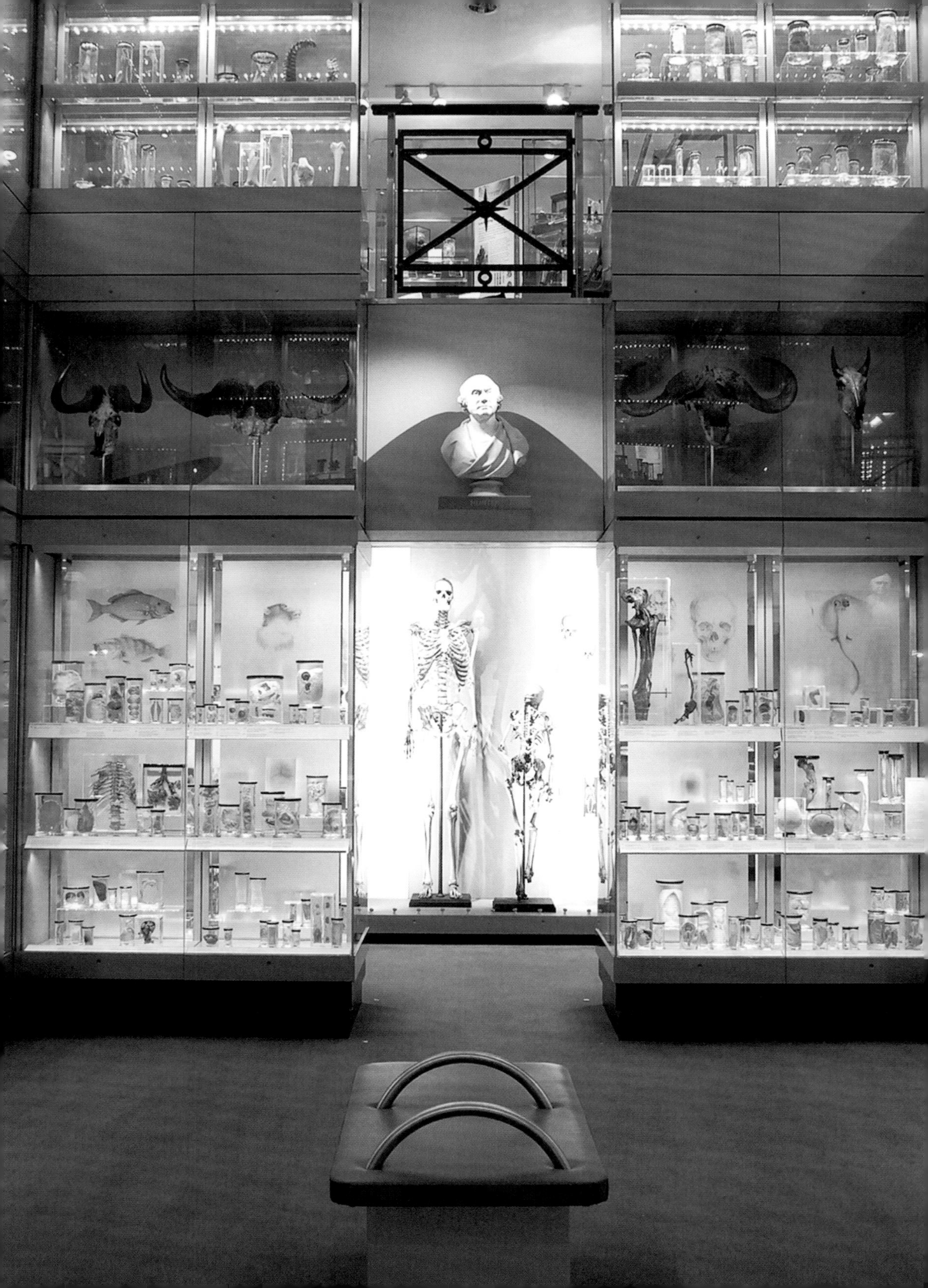

Medical Models in Britain 1750–1920

Samuel JMM Alberti

As a visitor to a medical museum, I might expect to encounter human remains – especially skeletons and spirit-preserved specimens (or preparations) in cylindrical jars (Figure 1). But these are often decayed or discoloured and I learn little from them. To make more sense of this deadened flesh and bone, medical museums also hold numerous illustrations, models and casts corresponding to the preparations – or replacing them entirely. In Britain, from the late 18th and through the 19th century, medical practitioners have worked especially with plaster and wax to design models of human anatomy.

Take, for example, the cast and image of a full-term fetus and a woman – her name lost to history – who died suddenly in 1750 in the ninth month of pregnancy (Figures 2 and 3).[1] They represent the dissection carried out by the famous physician and man-midwife William Hunter in London. The anatomised remains of the unfortunate mother and fetus are long since gone but these disturbing representations are preserved: one a lithograph in a book, the other in plaster of Paris in the collection Hunter bequeathed to the University of Glasgow. They are both arresting in different ways: the image breathtaking in its detailed fleshy folds and butchered thighs, the life-sized cast in colour and palpable three dimensions. Each provided different information and a different experience from dissected cadavers; cast and image complement and strengthen one another to aid in anatomical learning.

FIGURE 1 (OPPOSITE)
The Crystal Gallery in the Hunterian Museum at the RCS, opened in 2005.
Royal College of Surgeons of England.
Photograph by John Carr.

FIGURE 2 (BELOW)
Cast of 'The child in the womb, in its natural situation', made for William Hunter, 1750s.

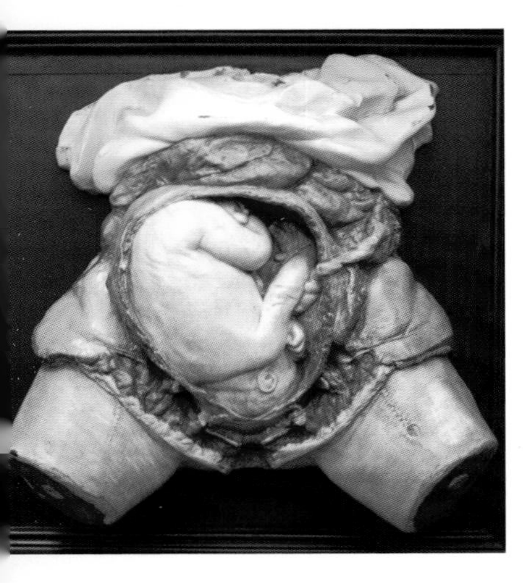

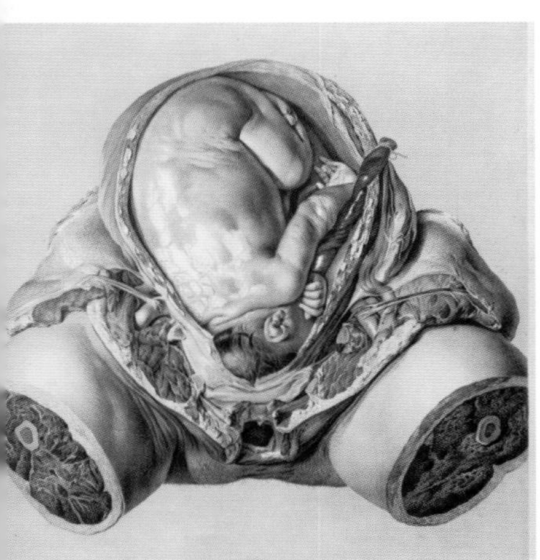

FIGURE 3 (ABOVE)
Jan van Rymsdyk
'The child in the womb, in its natural situation', from William Hunter, *The Anatomy of the Human Gravid Uterus* (Birmingham: Baskerville, 1774).
Wellcome Library, London.

The two were produced at the beginnings of a realist medical art practised in Britain, which did not shy away from its grisly origins. Every established teaching hospital, university, medical faculty and anatomy school in the later 18th, 19th and early 20th century had a medical collection, and models featured prominently in all of them. Durable and easier to procure and store than human bodies, they were important for research, medical teaching and in some cases – intentionally or otherwise – for entertainment. Although skilled European modellers, especially in Italy, France and latterly Germany, produced wares that are justifiably renowned (see Chapter 2), their British counterparts also merit historical and artistic attention.

Important as the models in William Hunter's collection were (in particular, his casts of pregnant women's uteri), this chapter focuses on those in the collection founded by his younger brother, John. While William's collection was transferred to Glasgow, John Hunter's museum remained in London, where they had both worked. As one of the most celebrated surgeons and anatomists of his generation, John Hunter gathered 14,000 specimens that formed the core of what became the pre-eminent medical museum in Victorian and Edwardian Britain. Housed in the RCS in central London, the Hunterian Museum played an important educational and research role for science and medicine. It eventually expanded across five large galleries, until three-quarters of the collection was destroyed during the Blitz in 1941.

Although now considerably smaller, the museum continues to thrive and is open to the public (see Figure 1). Among the surgical instruments, preserved human remains and zoological specimens that visitors can view are a number of medical models and casts, from early modern ivory mannequins to 21st-century simulations. These are all virtuoso sculptures in their own right, and have been displayed as such in art exhibitions.[2] But seeing them in the context of a medical museum helpfully reminds us of their clinical–educational origins, and their relationship with other media used in medical teaching and treatment. They present the dead body often in vivid colour and seem almost more alive than the faded specimens of fragmented preserved flesh. Some of these models manifest the intense and sometimes troubled relationship between clinician and modeller, artist and anatomist. Some showcase rare conditions that would not otherwise be seen, material snapshots of disease or injury. The place of these models in British medical culture up to the inter-war period is explored in this chapter, which concentrates on the materials used (principally wax and plaster), the practices of model-making and casting, and the practitioners themselves.

INTRICATE BODIES IN WAX

Although it is highly fragile, wax has been a popular choice for modelling the human body, for it is appealing in its malleability and its uncanny resemblance to moist human flesh. To exploit the eye-catching appeal of waxworks, continental European models were imported from the 18th century onwards for anatomy collections and commercial shows. Gradually, wax models were made in Britain to complement and challenge the imports – Marie Tussaud, for example, had arrived in England from Paris in 1802. In a more overtly medical context, Guy's Hospital Medical School in London found that importing waxes was so expensive and models were so important that a wax artist, Joseph Towne, was appointed.

Towne worked at Guy's for 53 years from 1826, producing more than 1,000 models.[3] His early efforts were of zoology and of human anatomy, based on dissections; later he turned to pathology, especially skin diseases (Figure 4). The majority were for use in the Guy's collection (now the Gordon Museum) but others were exported to India, the United States, Russia and elsewhere. At his London base, Towne worked closely with the surgeon Thomas Bryant, who was later President of the RCS.

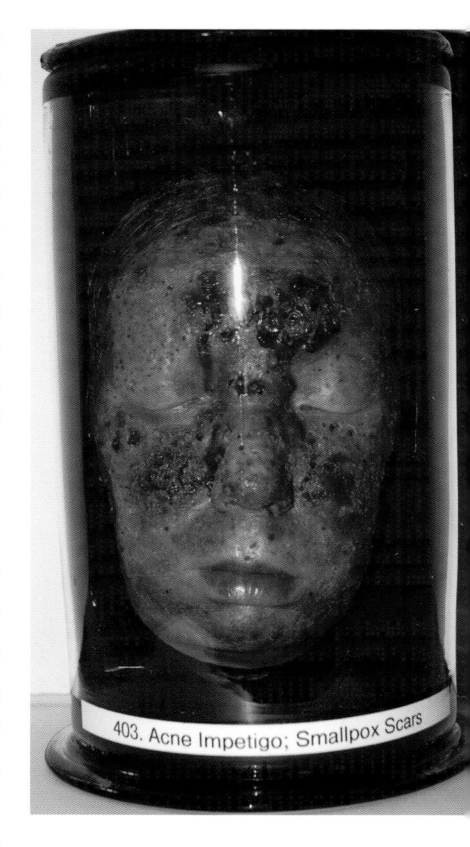

FIGURE 4
Joseph Towne
Wax model of smallpox, 1860s.
Gordon Museum, Guy's Campus, King's College London School of Medicine.

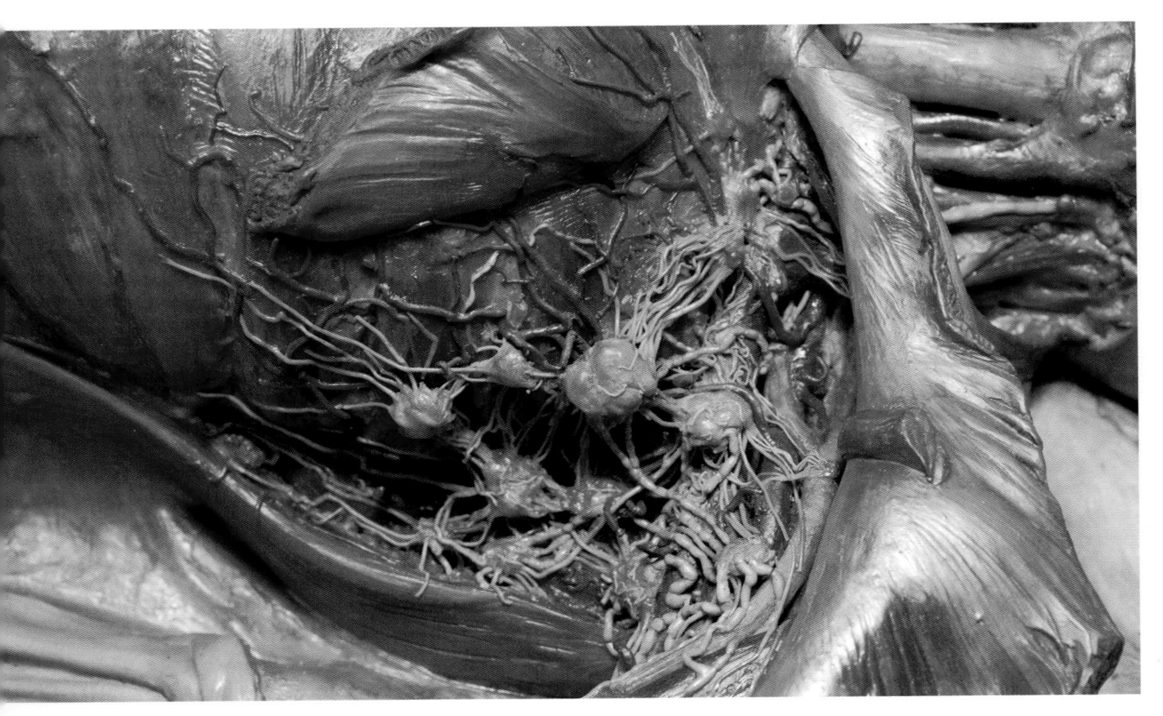

FIGURE 5
Joseph Towne
Wax model of the left arm showing veins and lymphatics in the axilla, 1860s.
Royal College of Surgeons of England. Photograph by John Carr.

Thanks to Bryant, a small selection of Towne's work travelled two miles across the Thames to the Hunterian Museum, where they survive today.

Among these models is a stunning rendering of an arm and shoulder, part torso and neck, showing the veins and lymphatic vessels (Figure 5). No preserved specimen of dissected flesh could retain these fine details; no image on paper could so vividly show the skin peeled away. Heavily informed by Towne's anatomical work on many cadavers, this is no idealised, universal body but rather a gritty representation of the corpse mid-dissection. So too is his arresting infant head and brain model, which is one of a series at the RCS (see Chapter 1). With this, Towne presented a snapshot of the lengthy dissecting process (Figure 6). And here, as in his many other anatomical models, he depicted the dead, including telling details of the corpse's lifeless appearance – in this case, the pallid face and the rolled eyes.

This grisly realism, this apparently true-to-death snapshot of a dissection, conceals the artistry and constructed nature of Towne's models. Very particular design decisions were made throughout the painstaking manufacture of these waxes. Towne worked with Bryant and other clinicians at Guy's to select particular elements of dissections and pathological conditions. For example, early in his career Towne struck up a productive working relationship with the pathologist Thomas Hodgkin (of lymphoma fame). He also worked closely with Thomas Addison (who also gave his name to a disease) and John Hilton, who later – like Bryant – became President of the RCS.

Towne was nonetheless highly secretive about his technique, locking himself in his studio and working on his models under a cloth. But from his surviving work and tools (which included a dull knife, wooden and bone spatulas, and a gouge) we can surmise that, like other modellers, he deployed three main methods – sculpting at room temperature, free modelling with warmed wax and moulding. Occasionally he would sculpt from a wax block; his larger models would have an underlying structure clothed in layers of wax tissue. A combination of plaster and wax moulding was often the most effective, however. If a body part was too delicate or complex to take a direct mould from, he would fashion a clay or coarse wax model, which would be covered in plaster to form a negative. After rubbing the inside with soft soap to block any pores and allow the cast to detach easily, the warmed wax was poured in; this was usually good quality beeswax, occasionally whale-based spermaceti. Initially two or three layers of superior wax were carefully applied, before they were stuffed with either a coarse core or, in the case of larger pieces, rags or wood chippings. Full-body models were constructed from an internal iron frame with cast limbs and/or organs overlaid. The surface was then polished and the finer details were introduced. If the model was intended to display lymphatic or blood vessels, these tended to be attached afterwards, and might be made using metal thread or wax-coated silk (see Figure 5).

FIGURE 6
Joseph Towne
Wax model of the head of a newborn infant, with the calvaria removed to show the brain in situ, 1860s.
Royal College of Surgeons of England. Photograph by John Carr.

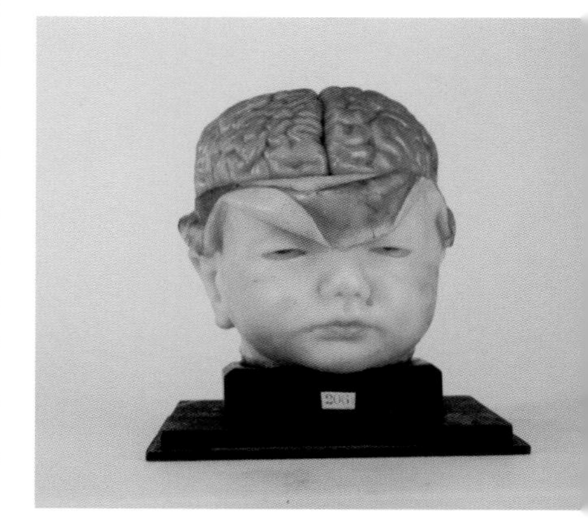

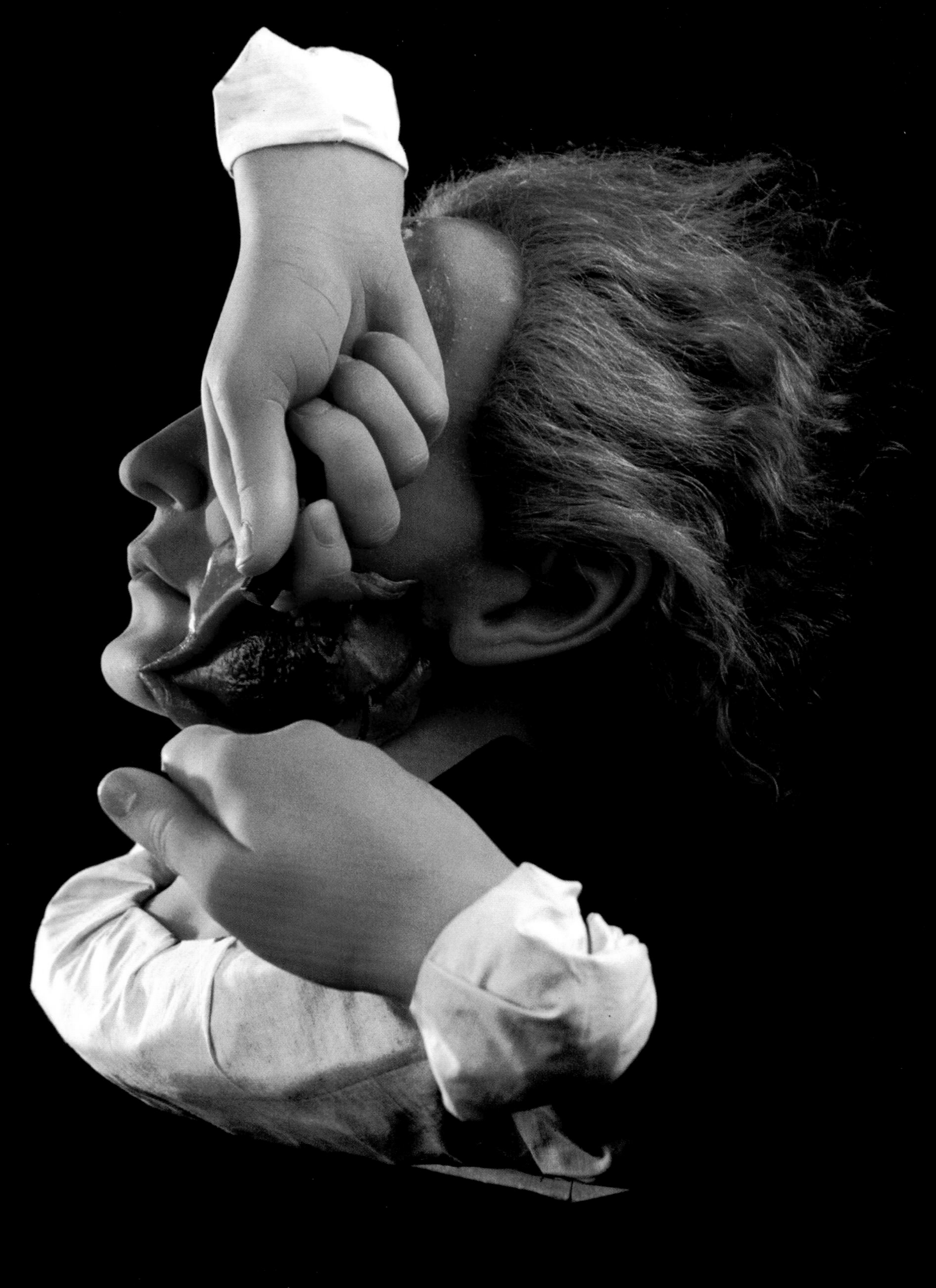

Dermatological (skin) moulds, by contrast, used the patient themselves as the initial positive, drawing on ancient methods of bronze casting for death masks (see Figure 4). Towne constructed a frame bordering the area in question, one or two inches proud of the surface. He then administered a thin layer of fine plaster until it was an inch thick overall. If the area included the nose or mouth, rubber tubes were inserted to avoid the necessity of the patient holding their breath for the time it took the plaster to dry. Once the plaster negative was removed, the wax could be poured into it, in a series of thin layers built up to around a quarter of an inch thick. Towne would then mount this impression on a wooden board, adding details of colour with pure oils and further details such as blisters, where necessary, copied directly from the patient.

By the later 19th century, at the end of Towne's long career at Guy's, wax models were common in British medical schools – especially dermatological moulages, which were vivid impressions of diseases of the skin. In contrast to Towne's individual works, many universities and colleges purchased sets of embryology models from the Ziegler factory (see Chapter 1). Such European imports remained important in British collections. For example, London's Hunterian Museum holds a late-19th-century model demonstrating a surgical procedure (Figure 7). The wax model of a human head has the left cheek opened to reveal an extensive necrosis of the mandible. Two hands work a Gigli saw, the blade of which has been wrapped around the mandible prior to resection. It is probably from continental Europe – the white fabric cuffs and floating hands are redolent of European surgical models and illustrations of this period.

MATERIAL IMPRINTS IN PLASTER

Although there was no strong tradition of wax modelling in Britain, the Victorians were much more confident in plaster, which was afforded greater cultural capital (by the late 19th century wax was

FIGURE 7 (OPPOSITE)
Wax model of the head of a man with the left cheek opened to show the excision of a mandibular tumour, 1890s.
Royal College of Surgeons of England. Photograph by John Carr.

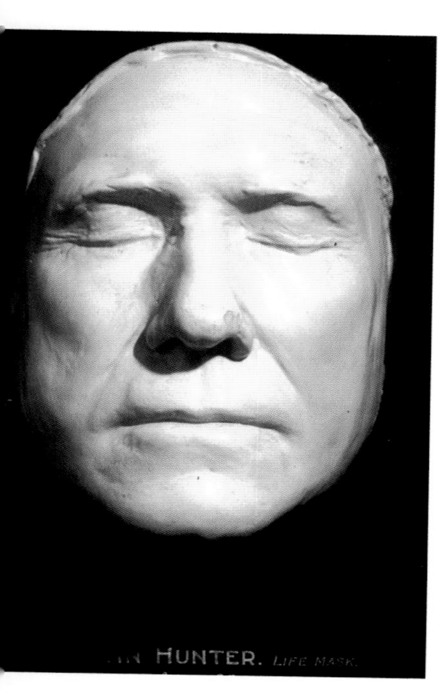

FIGURE 8
Joshua Reynolds
Life mask of John Hunter, 1786.
Royal College of Surgeons of England.
Photograph by John Carr.

often rather too closely associated with the fairground). From architecture to statuary, anything and everything could be cast in plaster. This material was cheap, robust and could be applied to the smallest statue or the largest of pillars. British cities may not have had the grand ancient and Renaissance architecture of some of their European peers but they could capture continental material culture in plaster and bring it back to Britain. Although collections of casts in museums and country houses are not always highly valued today, in the 19th and early 20th century the medium was in strong demand from classicists, architects, art historians, palaeontologists, archaeologists and anthropologists – and by medical practitioners.

Heads were particularly popular subjects. Casting faces of the living and the dead was a long-established tradition, and there was a trade in Britain and elsewhere in the faces of the famous and infamous. Sir Joshua Reynolds is alleged to have made the cast of John Hunter while he was preparing his portrait (Figure 8); Hunter later described how the suction when the plaster was removed caused a blood-blister on his nose. Death masks were also appealing to the macabre tastes of many Victorians; if one was especially famous, the casting might extend to the inside of the head as well as its surface

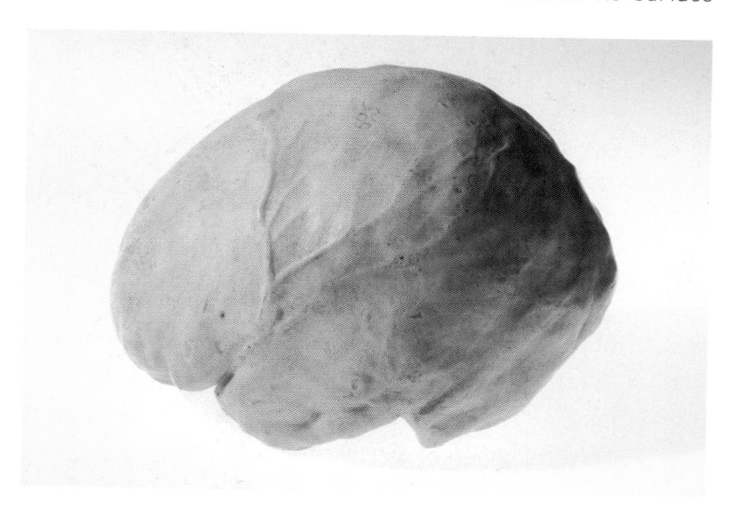

FIGURE 9
Cast of the cranial cavity of the skull of the writer Jonathan Swift, 1864.
Royal College of Surgeons of England.
Photograph by John Carr.

(Figure 9). Such 'endocranial' casting was a common technique across anthropology and primatology.

While classicists were casting the limbs of statues, surgeons used plaster to make impressions of flesh and bone. Casts of deformities had featured in early modern *Wunderkammern* (cabinets of curiosities); they were also to be found in the Victorian hospital. The Great Ormond Street children's hospital was a site for the treatment of orthopaedic conditions, and a series of arms and legs were cast as a 3D clinical record. Figure 10 shows the cast of the leg of 'Amy P.', a child suffering with rickets, whose condition was assessed by the Great Ormond Street surgeon Edmund Owen. The plaster captured the child's physical condition prior to medical treatment, which involved fracturing the leg, and was used presumably for comparison and for record (it was one of a large collection, now housed at University College London). A cast like this could be used to demonstrate the progress (or deterioration) of a condition or injury. Plaster froze fleeting moments in time, before or after death; the gravid uterus cast (see Figure 2) is one of a series showing the progress of a dissection. Whereas waxes were often composites of many dissections, many casts could be made of one dissection.

FIGURE 10
Cast of the leg of 'Amy P.', a rickets patient at Great Ormond Street Hospital, 1885.

Photograph by John Carr.

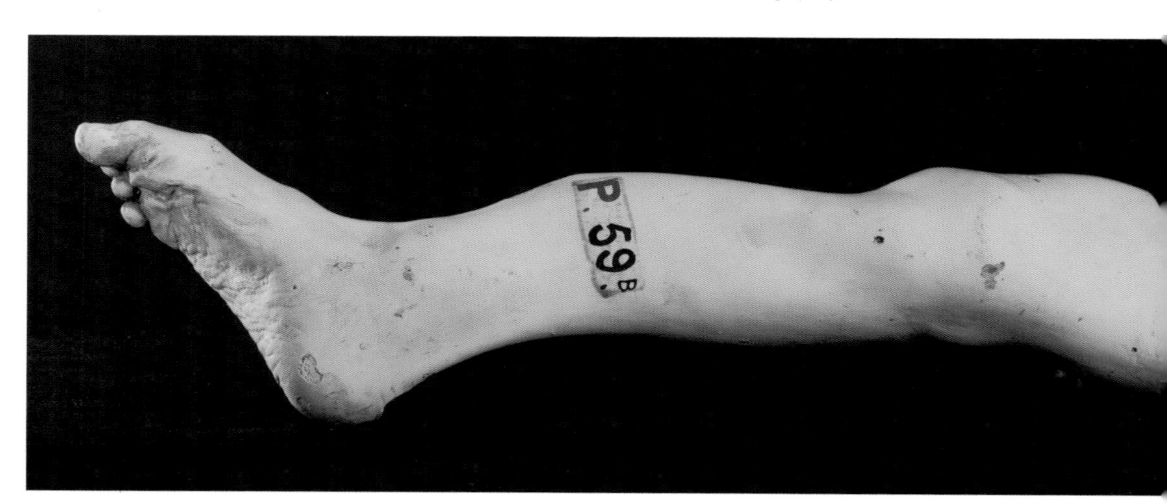

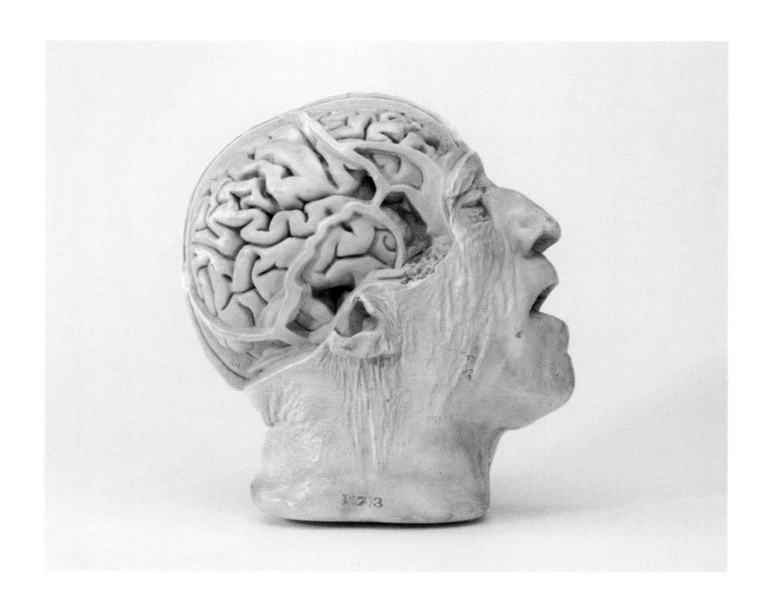

FIGURE 11
Daniel Cunningham
Cast of the head of a 75-year-old man, with the left side of the skull removed to show the brain, 1892.
Royal College of Surgeons of England. Photograph by John Carr.

Continuing the cranial theme in the RCS collections, the College also holds several casts of the skull and brain by the renowned Scottish anatomist Daniel John Cunningham (Figure 11).[4] At the time of their manufacture, Cunningham was teaching at Trinity College Dublin, and contributing to the debate about the relationship between the shape of the brain and the shape of the skull (an extension of the same intellectual endeavour that generated many of the life and death masks mentioned above). Like Hunter's gravid uterus and even more like Towne's waxes, this is a ghastly impression of the cadaver, with the age of the patient emphasised by his wrinkles and a post-mortem cry of anguish on his lips.

Despite such brutal-looking results, casting was always a delicate process and anatomical casts were even more so, given their clinical or post-mortem contexts. Plaster can burn the skin of the living and stick to the corpse. For casts like Cunningham's (and he produced a series of them), the whole head was preserved before sections of the skull were chiselled away. Although the brain was injected with preservative fluid, the anatomist only had a 24-hour window in which to make a mould before this most delicate of organs began to shrink. Cunningham found the best method was to use plaster of Paris in five or six parts to generate the mould, filling the gaps between with gelatine, having applied a thin layer of oil to prevent the plaster sticking. This flimsy negative was used to cast the more robust positive. The result doesn't have quite the same bulbous quality as wax and seems flatter, more deadened than its glistening counterpart. In the end, Cunningham accumulated the impressions of the heads of 6 primates and 22 humans for this comparative study. The data may no longer be of great interest but the material objects remain in the Hunterian Museum's collection – reminders of the Victorian/Edwardian fascination with plaster.

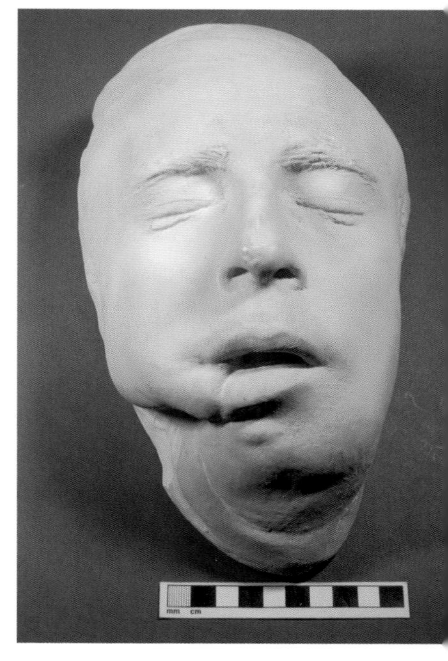

FIGURE 12
Replica of John Walkley Edwards' cast of the face of Private Pritchard, 1917.
Royal College of Surgeons of England; original at the Royal Australasian College of Surgeons.

ENDURING MODELS – INTO THE 20TH CENTURY

Plaster continued to be used in the 20th century. The First World War presented a range of horrific new injuries, which surgeons tried their best to record in both two dimensions and three. At the plastic surgery unit at the Queen's Hospital in Sidcup, Kent, for example, surgeon–artist Henry Tonks drew pastel portraits of facially wounded soldiers while sculptor John Walkley Edwards cast their damaged faces (Figure 12). The process must have been unsettling and painful for the patient, with the fluid running deep into their wounds. The results are extraordinary – and emotionally moving – material records of these extensive, life-changing injuries.[5]

The facial cast in the RCS collection is actually a reproduction of the 1917 original that accompanied the clinicians and patients of the Australian Imperial Force to Australia after the war, for plaster casts were eminently reproducible and there was thriving trade in some areas of plaster work (although this was a one-off). Albeit more cumbersome and breakable, plaster casts could be reproduced and circulated like books: they were material publications.

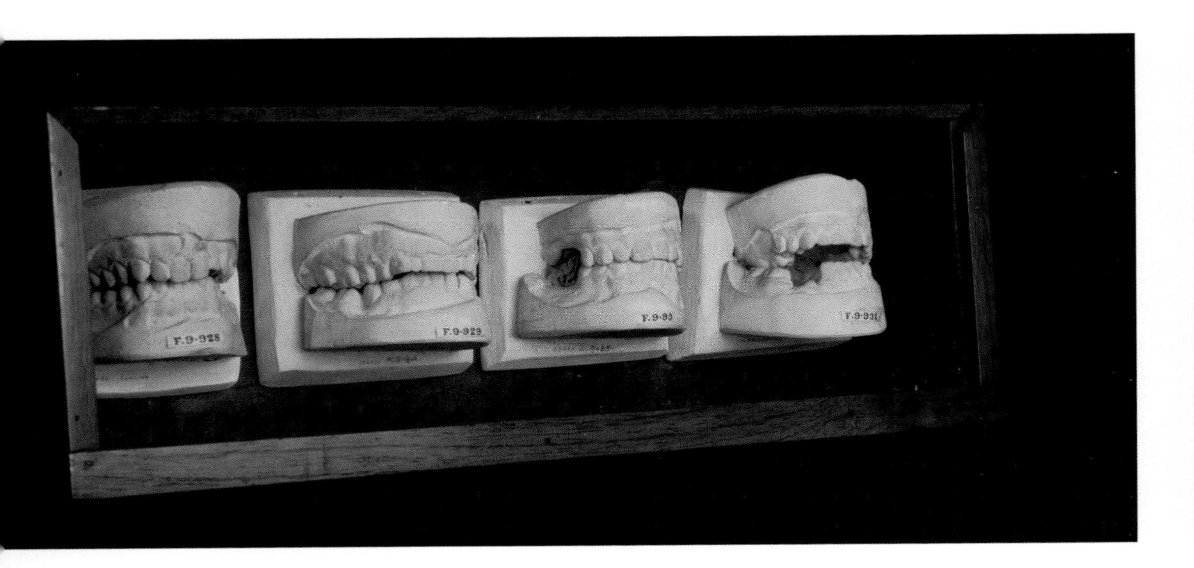

FIGURE 13
Dental casts of maxillae and mandibles showing gunshot wounds, 1916.
Royal College of Surgeons of England. Photograph by John Carr.

More subtle casts also revealed horrific injuries. Dental casts were used throughout the 19th century and still are today. Figure 13 may not appear unusual, except for the chasm caused by a gunshot injury. Dental surgeon J Frank Colyer worked with patients at Sidcup, at the war hospital in Croydon (where this cast was made) and was Honorary Curator of the Odontological Collection at the RCS (where Colyer deposited the casts after the war).[6] Plaster casts were an important element of clinical assessment, in planning dental reconstruction and in the manufacture of prosthetics.

Wax also remained in use during the First World War, not only for facial moulages but also for training models. Like the facial plasters, the wax in Figure 14 is well-travelled, having been crafted in Britain by the New Zealand sculptor Thomas Kelsey, a sergeant in the New Zealand Medical Corps. After the war, the model travelled back to Dunedin to join the large collection of casts and models in plaster and wax that Kelsey generated for the University of Otago. This model was sent back to Sidcup in 1990 and it is now in the RCS collection. Kelsey has demonstrated the different techniques developed by plastic surgeons in

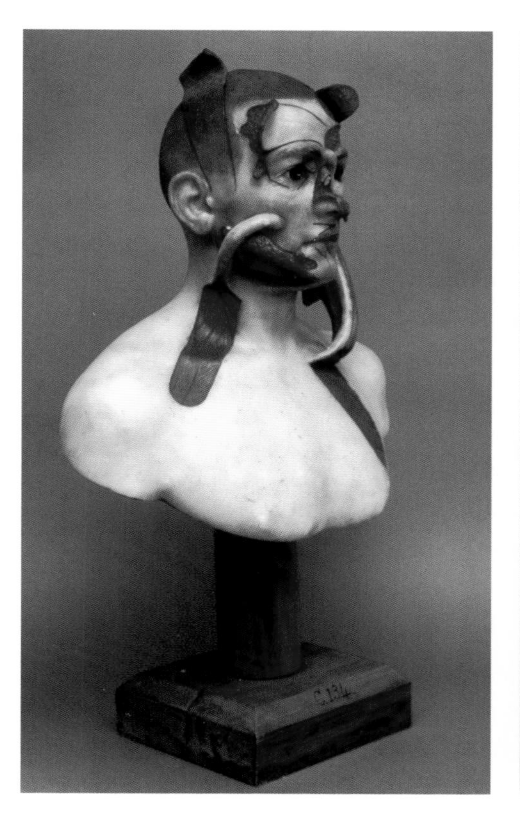

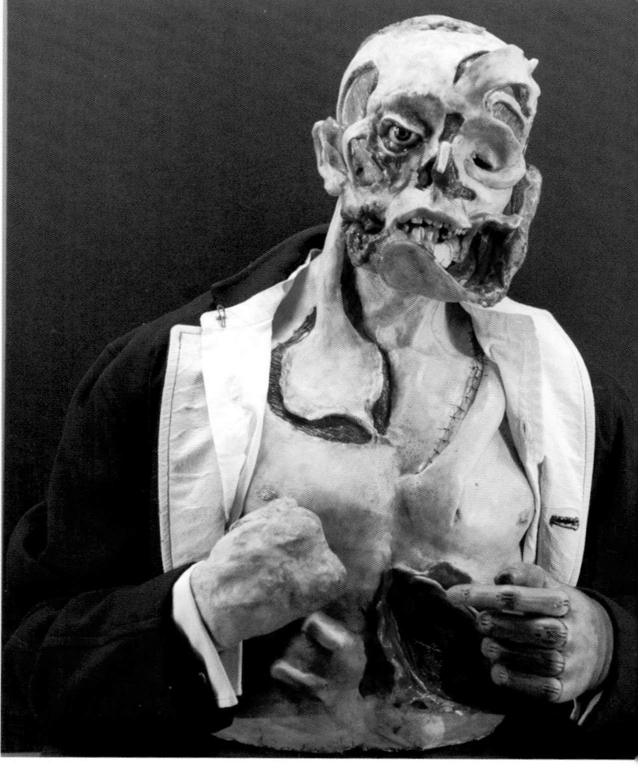

response to the injuries generated by trench warfare, including the tube pedicle. It was intended for use in training but no doubt it had as dramatic an emotional impact then as it has now. It also inspired sculptor Eleanor Crook to craft a successor, 'that red wet Thing I must somehow forget', to mark the re-opening of the Hunterian Museum in 2005 (Figure 15). Models can have strange and unpredictable afterlives and new meanings.

The First World War models and casts were specific to their military context but in the early 20th century the manufacture and trade in anatomical models thrived (Figure 16). European companies including Auzoux and Somso sold their wares widely in Britain: most anatomy departments would have had a series of them, even if they were only deployed for basic instruction. By the

FIGURE 14 (ABOVE LEFT)
Thomas H Kelsey
Model showing reconstructive techniques crafted for the New Zealand Medical Corps, 1917.
Royal College of Surgeons of England. Photograph by John Carr.

FIGURE 15 (ABOVE RIGHT)
Eleanor Crook
'...that red wet Thing I must somehow forget', 2005.
Royal College of Surgeons of England. Photograph by John Carr.

middle of the century, model-making companies began to develop more robust models using new plastics, as noted in Chapter 1.

From plaster to plastic, then, the historic clinical value and aesthetic appeal of medical models is evidenced by those that remain in museum collections today. Individually crafted waxes were museums' central showpieces from the late 18th century in Britain as they were on the Continent, and they endured well into the Victorian period. Towards the end of the 19th century, however, factory-produced models (for example, those by Auzoux's firm) outnumbered those made by craftsmen employed by medical teaching institutions (of which the most celebrated is Towne). By this time, however, plaster emerged as a medium of choice for scientific and medical record-making, and casts proliferated in anatomical and anthropological museums, as they did in other collections. Bodies and faces were cast in their thousands, then reproduced and circulated well into the inter-war period.

Plaster and wax alike were important in durably recording bodies in the third dimension and teaching students how to see those bodies, inside and out. These modelled bodies could be scaled up, coloured, transported and reproduced. They may now seem mute, often having lost their documentation and traces of their original use, but we can nonetheless glean from them their past importance and the skills deployed in their manufacture. Senior clinicians may have originally requested their construction but they were often crafted by humble artisans, technicians whose skills remain on display in these extraordinary models and casts. Indigenous skills developed in Britain through model design with a variety of materials were to continue at the RCS and other medical institutions into the 21st century, as displayed by models in the next section of this book.

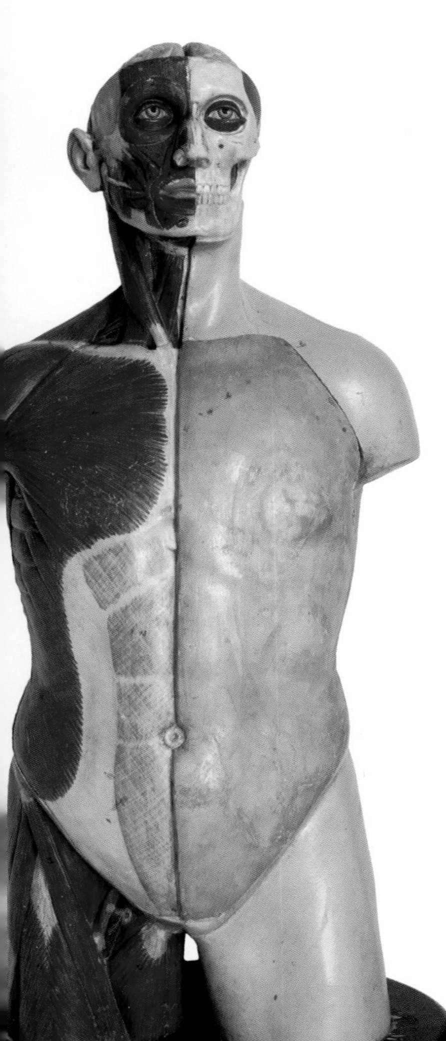

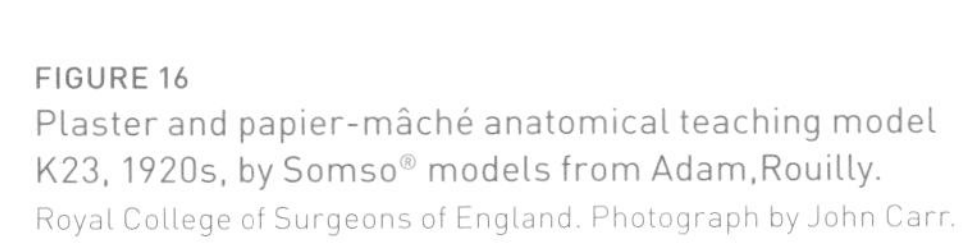

FIGURE 16
Plaster and papier-mâché anatomical teaching model K23, 1920s, by Somso® models from Adam,Rouilly.
Royal College of Surgeons of England. Photograph by John Carr.

NOTES

1. Ludmilla J Jordanova, 'Gender, generation and science: william hunter's obstetrical atlas', in William F Bynum and Roy Porter, eds, *William Hunter and the Eighteenth-Century Medical World* (Cambridge: Cambridge University Press, 1985), pp. 386–412; NA McCulloch, D Russell and Stuart W McDonald, 'William Hunter's casts of the gravid uterus at the University of Glasgow', *Clinical Anatomy*, 14 (2001), 210–17.
2. Martin Kemp and Marina Wallace, *Spectacular Bodies: The Art and Science of the Human Body from Leonardo to Now* (London: Hayward Gallery, 2000).
3. Samuel JMM Alberti, 'Wax bodies: art and anatomy in Victorian museums', *Museum History Journal*, 2 (2009), 7–36.
4. Daniel J Cunningham, *Contribution to the Surface Anatomy of the Cerebral Hemispheres* (Dublin: Academy House, 1892).
5. Samuel JMM Alberti, ed., *War, Art and Surgery: The Work of Henry Tonks and Julia Midgley* (London: Royal College of Surgeons, 2014).
6. Kristin Hussey, 'The Colyer Collection of First World War dental radiographs and casts at the Hunterian Museum', *Dental Historian*, 59 (2014), 66–73.

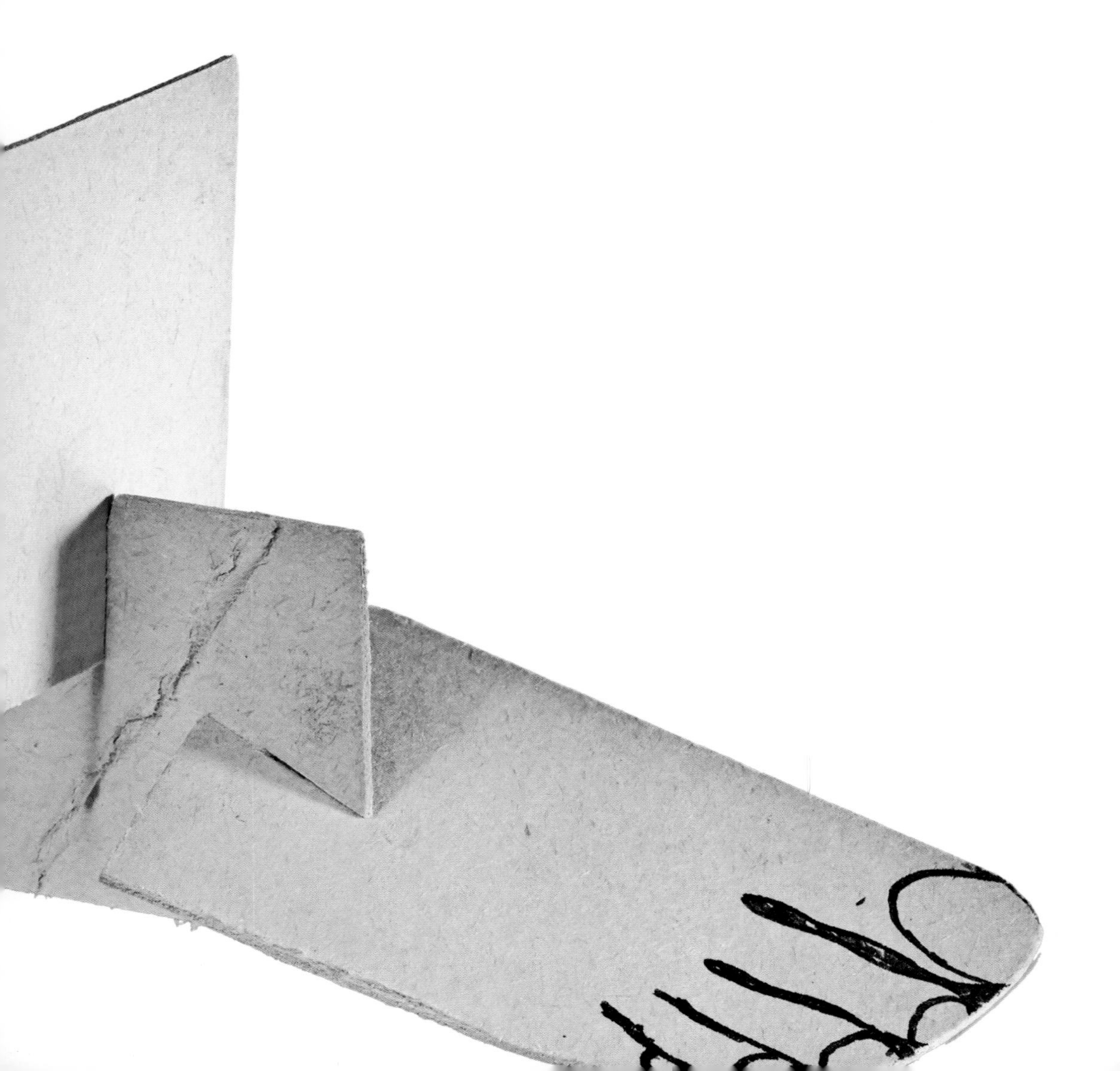

MODELS

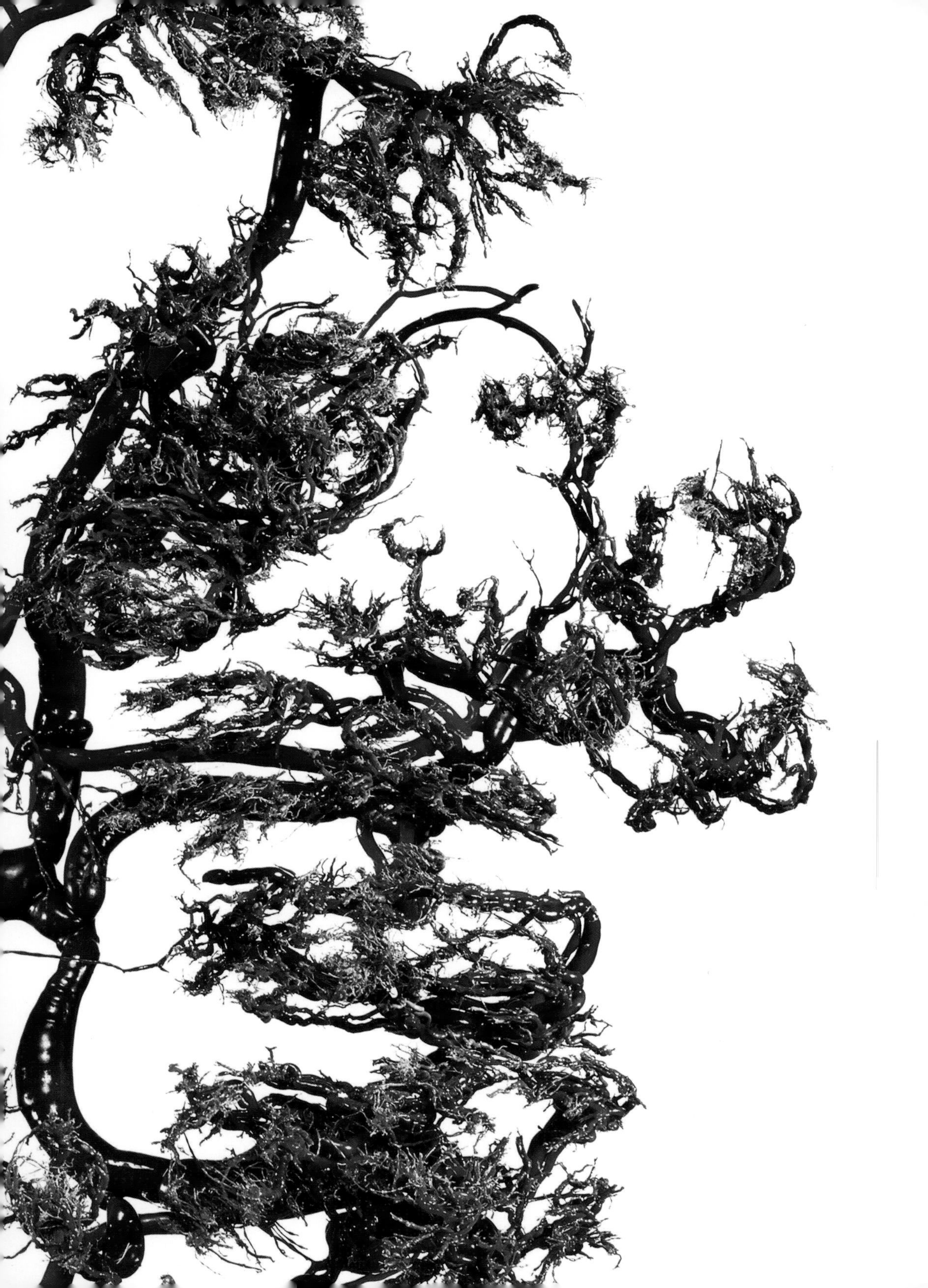

Corrosion casts: David Hugh Tompsett

CATALOGUE 1
David Hugh Tompsett
Corrosion cast of the major arteries supplying the brain, 1957, resin, 10 x 15 x 7 cm.
RCSAC/170b.
Photograph by Michael Frank.

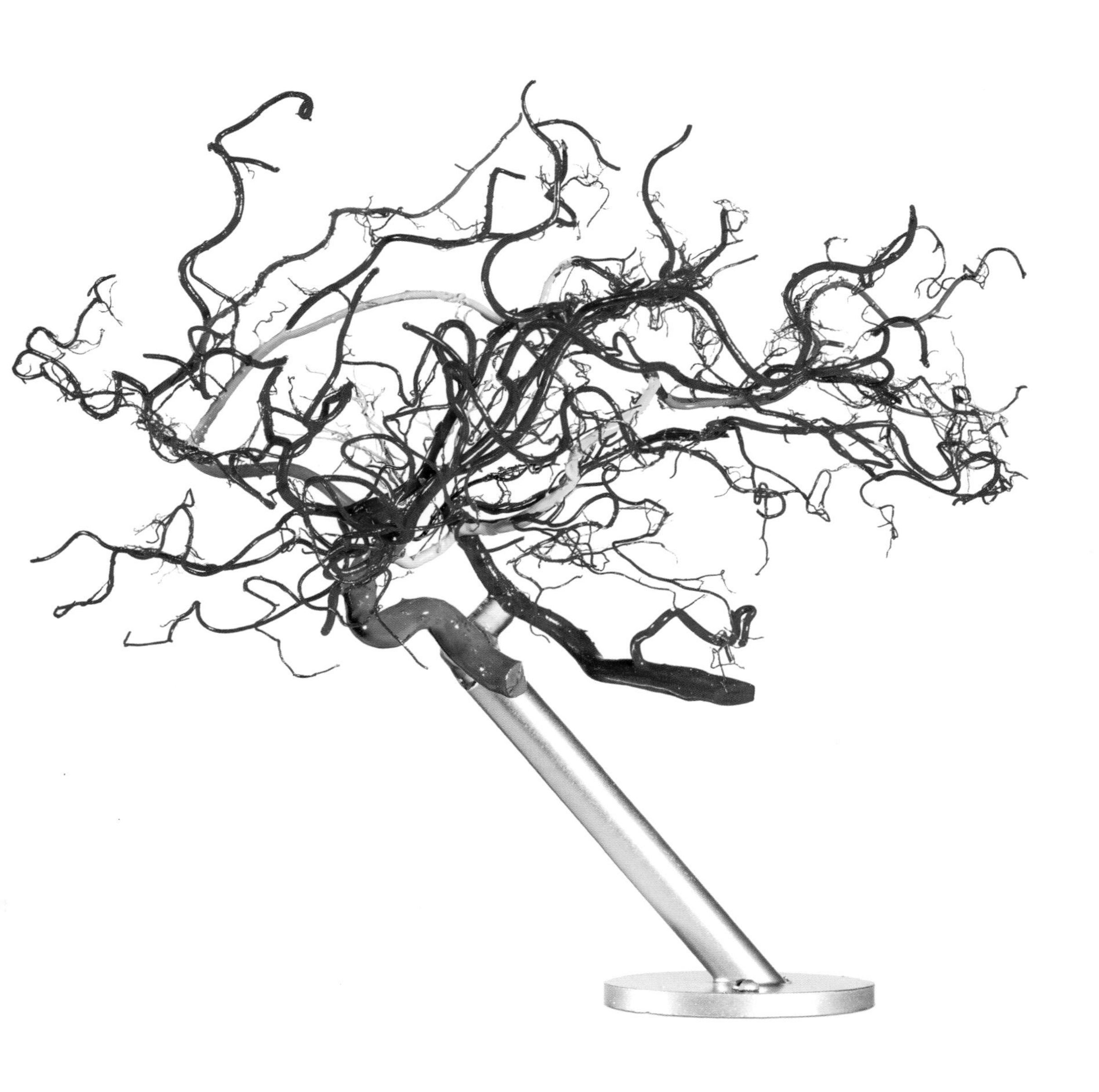

CATALOGUE 2
David Hugh Tompsett
Corrosion cast of the blood vessels in the brain, 1957, resin, 9 x 14 x 15 cm.
RCSAC/170e.
Photograph by Michael Frank.

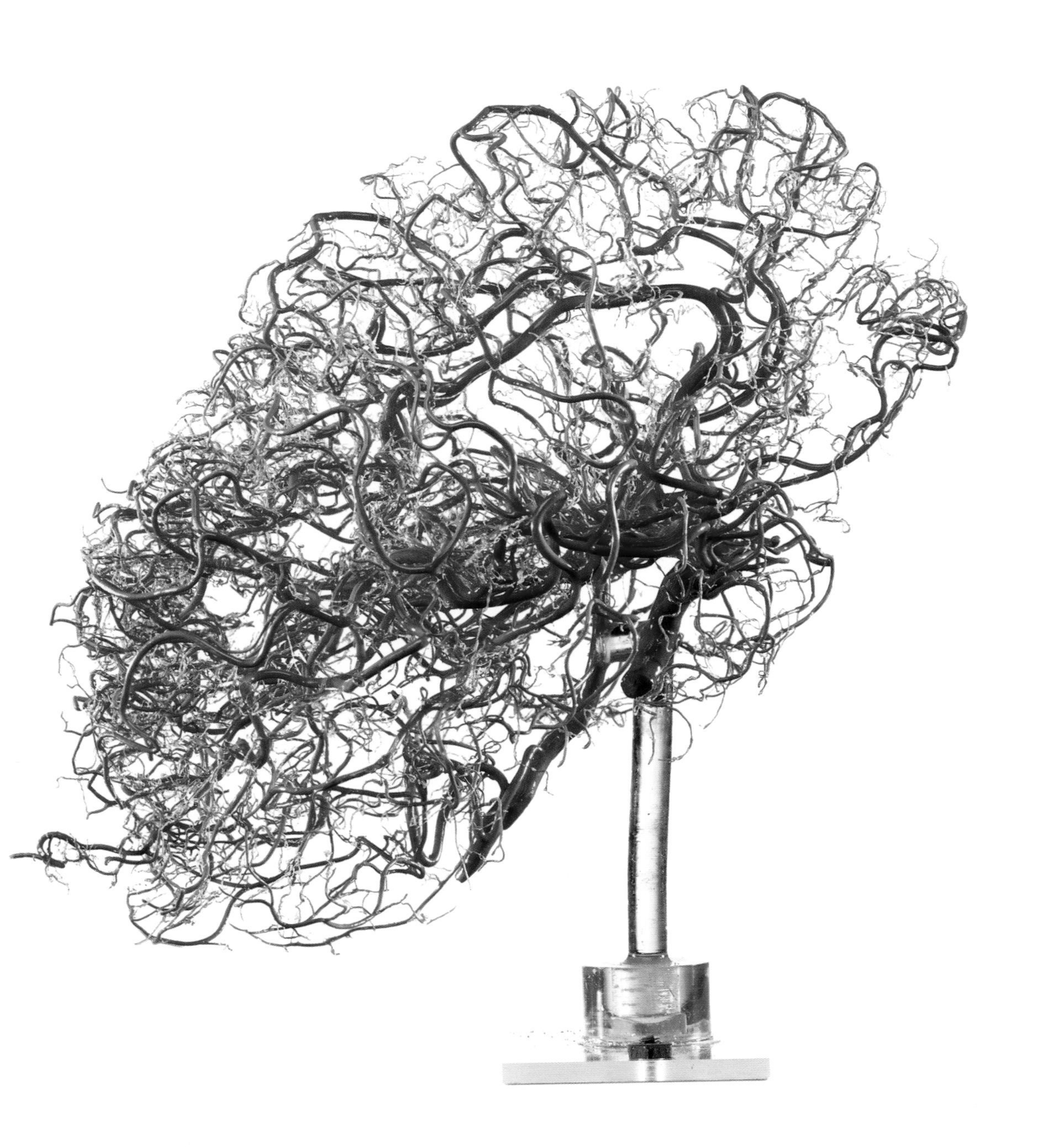

CATALOGUE 3
David Hugh Tompsett
Corrosion cast of blood vessels in the brain (the different colours show different major vessels and their branches, and were highly technically difficult to produce in this way), 1957, resin, 17 x 19 x 13 cm.
RCSAC/170c.
Photograph by Michael Frank.

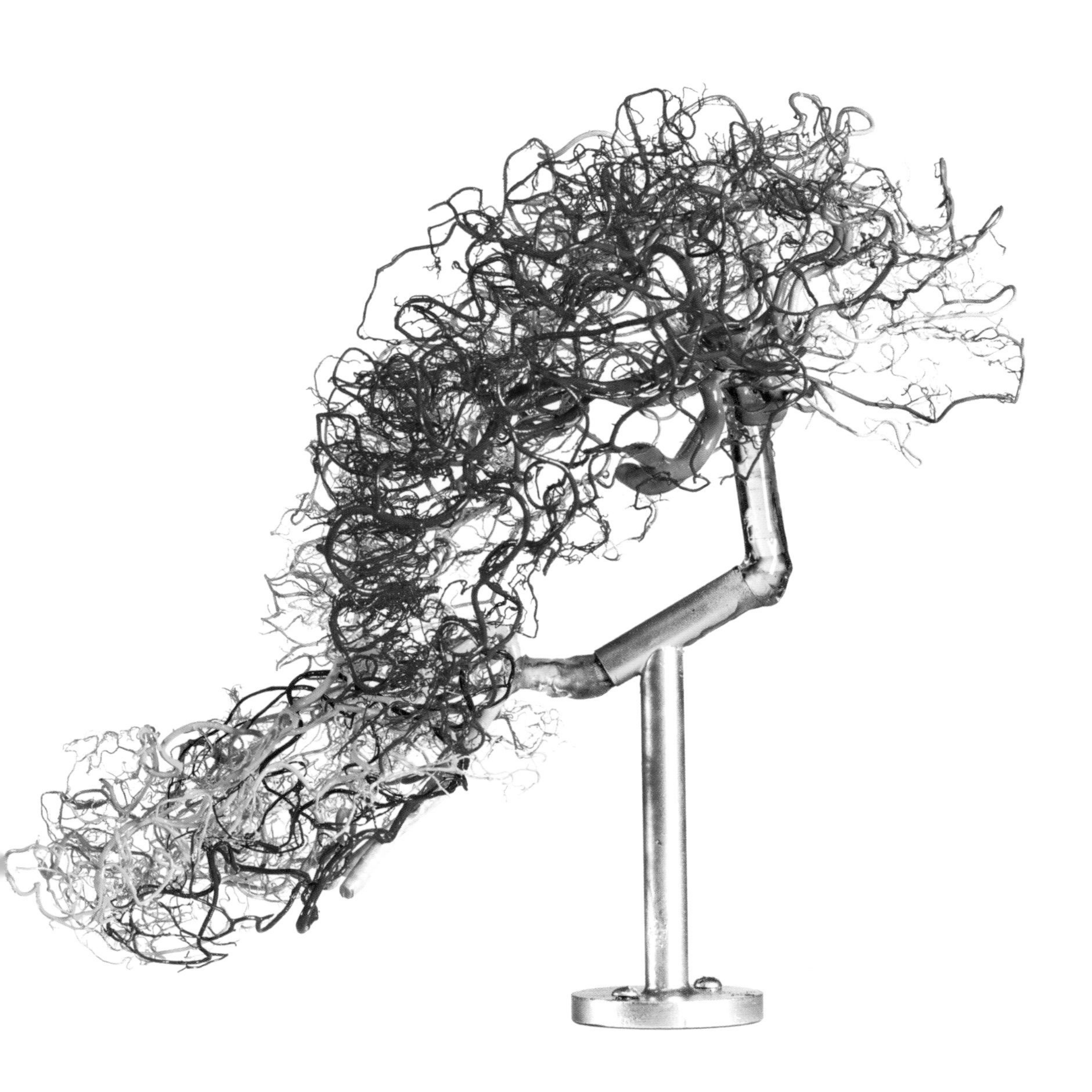

CATALOGUE 4
David Hugh Tompsett
Corrosion cast of blood vessels in the brain, 1960, resin, 10.5 x 16 x 11 cm.
RCSAC/170i.
Photograph by Michael Frank.

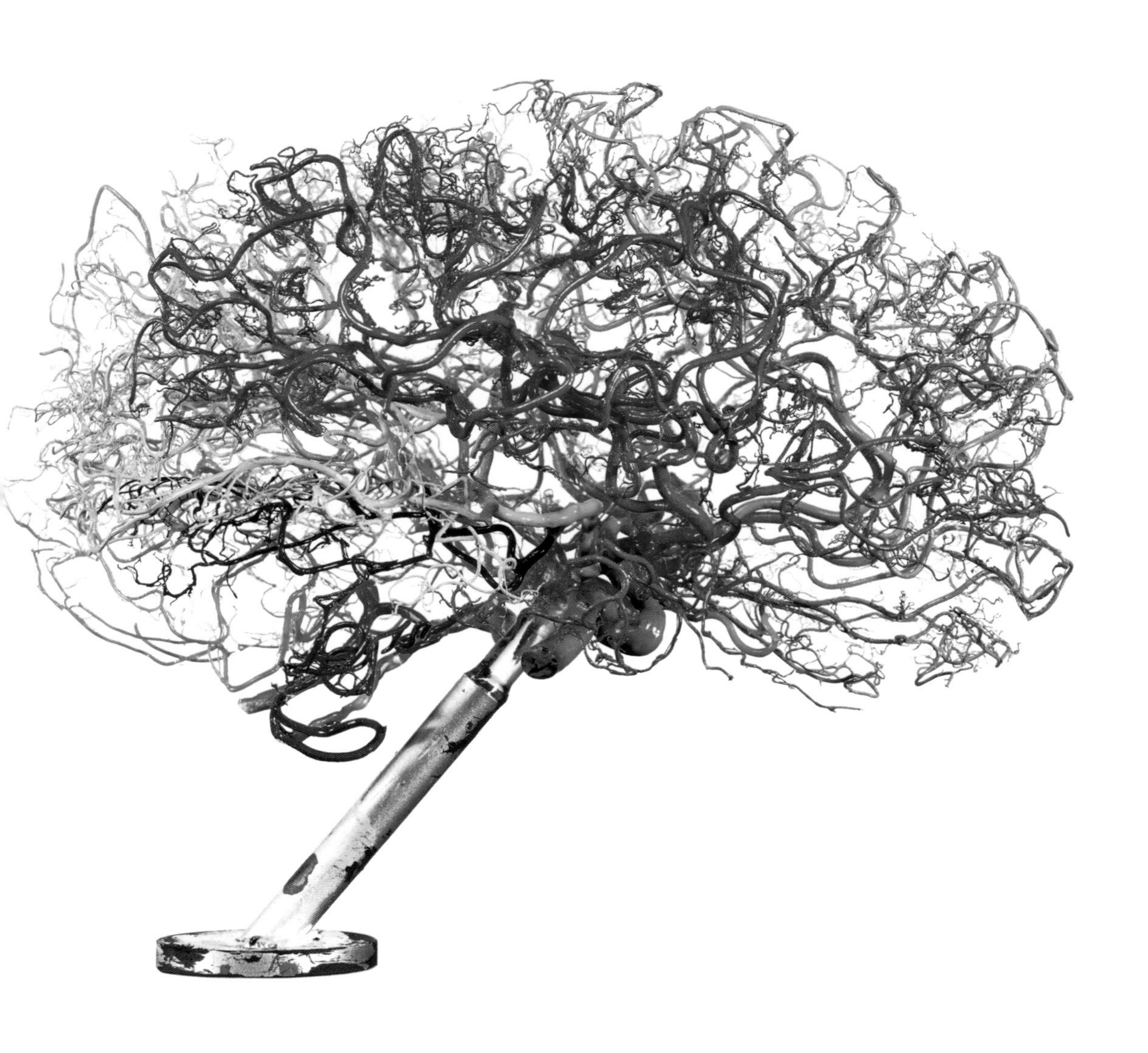

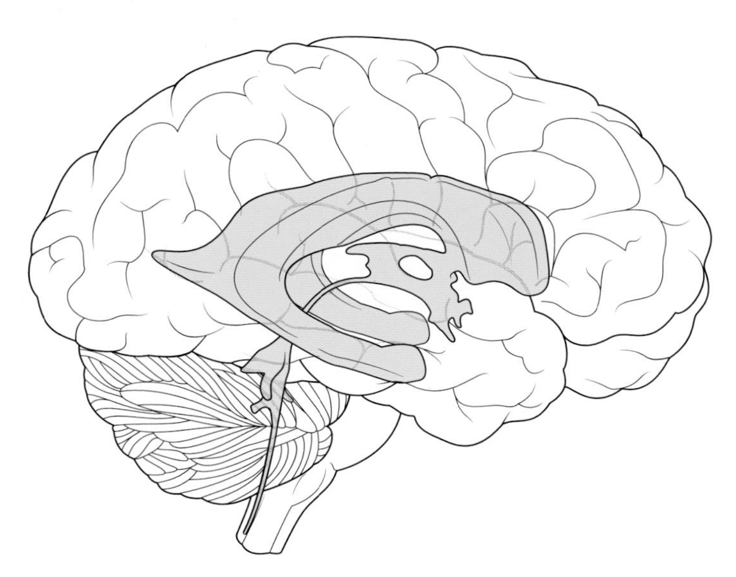

Diagram of the ventricles (in yellow) in the human brain, by Francesca Corra.

CATALOGUE 5
David Hugh Tompsett
Casts of ventricles in three brains and detail of number four (above) (display stand removed), 1950s–60s, resin, 8.5 x 7.5 x 7 cm; 10 x 6.5 x 7 cm; 10.5 x 6.5 x 7 cm.
RCSHM/D 717d.
Photograph by Michael Frank.

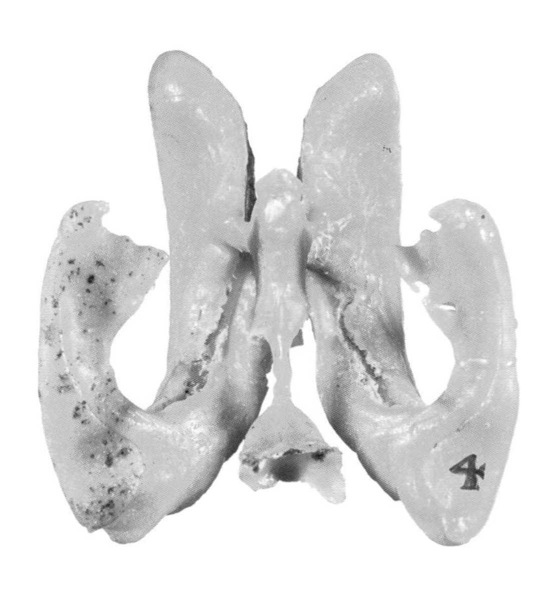
4

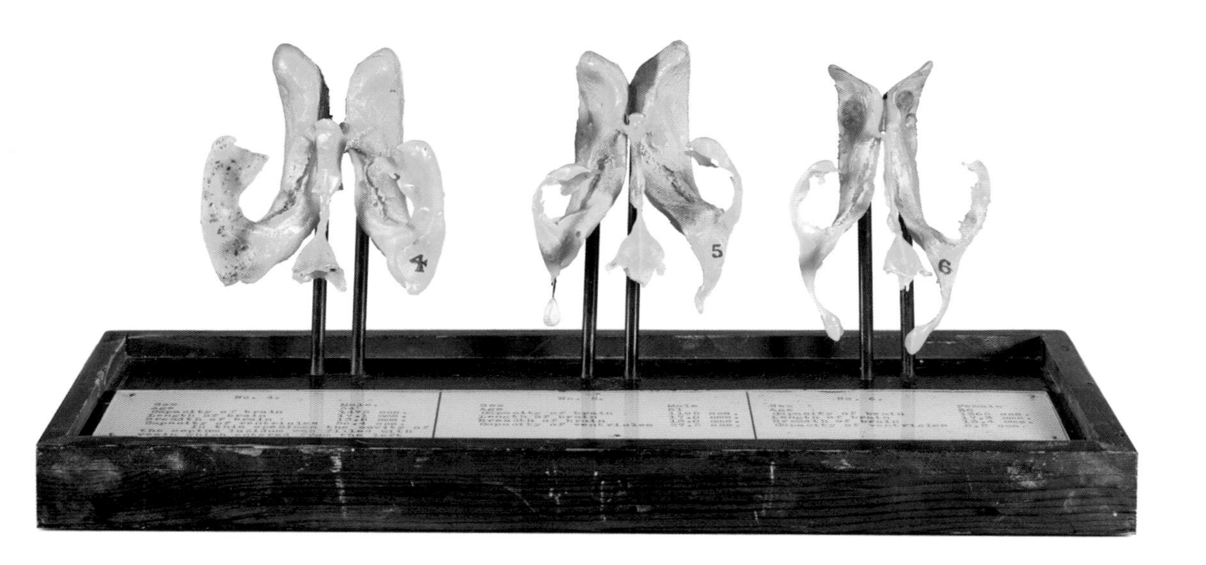
4
5
6

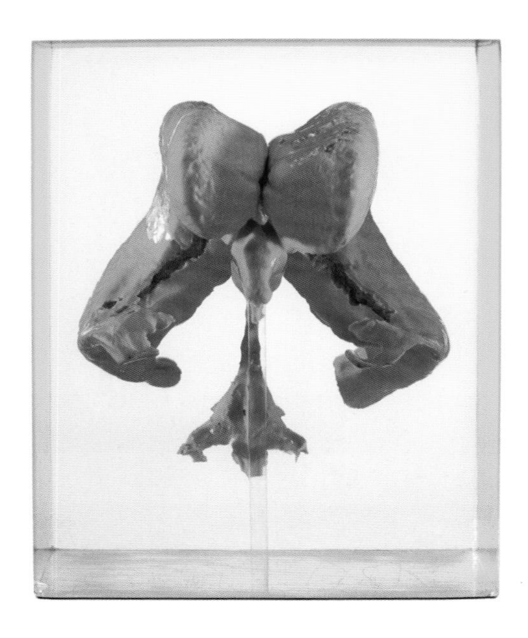

CATALOGUE 6
David Hugh Tompsett
Corrosion cast of the ventricles in the brain, set in a transparent block, side view (right), front view (left), 1965, resin, 12 x 12.5 x 10 cm.
See diagram with Catalogue 5.
RCSAC/219f.
Photographs by Michael Frank.

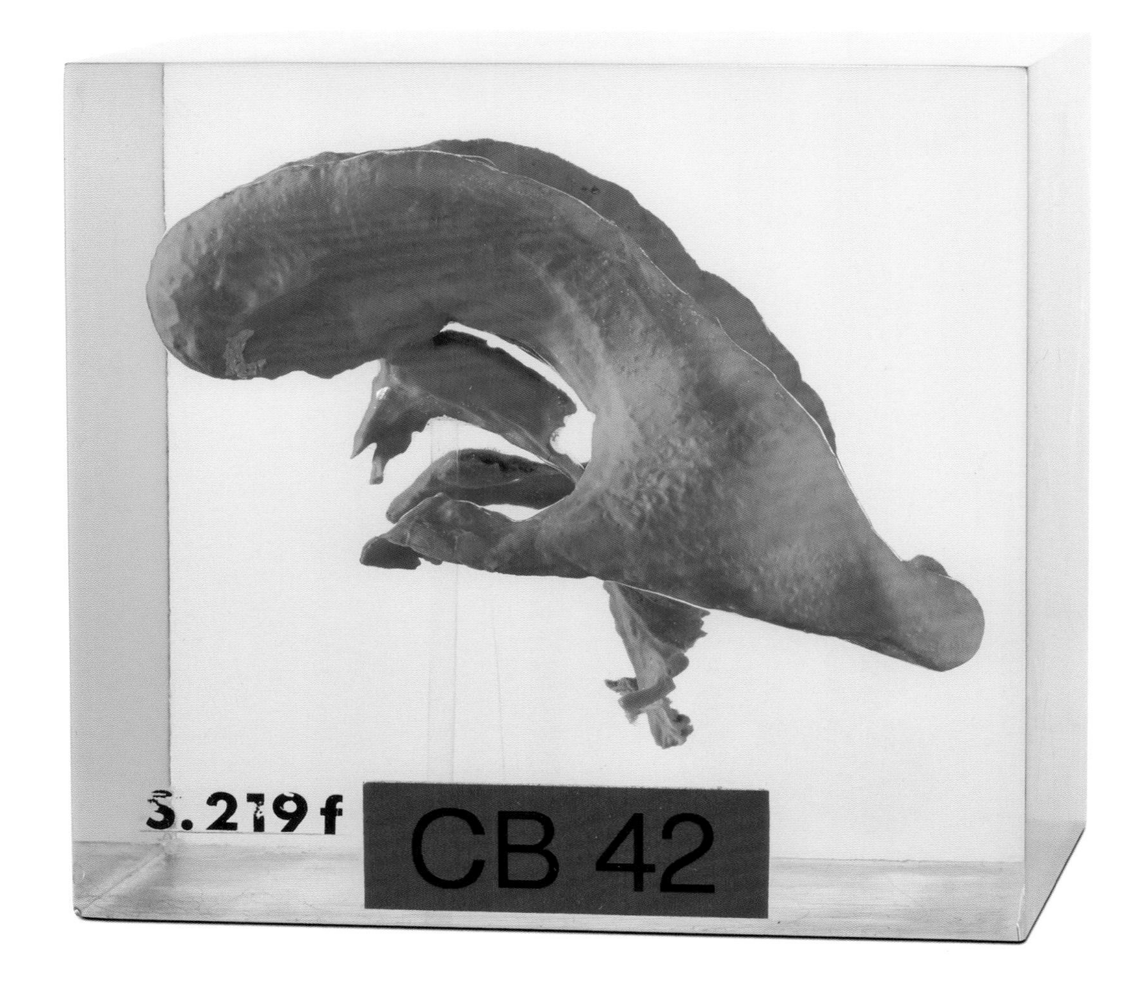
S.219f
CB 42

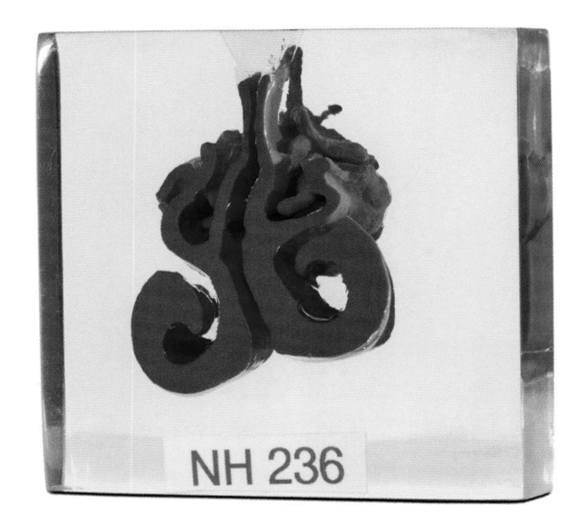

CATALOGUE 7
David Hugh Tompsett
Corrosion cast of the nasal fossae (cavities) set in five transparent blocks, side view (right), and front view of a single block (left) 1962, resin, 6 x 6 x 1 cm (each block).
RCSHM/M 2085.
Photographs by Michael Frank.

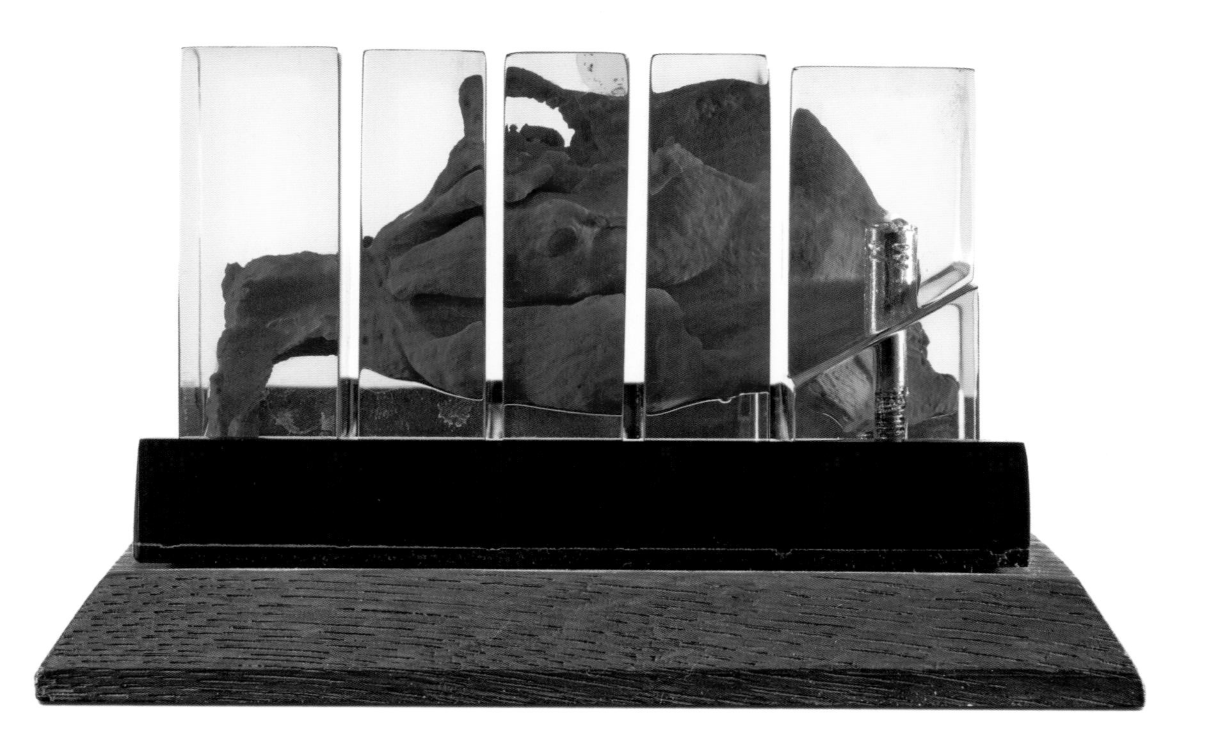

CATALOGUE 8
David Hugh Tompsett
Four casts of the middle and inner ear, set in transparent blocks, 1960s, resin, 6 x 7 x 5.5 cm (each block).
RCSAC/410.1.
Photographs by Michael Frank.

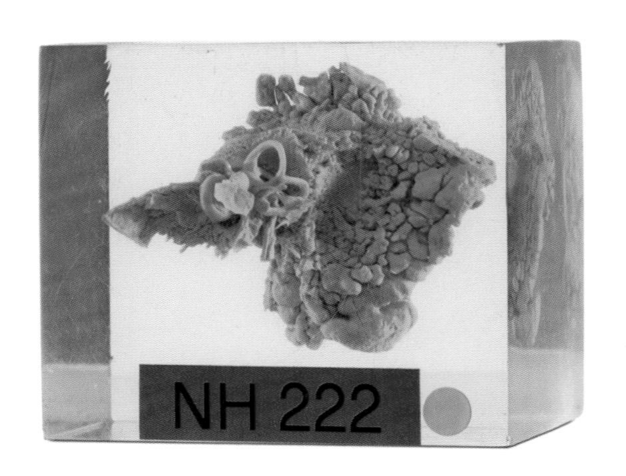
NH 222

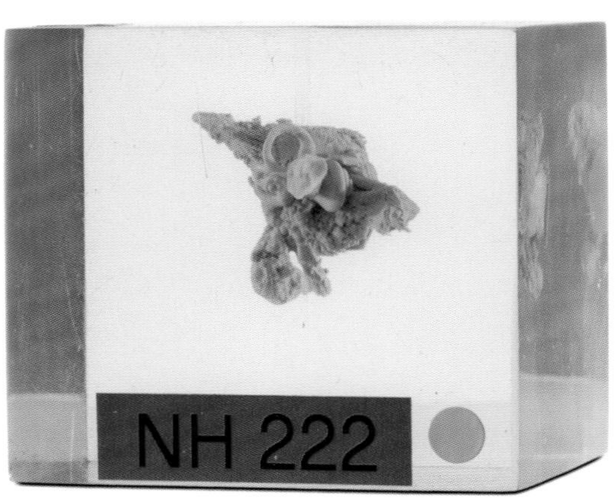
NH 222

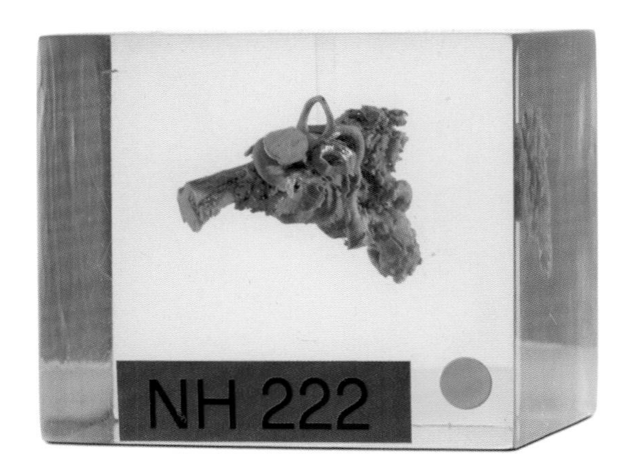
NH 222

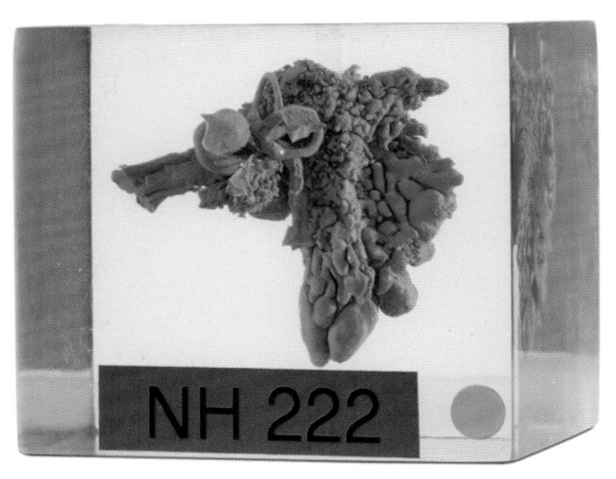
NH 222

CATALOGUE 9
David Hugh Tompsett
Five casts of the middle and inner ear, 1950s-60s, resin, 9 x 8.5 x 8 cm (each box).
RCSAC/D1b, RCSAC/D2b, RCSA/D3, RCSAC/D4, RCSAC/D5
Photographs by Michael Frank.

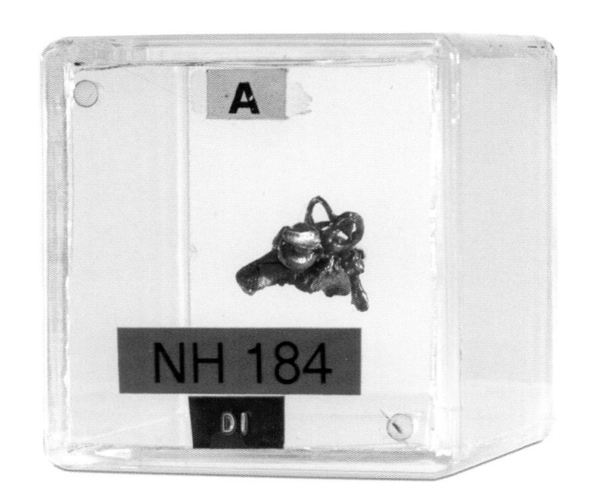
A
NH 184
D1

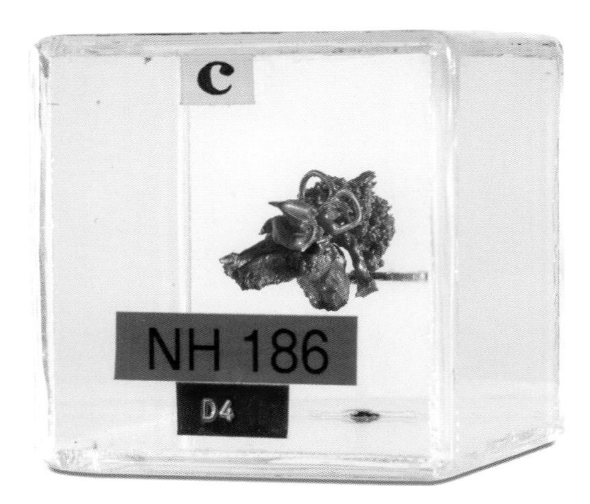
C
NH 186
D4

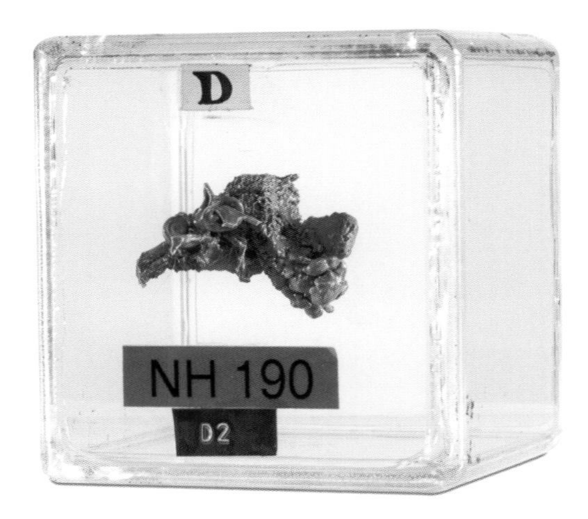
D
NH 190
D2

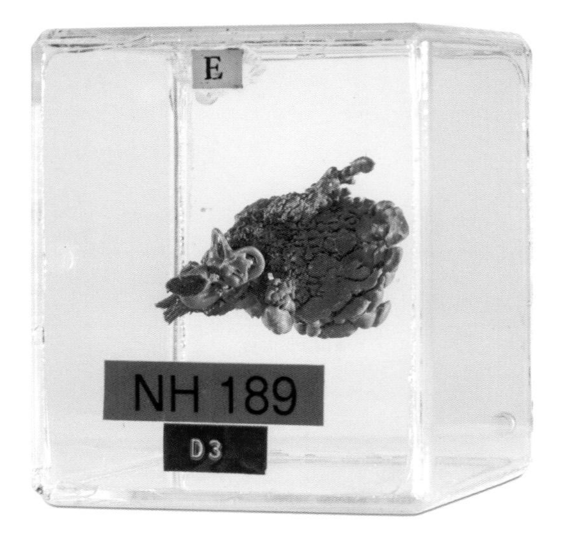
E
NH 189
D3

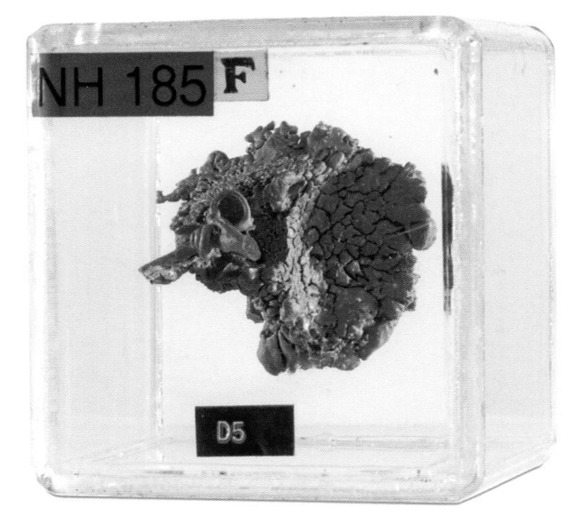
NH 185
F
D5

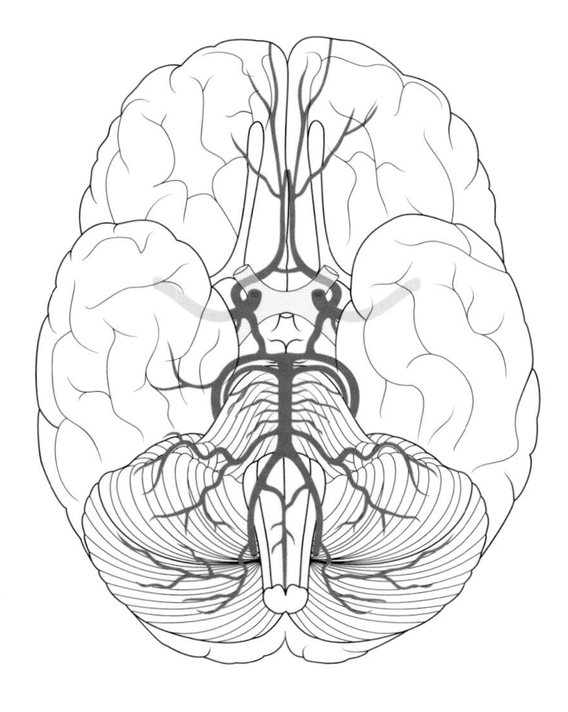

Diagram of the circle of Willis (in red) in the human brain, by Francesca Corra.

CATALOGUE 10
David Hugh Tompsett
Corrosion cast of the arterial circle of Willis, 1964, resin, 90 x 5.5 x 6.5 cm.
The diagram is viewed from the base of the brain, the cast from the front.
RCSAC/170m.
Photograph by Michael Frank.

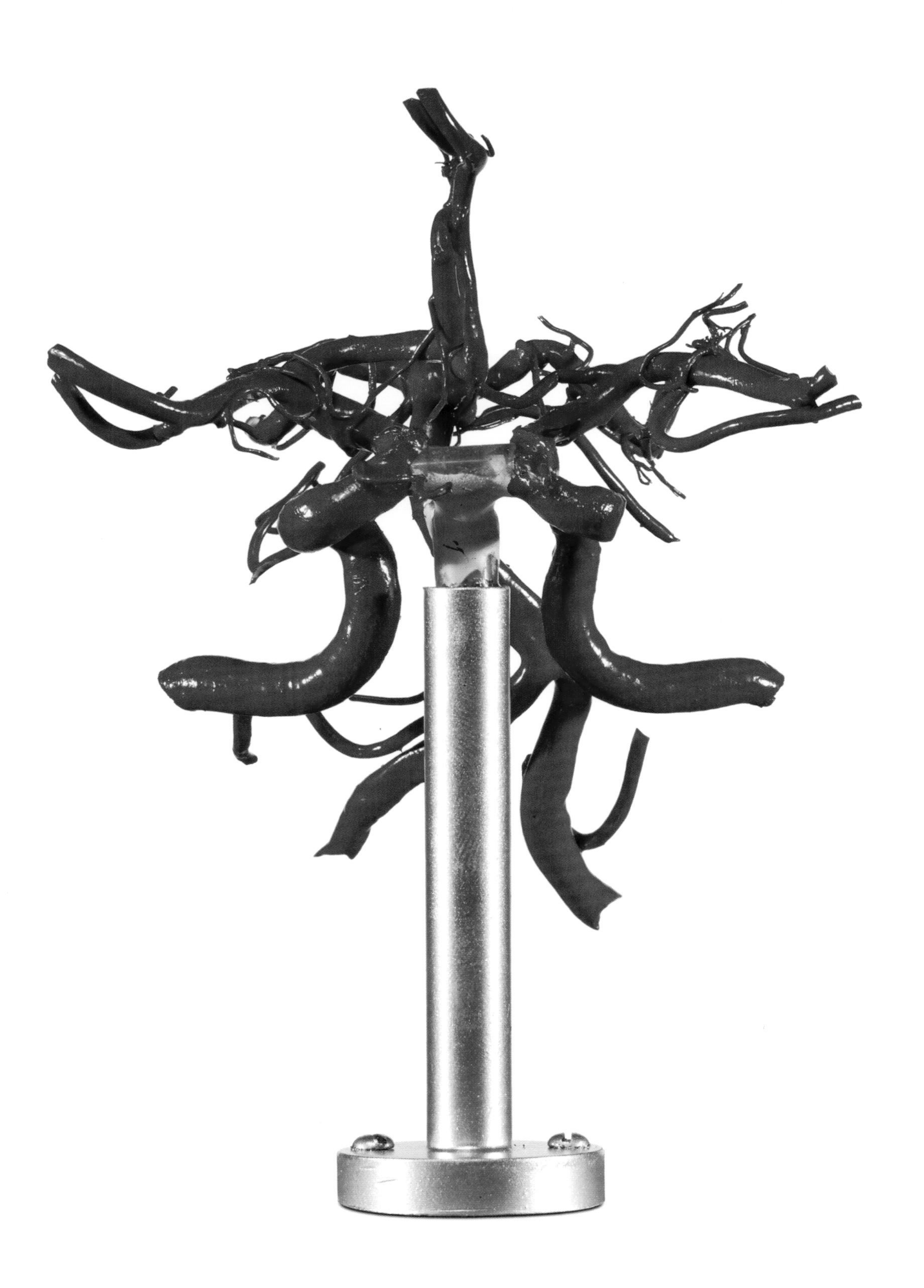

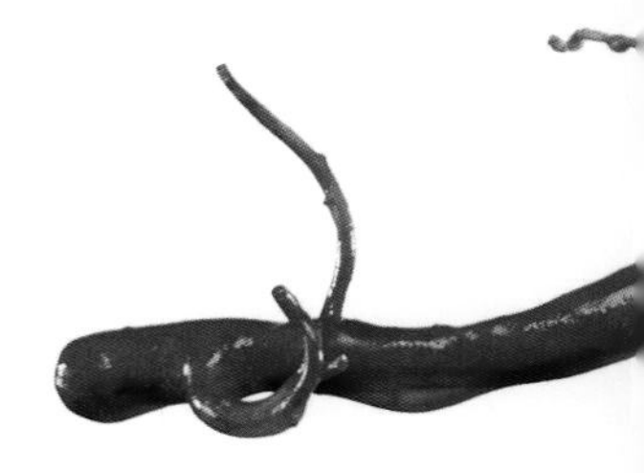

CATALOGUE 11
David Hugh Tompsett
Corrosion cast of the arch of the aorta and the great vessels arising from the aorta, 1972, resin, 14 x 20 x 9.5 cm.
RCSAC/263.12.
Photograph by Michael Frank.

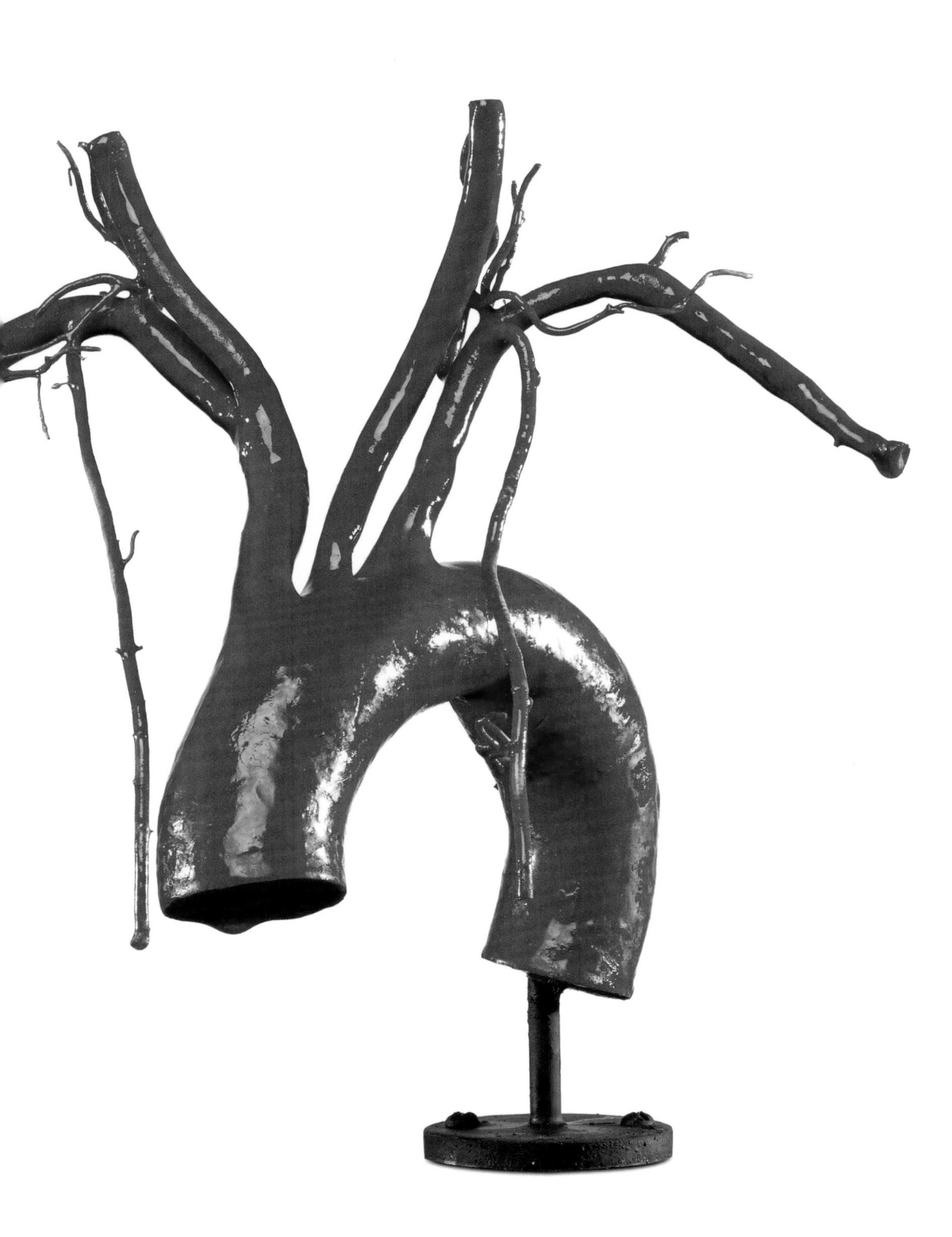

CATALOGUE 12
David Hugh Tompsett
Corrosion cast of left ventricle of the heart and aorta, showing the origin of the aorta and its main branches into the neck, 1960, resin, 36 x 11.5 x 10 cm.
RCSAC/268a.
Photograph by Michael Frank.

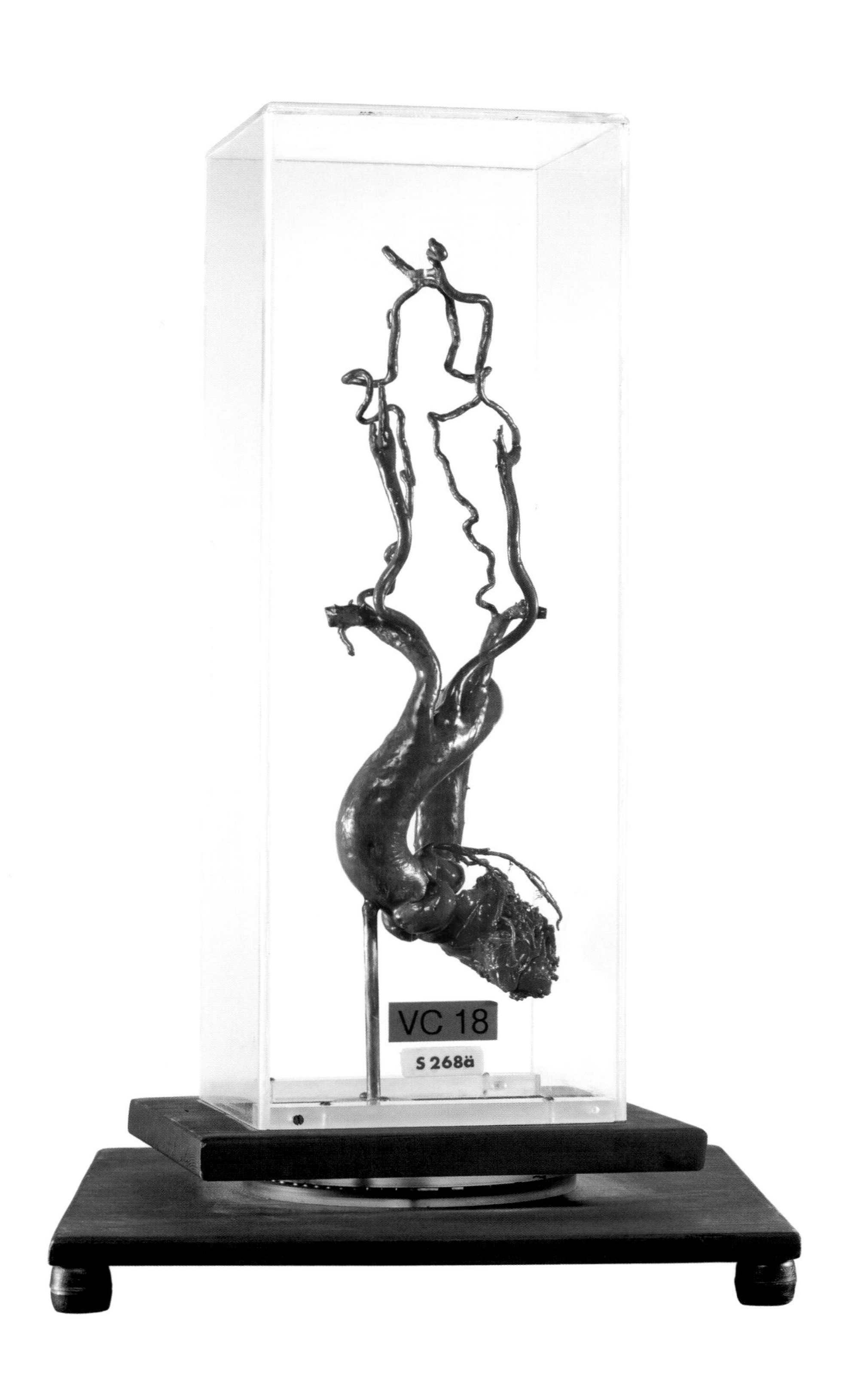
VC 18
S 268ä

CATALOGUE 13
David Hugh Tompsett
Corrosion cast of blood vessels supplying the spinal cord from a patient with curvature of the spine, 1950s-60s, resin, 65 x 17.5 x 19 cm.
RCSHM/K 429.1.
Photograph by Michael Frank.

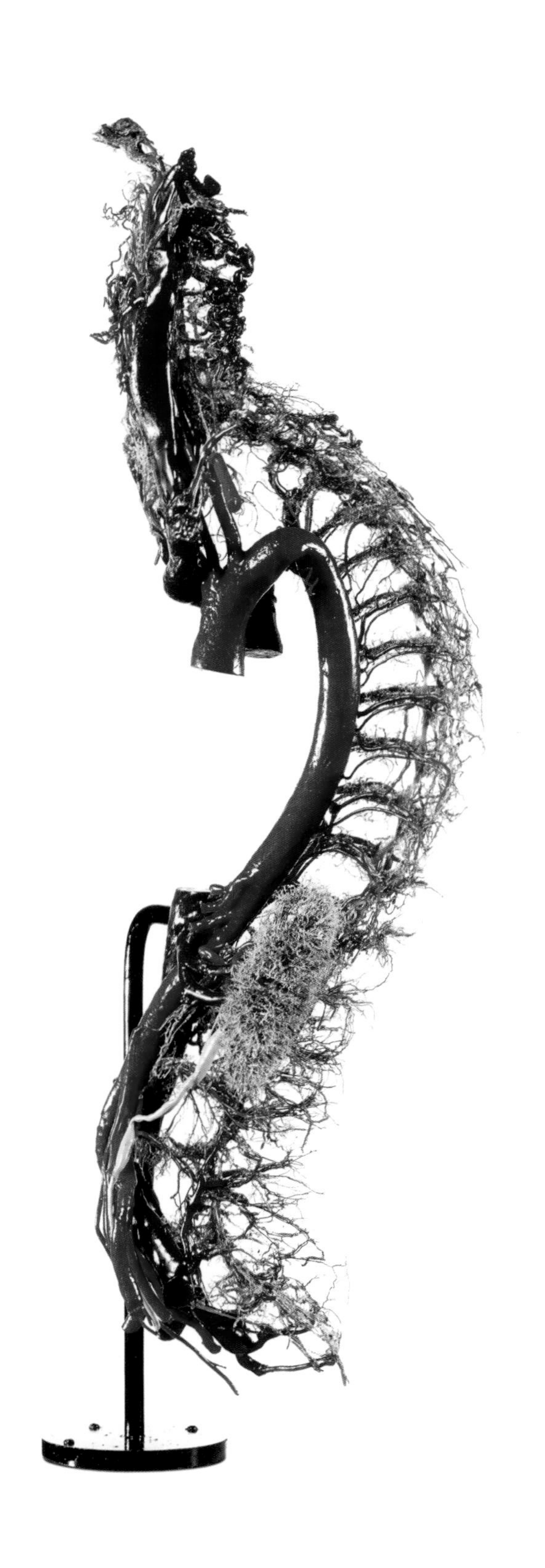

CATALOGUE 14
David Hugh Tompsett
Corrosion cast of coronary blood vessels in the heart, including ascending aorta (red) and pulmonary trunk (blue), 1955, resin, 17.5 x 9.5 x 7.5 cm.
RCSAC/263.2.
Photograph by Michael Frank.

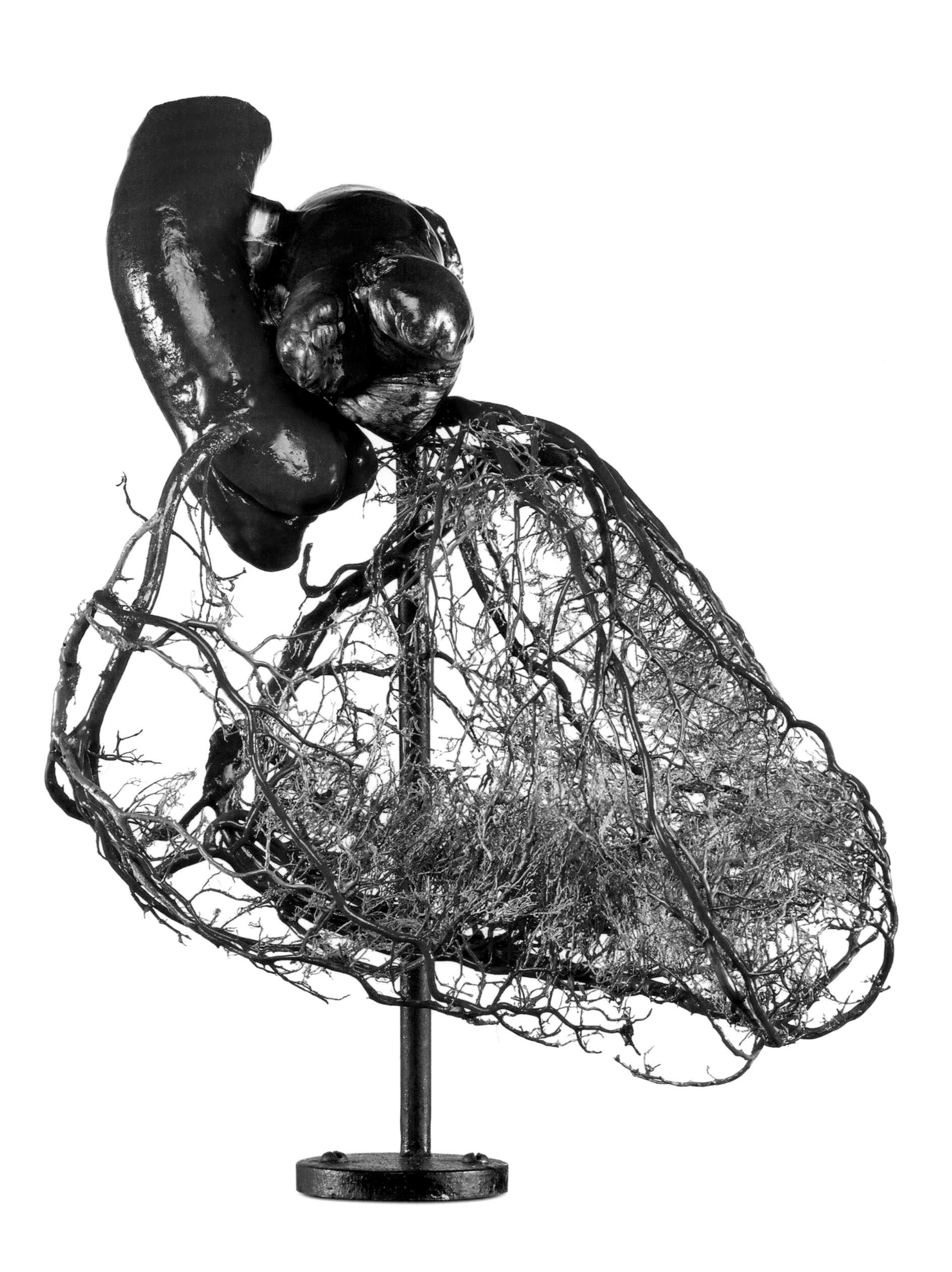

CATALOGUE 15
David Hugh Tompsett
Corrosion cast of blood vessels in the heart (display stand removed), 1958, resin, 14 x 8.5 x 9.5 cm.
RCSAC/264aa.
Photograph by Michael Frank.

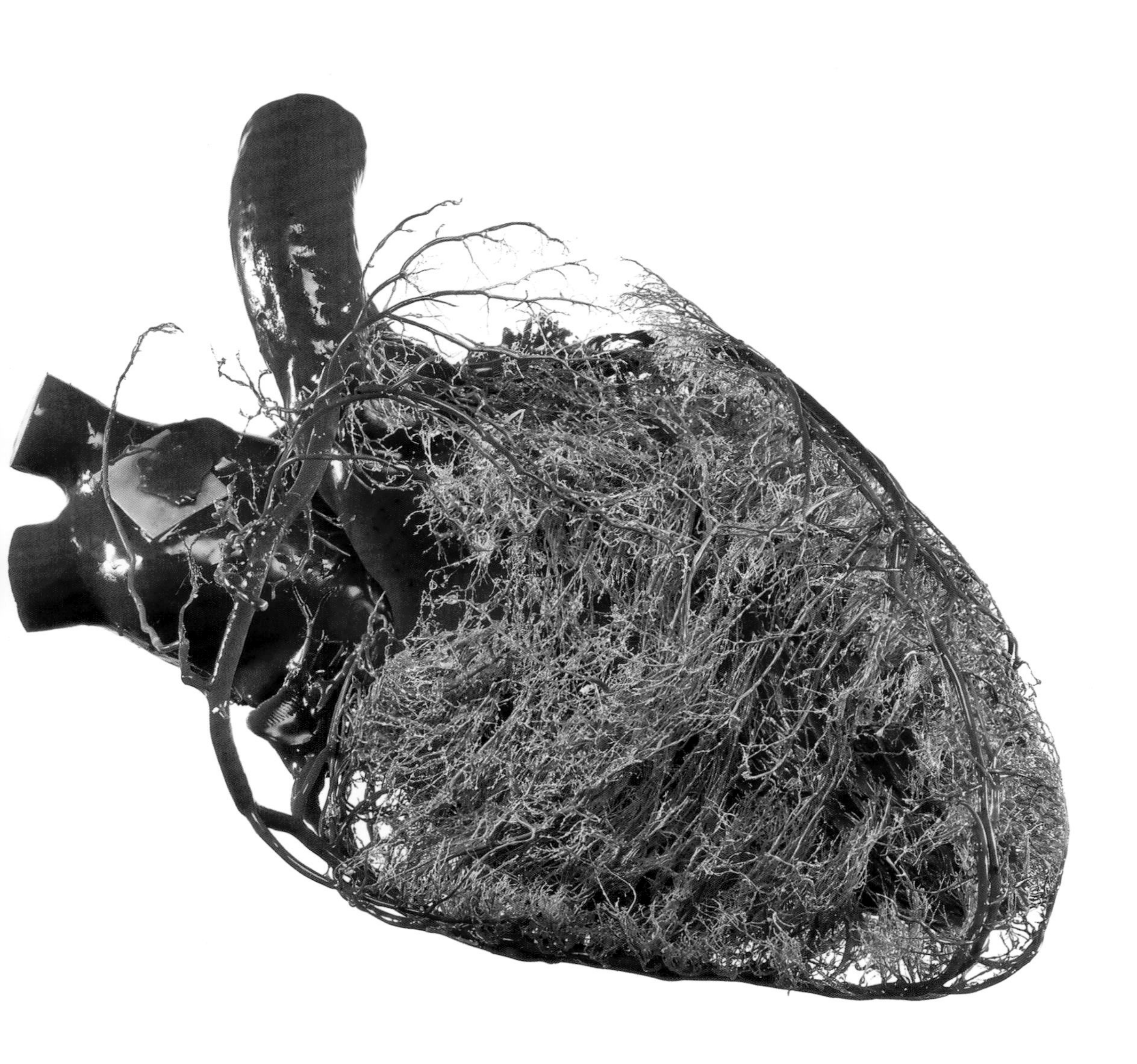

CATALOGUE 16
David Hugh Tompsett
Corrosion cast of the heart showing roots of major vessels and cardiac vasculature (display stand removed), 1950s-60s, resin, 19 x 11 x 11 cm.
RCSAC/263.1.
Photograph by Michael Frank

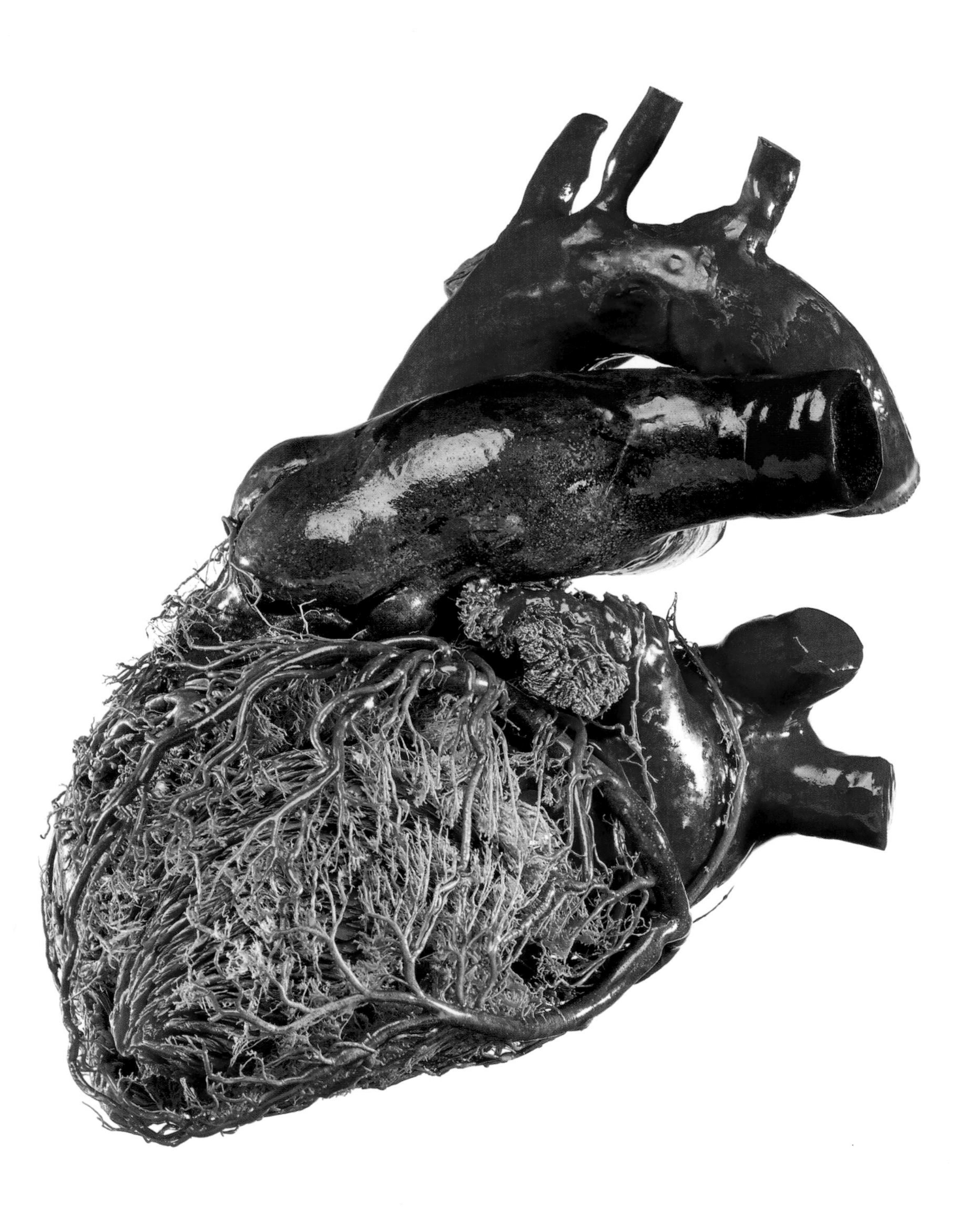

CATALOGUE 17
David Hugh Tompsett
Corrosion cast of the coronary arteries arising from the aortic sinus, set in a transparent block, 1965, resin, 13 x 13 x 12.5 cm.
RCSAC/264s.
Photograph by Michael Frank.

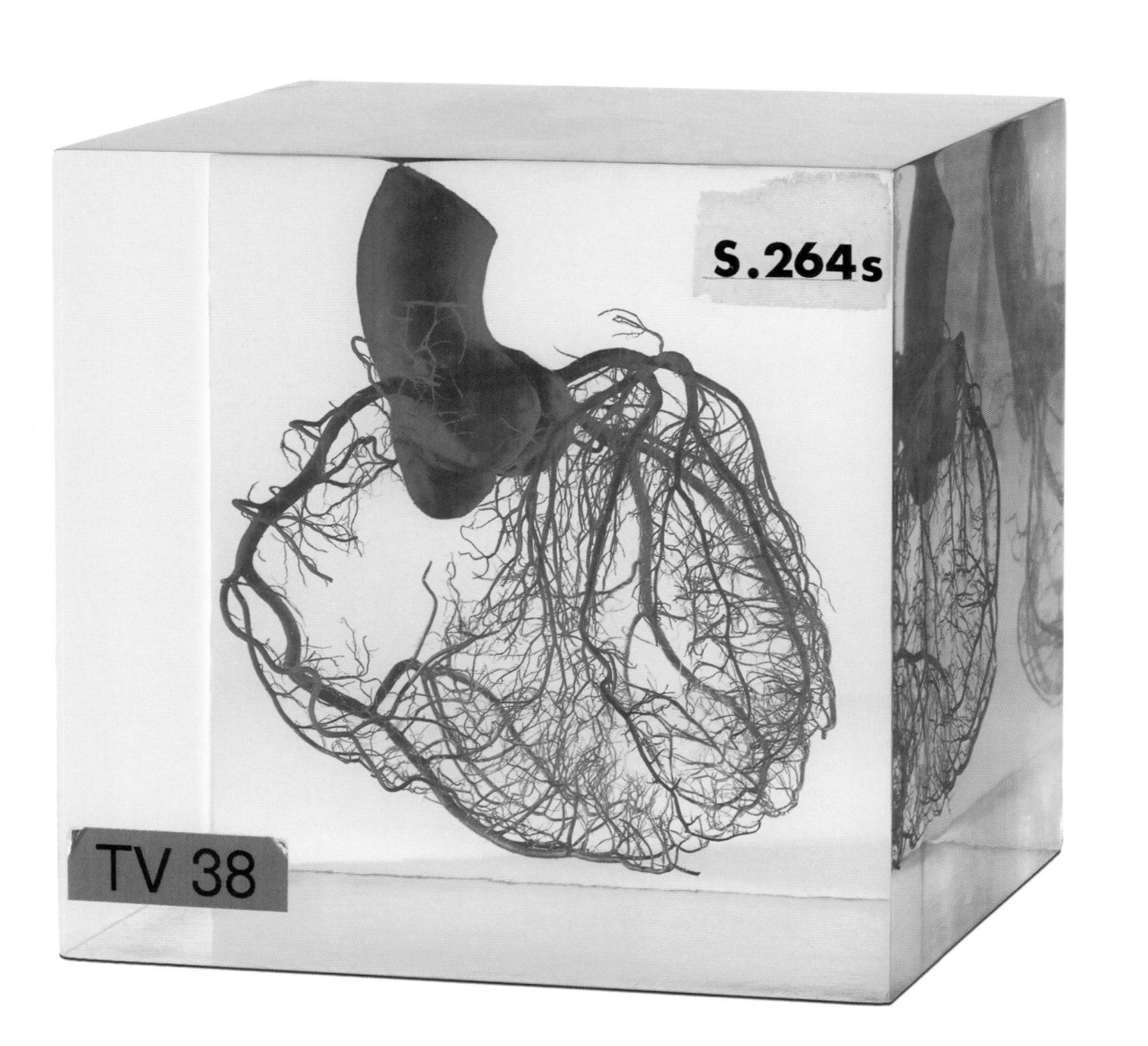
S.264s
TV 38

CATALOGUE 18
David Hugh Tompsett
Coloured corrosion cast of both lungs demonstrating bronchopulmonary segments (display stand removed), 1965, resin and paint, 23 x 2 x 14.5 cm.
RCSAC/254p.
Photograph by Michael Frank.

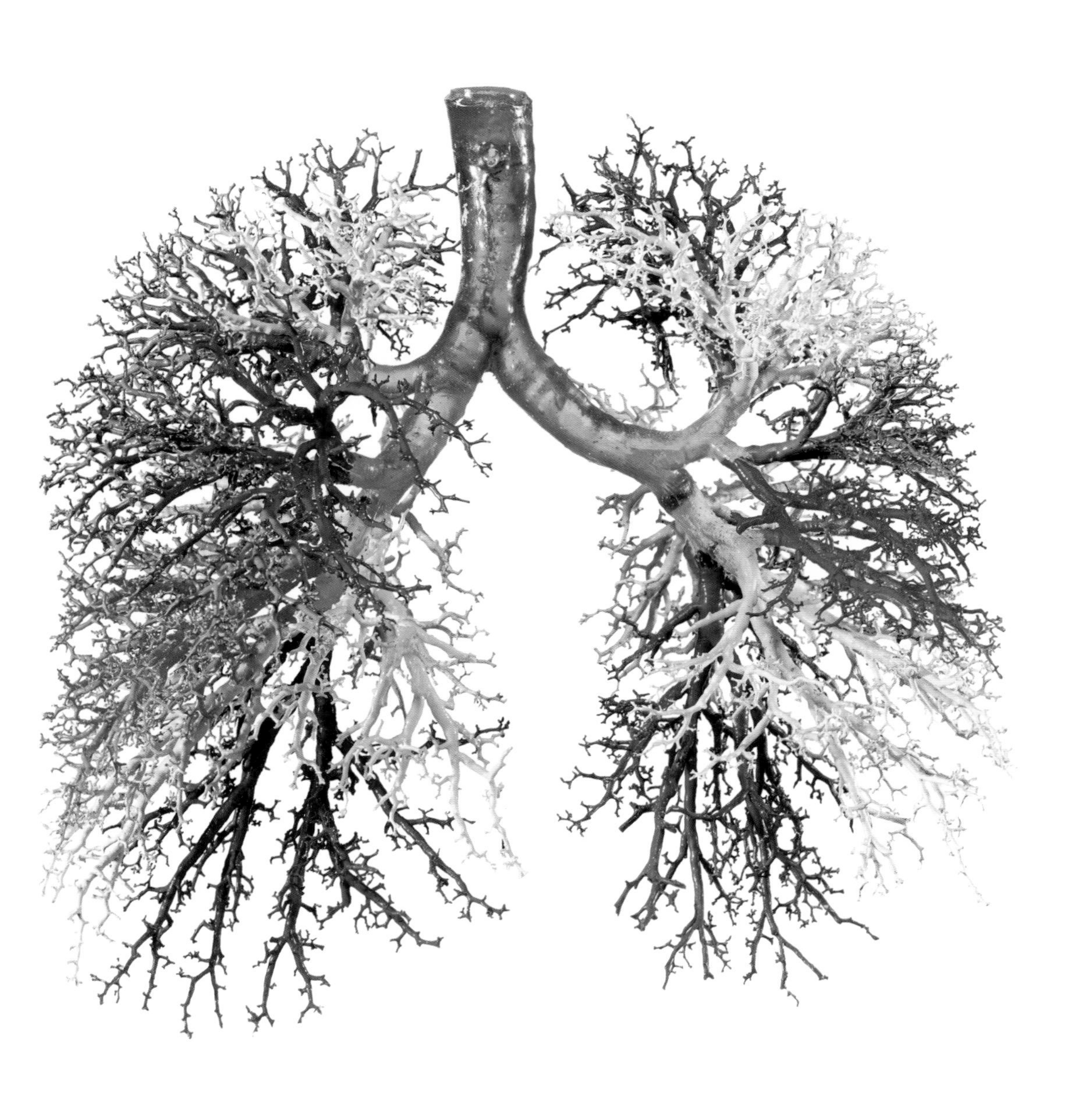

CATALOGUE 19
David Hugh Tompsett
Corrosion cast of bronchial tree in the lungs and pulmonary arteries (red) (display stand removed), 1971, resin, 21.5 x 21 x 13 cm.
RCSAC/253.53.
Photograph by Michael Frank.

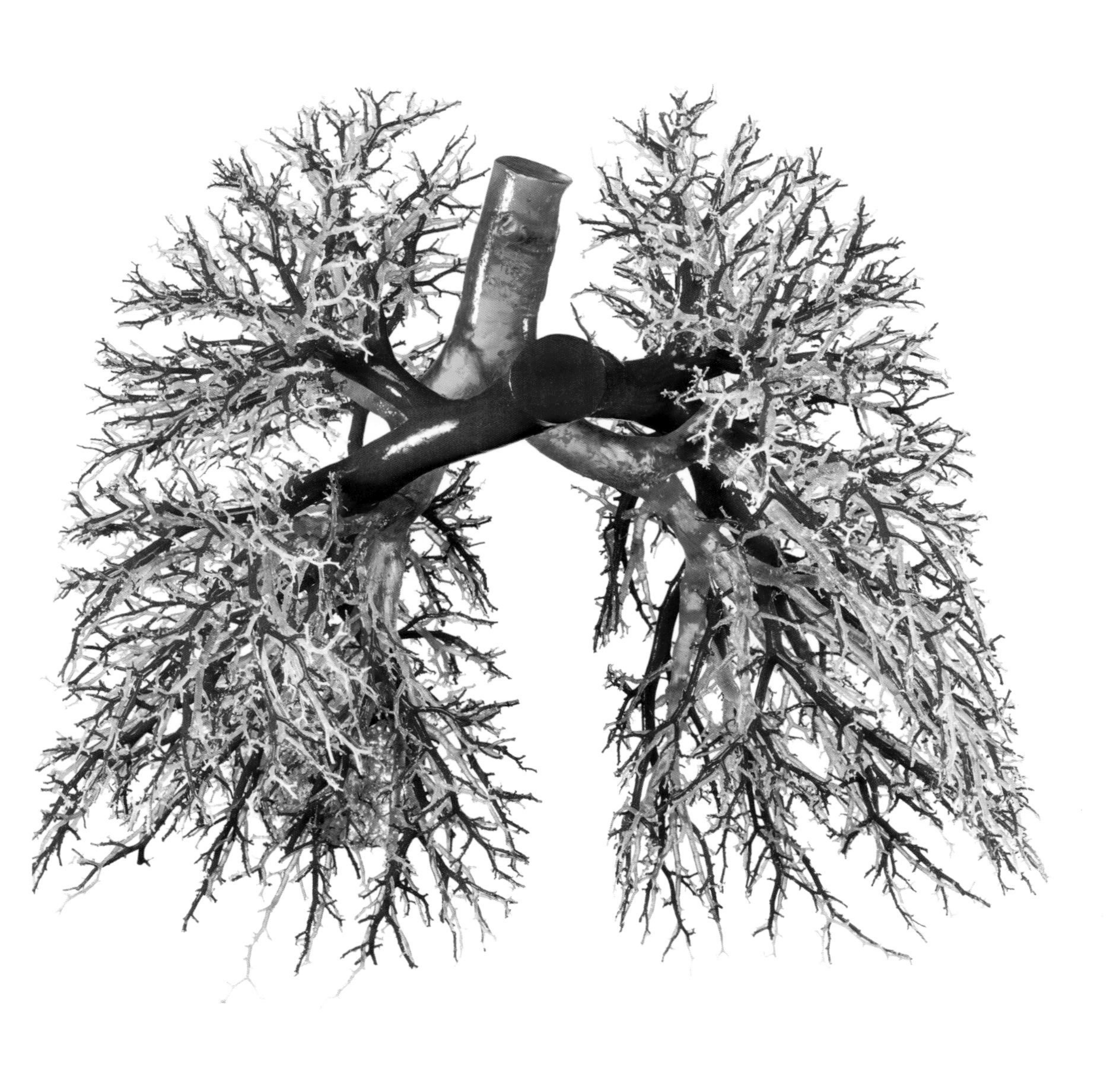

CATALOGUE 20
David Hugh Tompsett
Corrosion cast of bronchial tree before 'pruning' (from a female aged 24 years) (display stand removed), 1950s-60s, resin, 25 x 20 x 15 cm.
RCSAC/253.6a.
Photograph by Michael Frank.

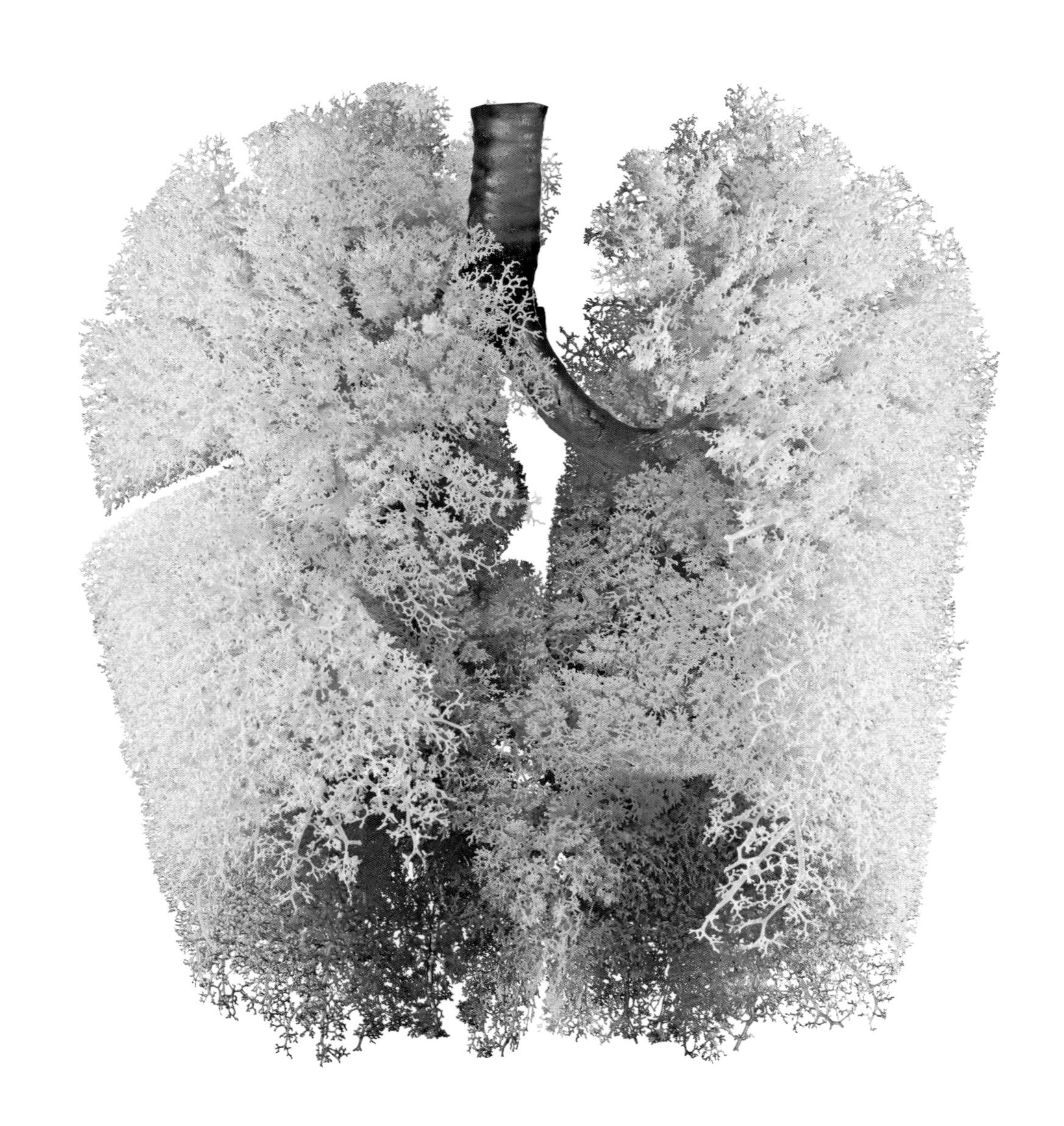

CATALOGUE 21
David Hugh Tompsett
Corrosion cast of the bronchial tree (from an neonate aged 1 day), 1961, resin, 7 x 9.5 x 7.5 cm.
RCSAC/253.3.
Photograph by Michael Frank.

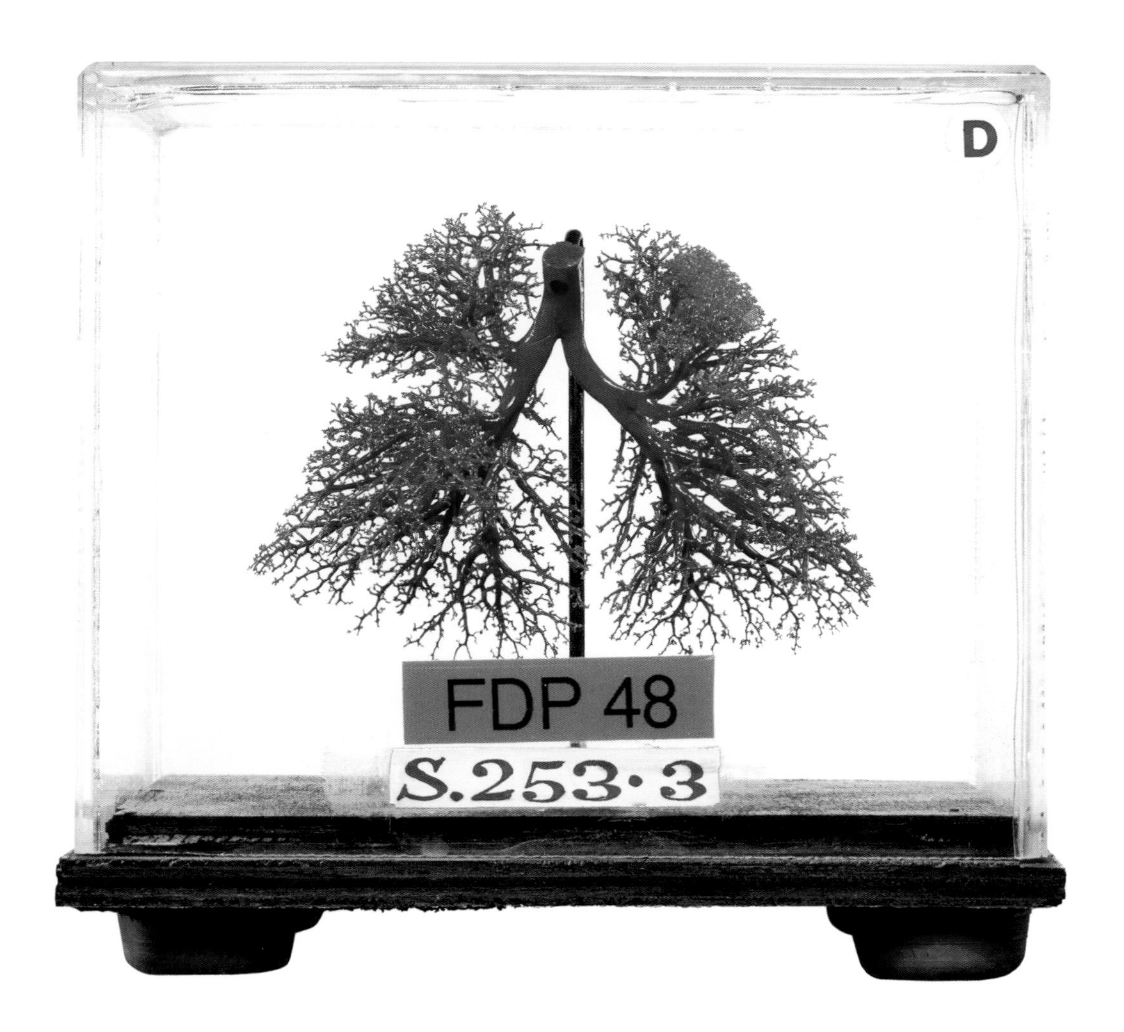
D
FDP 48
S.253·3

CATALOGUE 22
David Hugh Tompsett
Coloured segmental cast of the bronchial tree, painted and set in a transparent block, 1971, resin, 15 x 16 x 12 cm.
RCSAC/253.54.
Photograph by Michael Frank.

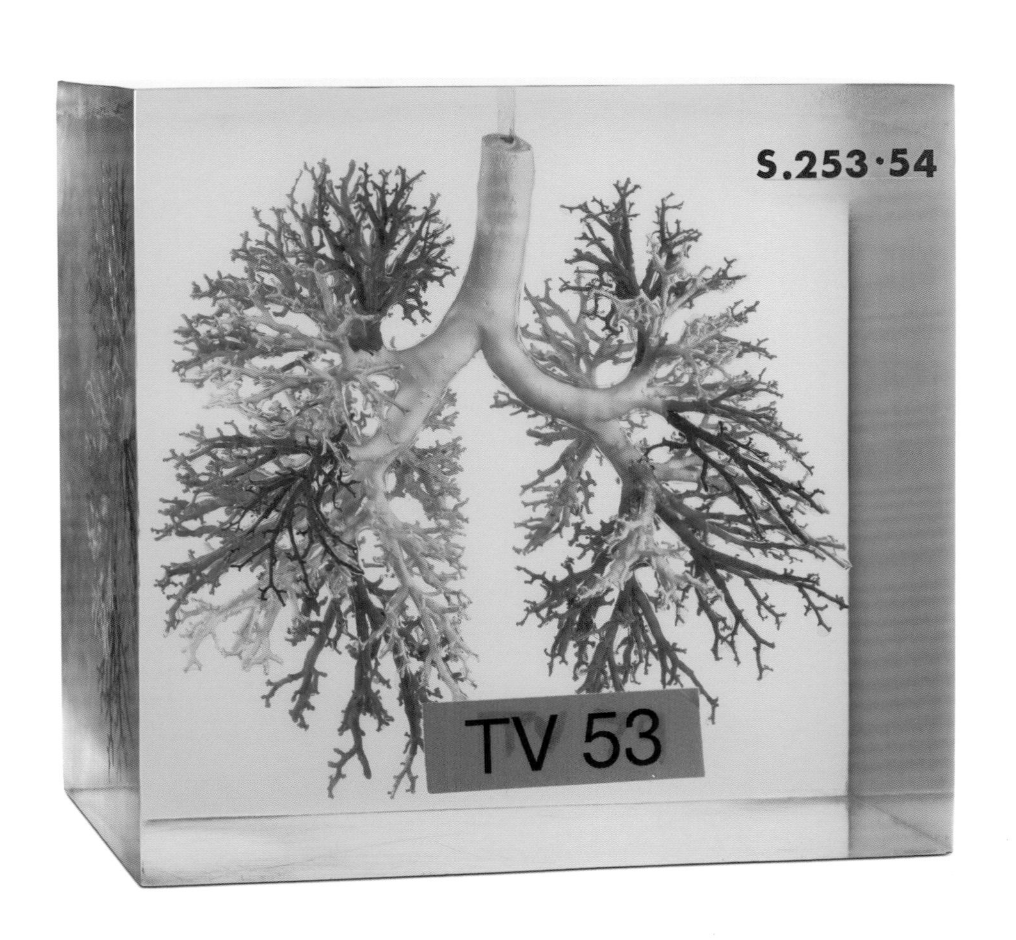
S.253·54
TV 53

CATALOGUE 23
David Hugh Tompsett
Corrosion cast of the bronchial tree and pulmonary vessels in the lungs and blood vessels in the heart (display stand removed), 1950s-60s, resin, 24 x 22 x 16 cm.
RCSAC/254k.
Photograph by Michael Frank.

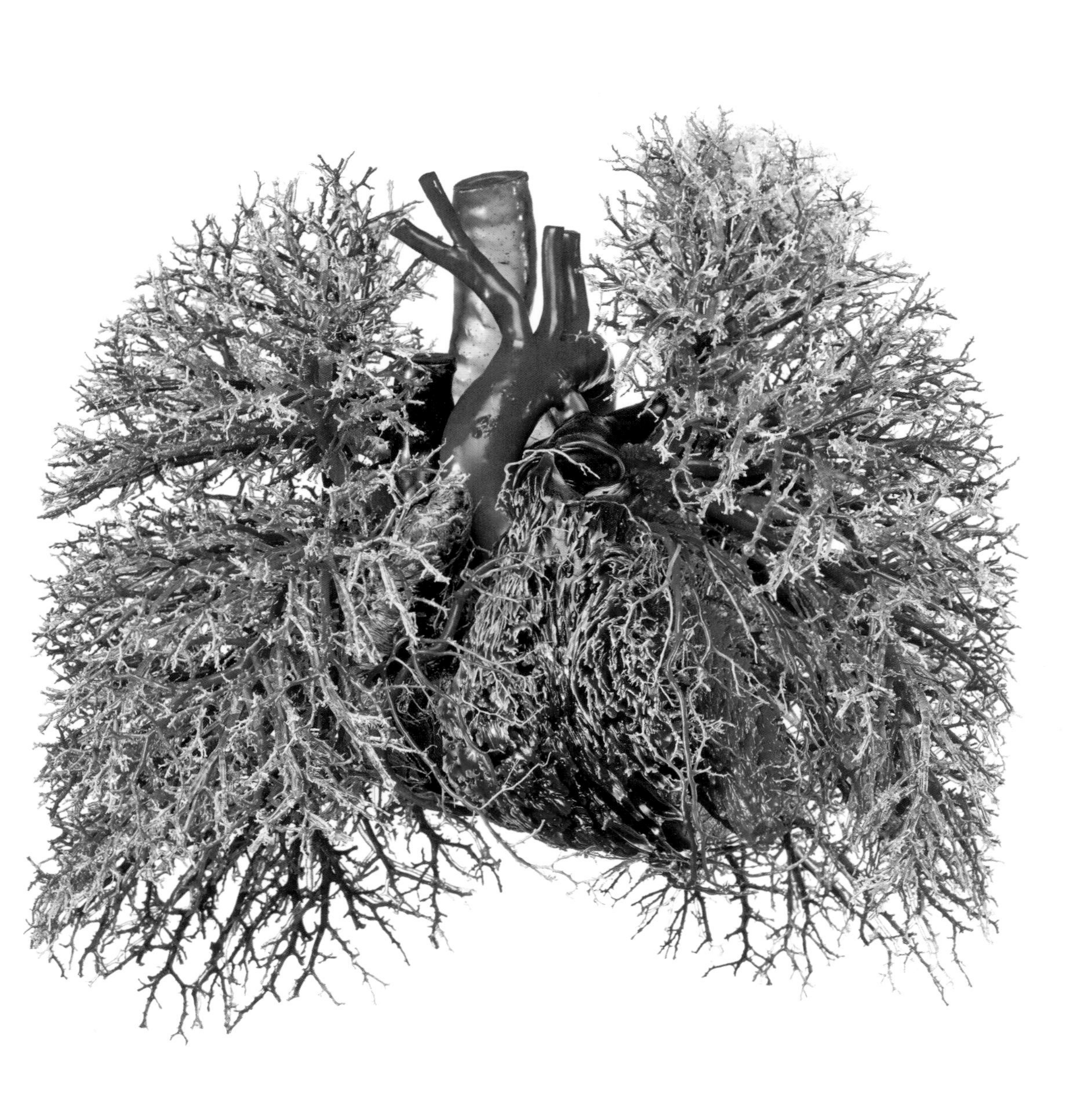

CATALOGUE 24
David Hugh Tompsett
Corrosion cast of a segment of aorta and arteries of the kidneys (red), and ureters (yellow) duplex on the left (display stand removed), 1950s-60s, resin, 13.5 x 15.5 x 8 cm.
RCSAC/289i.
Photograph by Michael Frank.

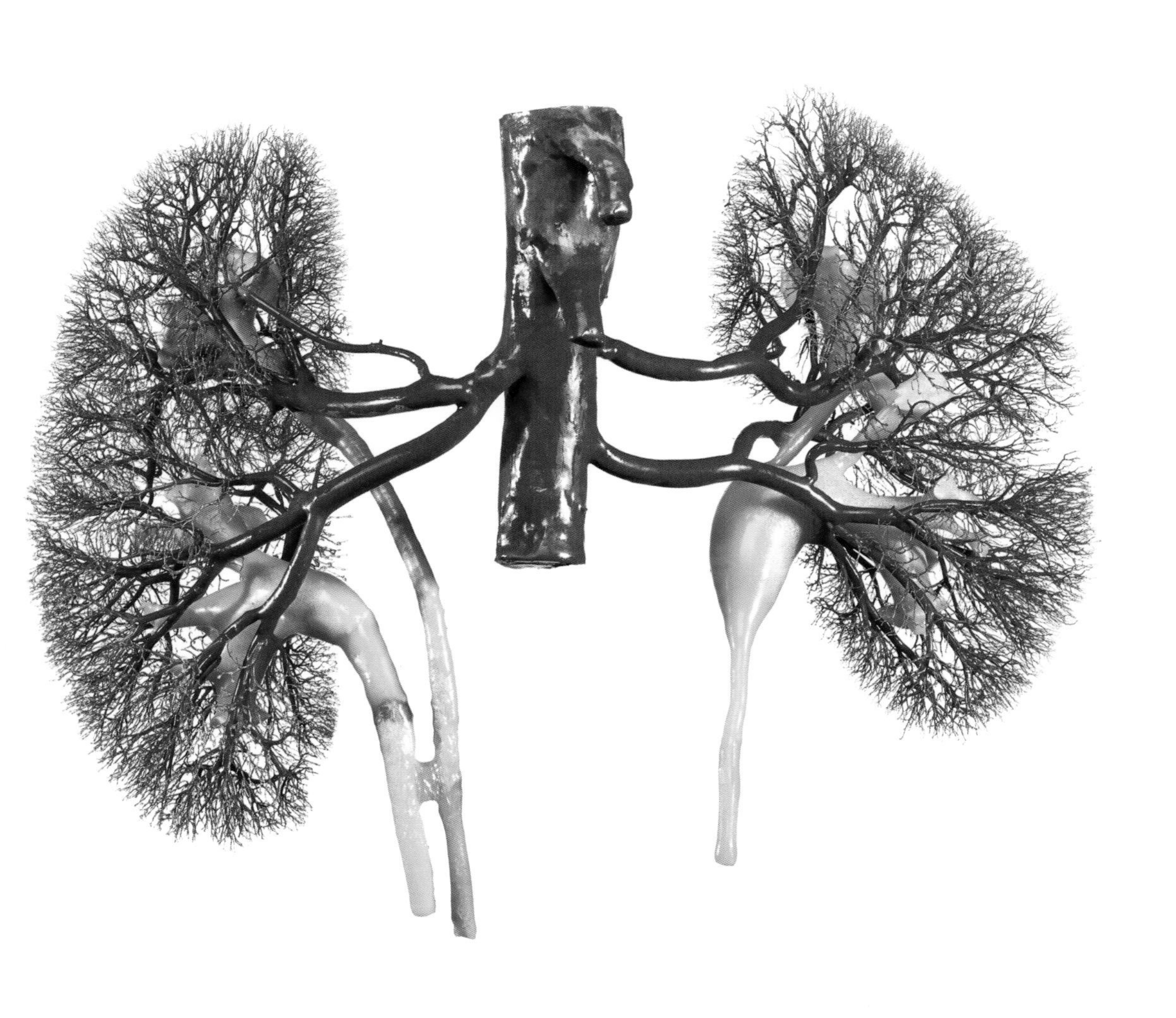

CATALOGUE 25
David Hugh Tompsett
Corrosion cast of the vessels in the kidneys, the aorta (red) and inferior vena cava (blue), with unusual double ureters (yellow) on both sides (display stand removed), 1950s-60s, resin, 14 x 19.5 x 8 cm.
RCSAC/289j.
Photograph by Michael Frank.

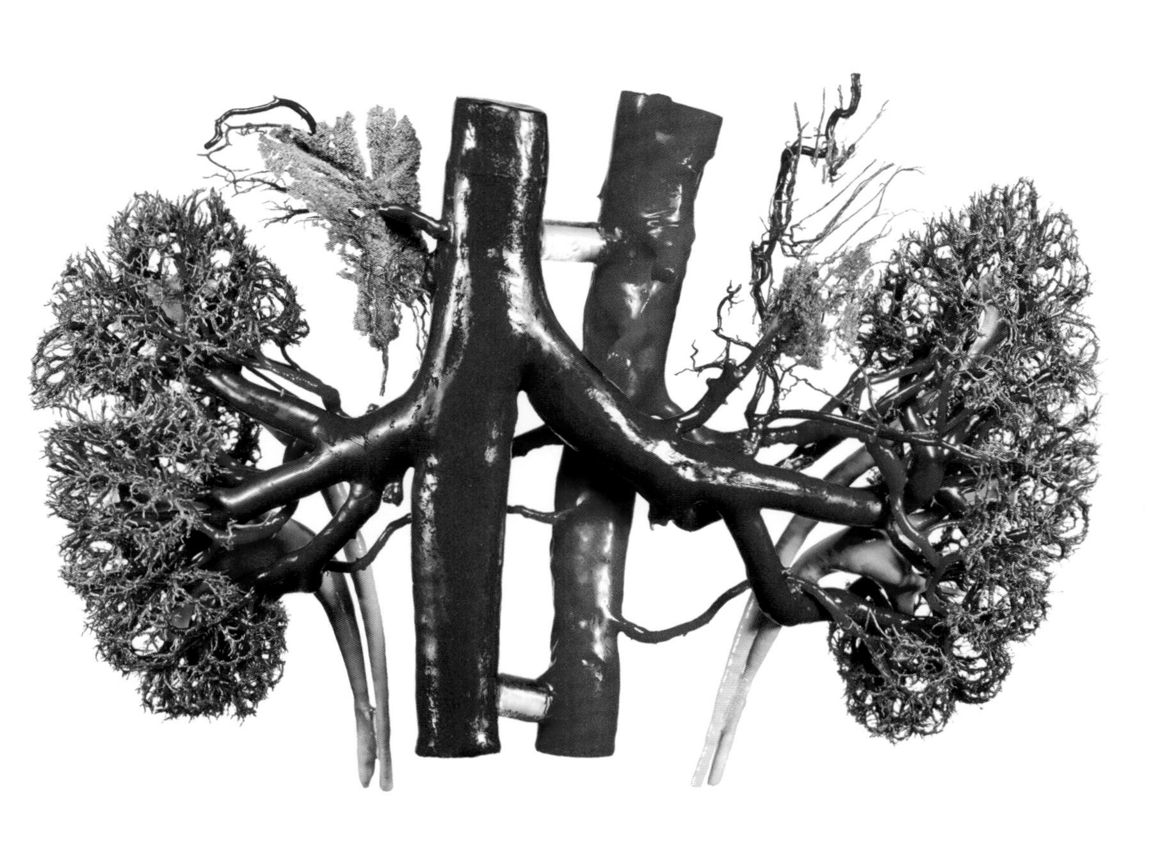

CATALOGUE 26
David Hugh Tompsett
Corrosion cast of the kidneys showing the ramification of the blood vessels (red) and their connection with the main trunks of the ureters (yellow), 1950s-60s, resin, 22 x 20.5 x 45 cm.
RCSAC/289c.
Photograph by Michael Frank.

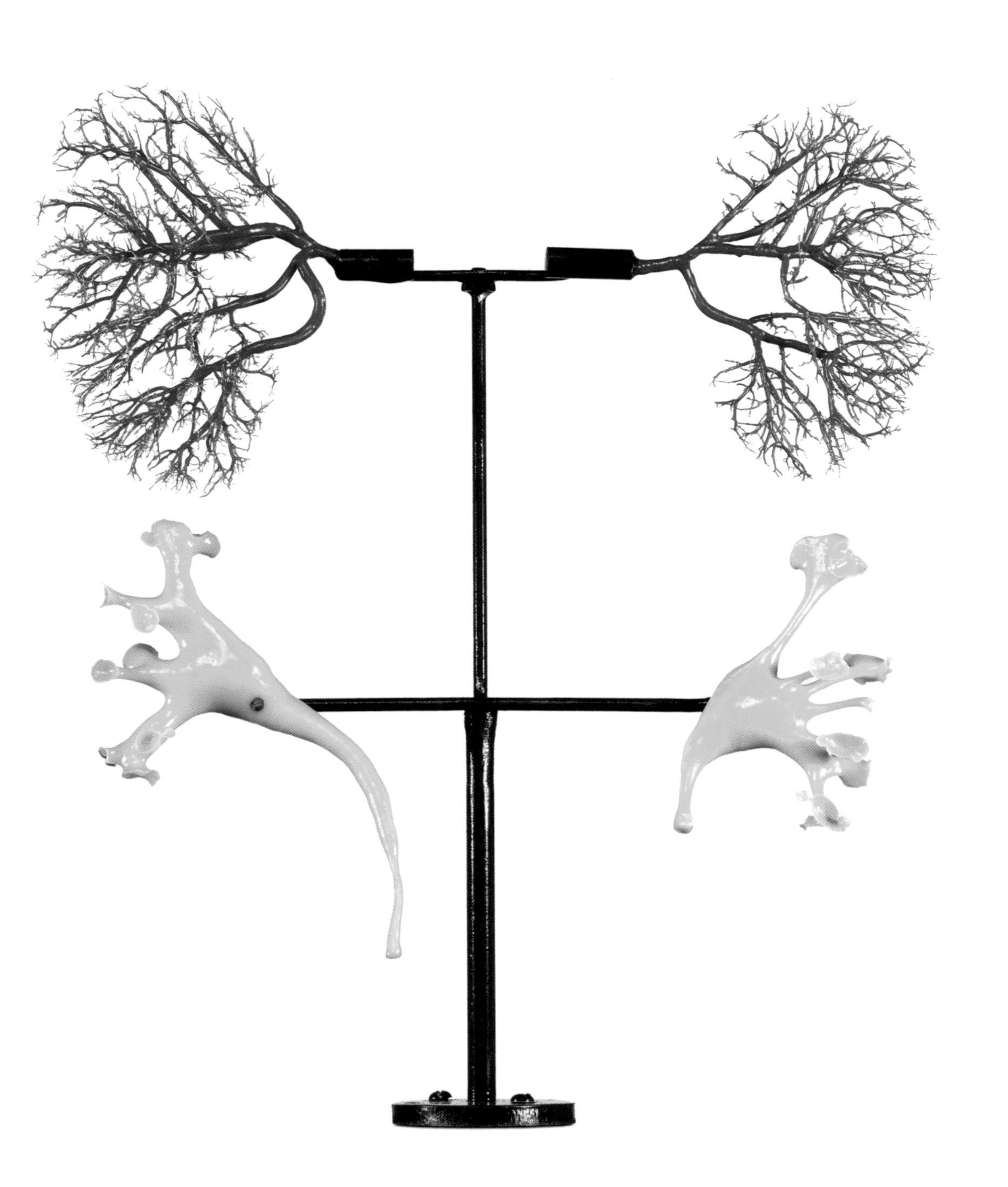

CATALOGUE 27
David Hugh Tompsett
Corrosion cast of the left kidney, with ureter (yellow) showing the finest vessels that it is possible to display with this method of injection, 1950s-60s, resin, 11 x 9 x 5 cm.
RCSAC/289.5.
Photograph by Michael Frank.

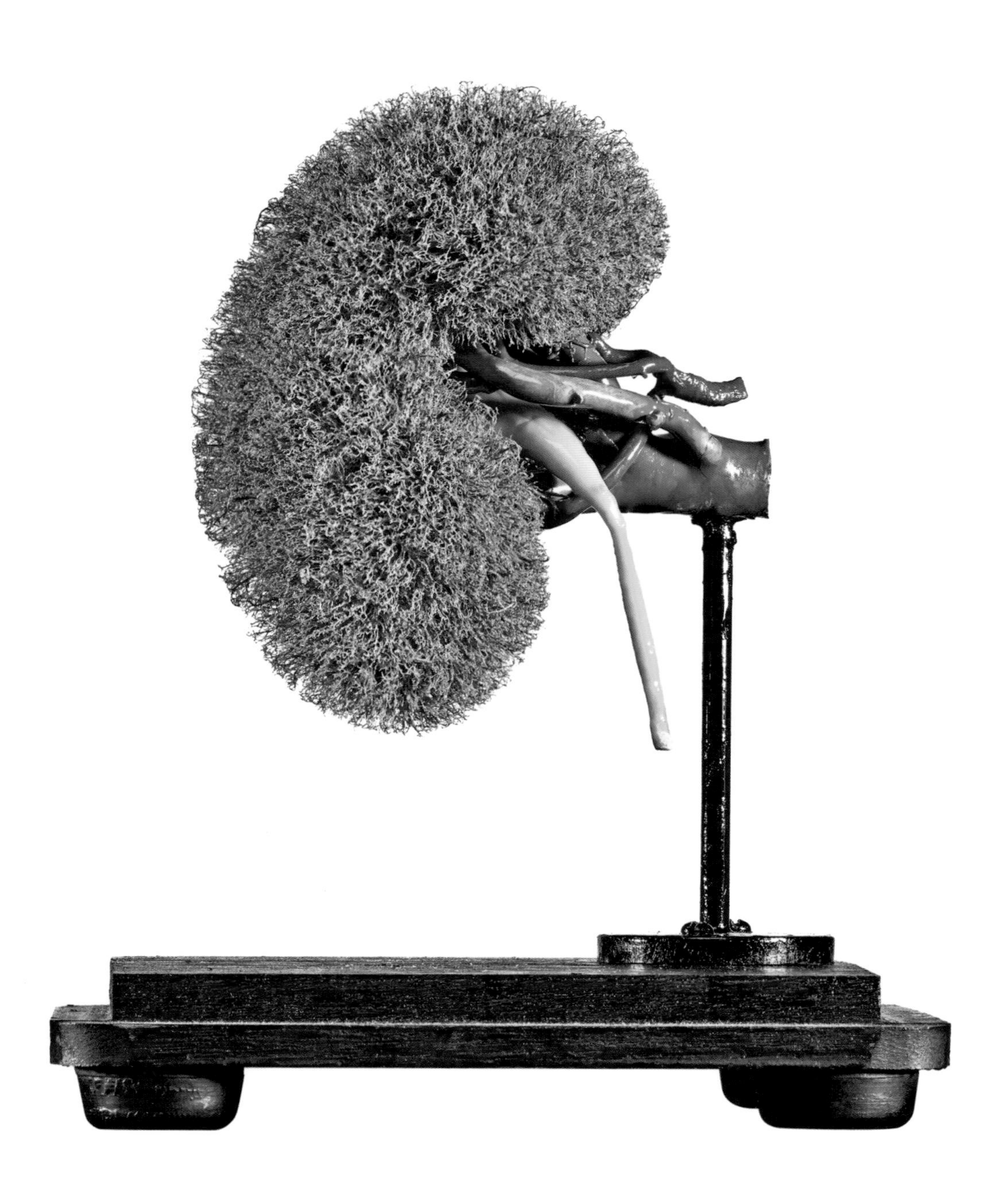

CATALOGUE 28
David Hugh Tompsett
Corrosion cast of the arteries
(red) and veins (blue) in the spleen,
1950s-60s, resin, 10 x 7 x 7 cm.
RCSAC/279.
Photograph by Michael Frank.

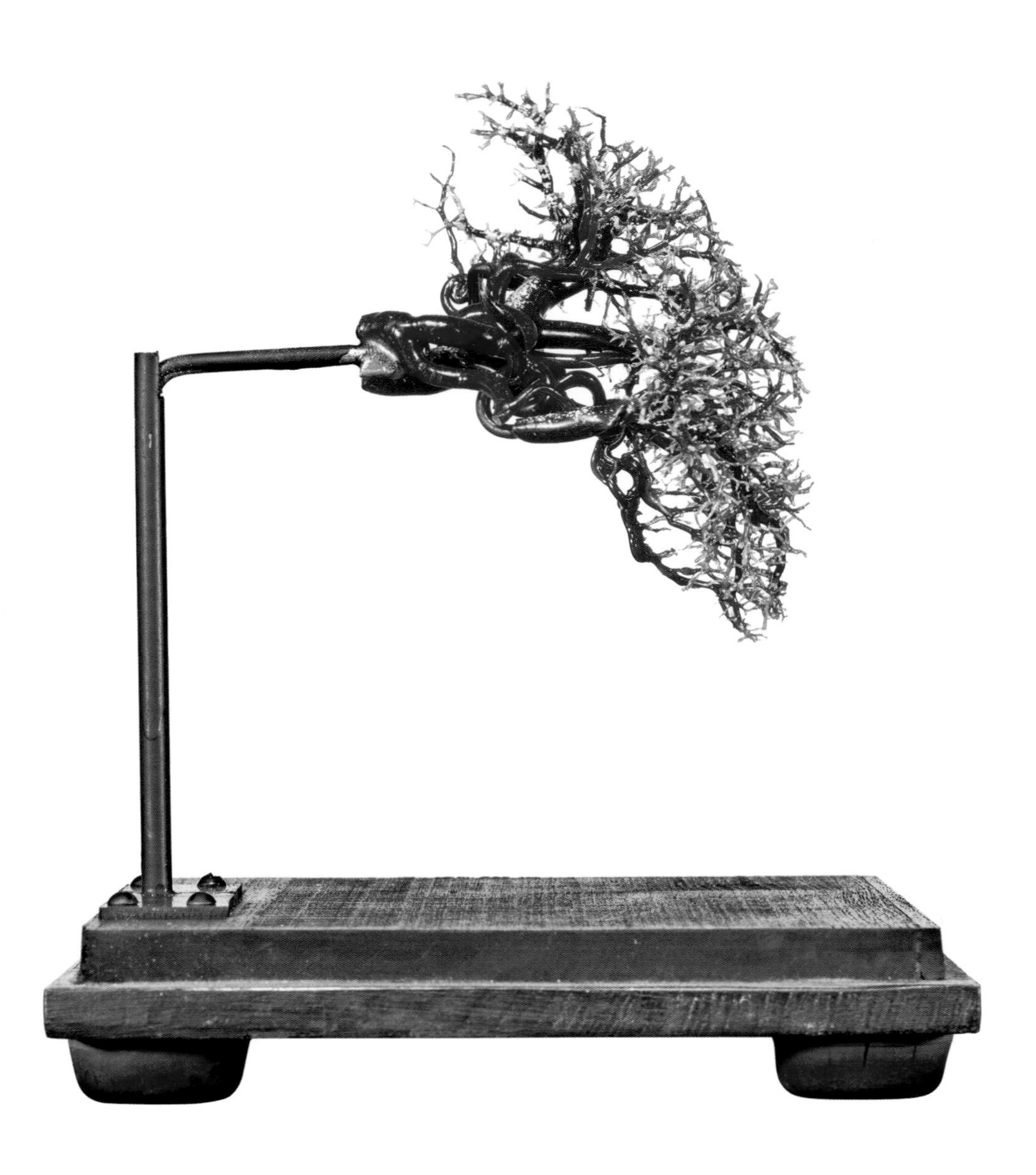

CATALOGUE 29
David Hugh Tompsett
Corrosion cast of the liver after injection of the hepatic artery (red), biliary tract and gallbladder (yellow) and inferior vena cava (blue), 1955, resin, 20 x 25 x 14 cm.
RCSAC/278a.
Photograph by Michael Frank.

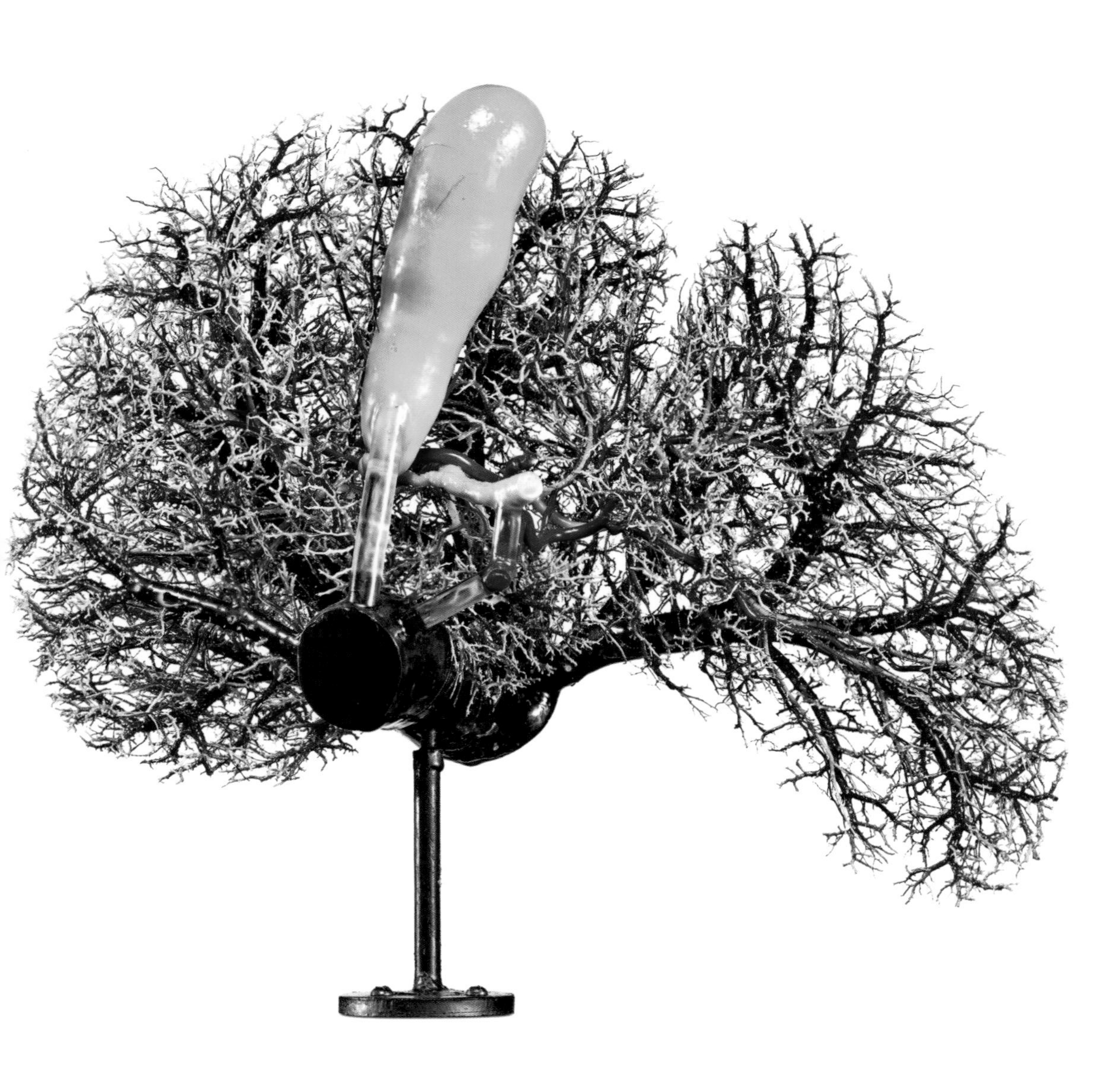

CATALOGUE 30
David Hugh Tompsett
Corrosion cast of the biliary system and pancreatic ducts, 1959, resin, 18 x 27 x 17 cm.
RCSAC/275b.
Photograph by Michael Frank.

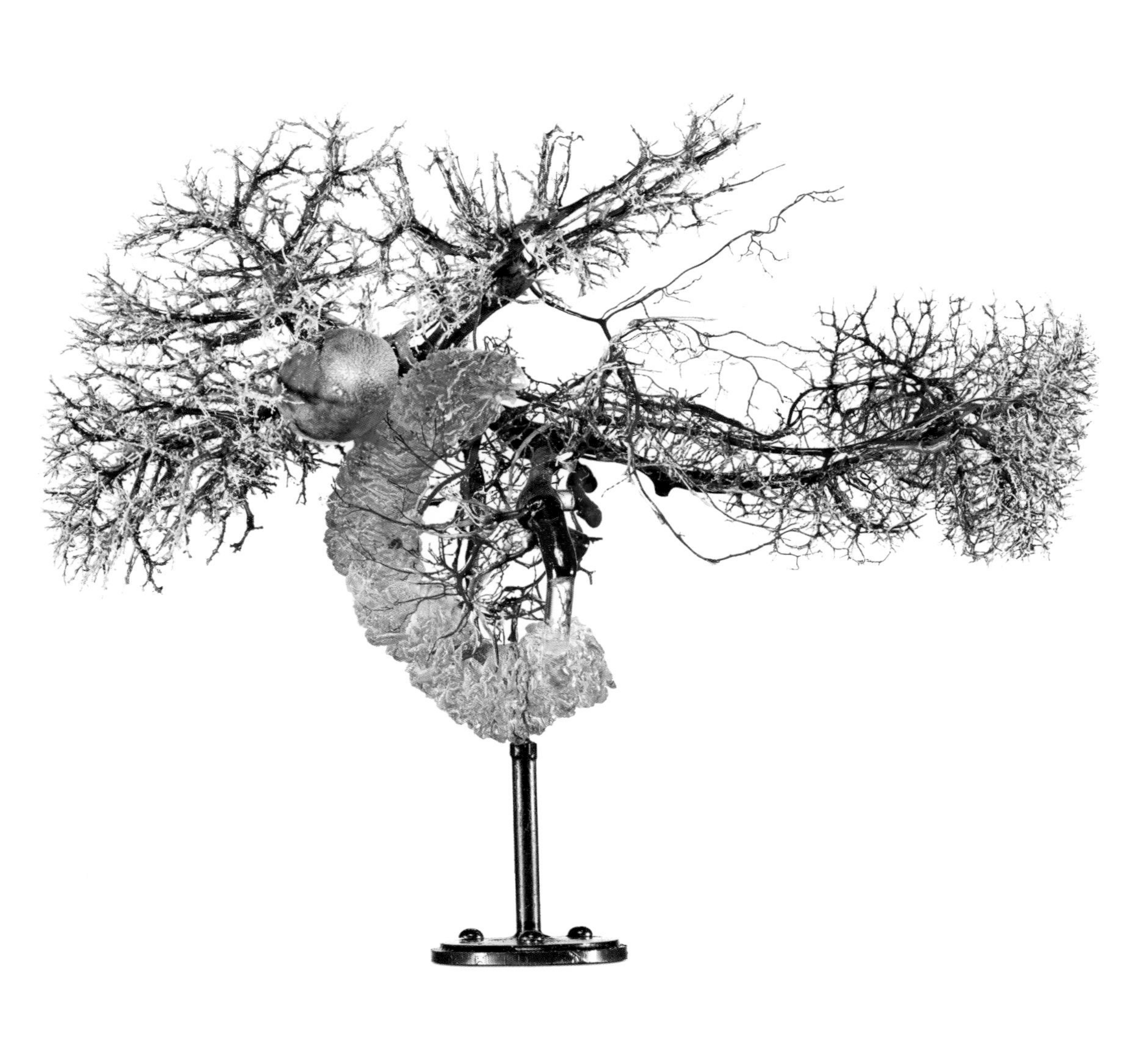

CATALOGUE 31
David Hugh Tompsett
Corrosion cast of the vessels of upper abdominal viscera, with resin in the duodenum and distal end of the pyloric antrum (yellow), 1959, resin, 23 x 29.5 x 18 cm.
RCSAC/275c.
Photograph by Michael Frank.

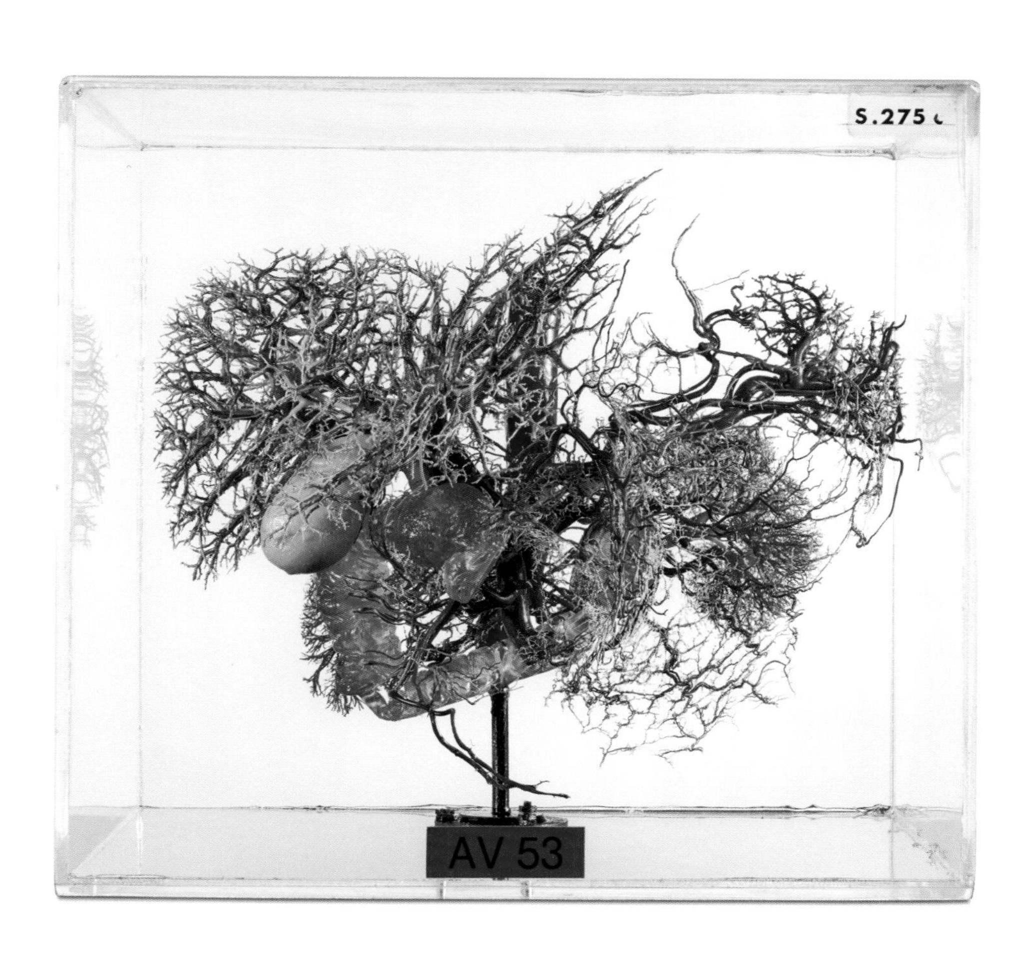
S.275
AV 53

CATALOGUE 32
David Hugh Tompsett
Corrosion cast of vessels in the liver, stomach, pancreas and duodenum (from a child aged 10 years), 1965, resin, 13 x 19 x 14 cm.
RCSAC/275d.
Photograph by Michael Frank.

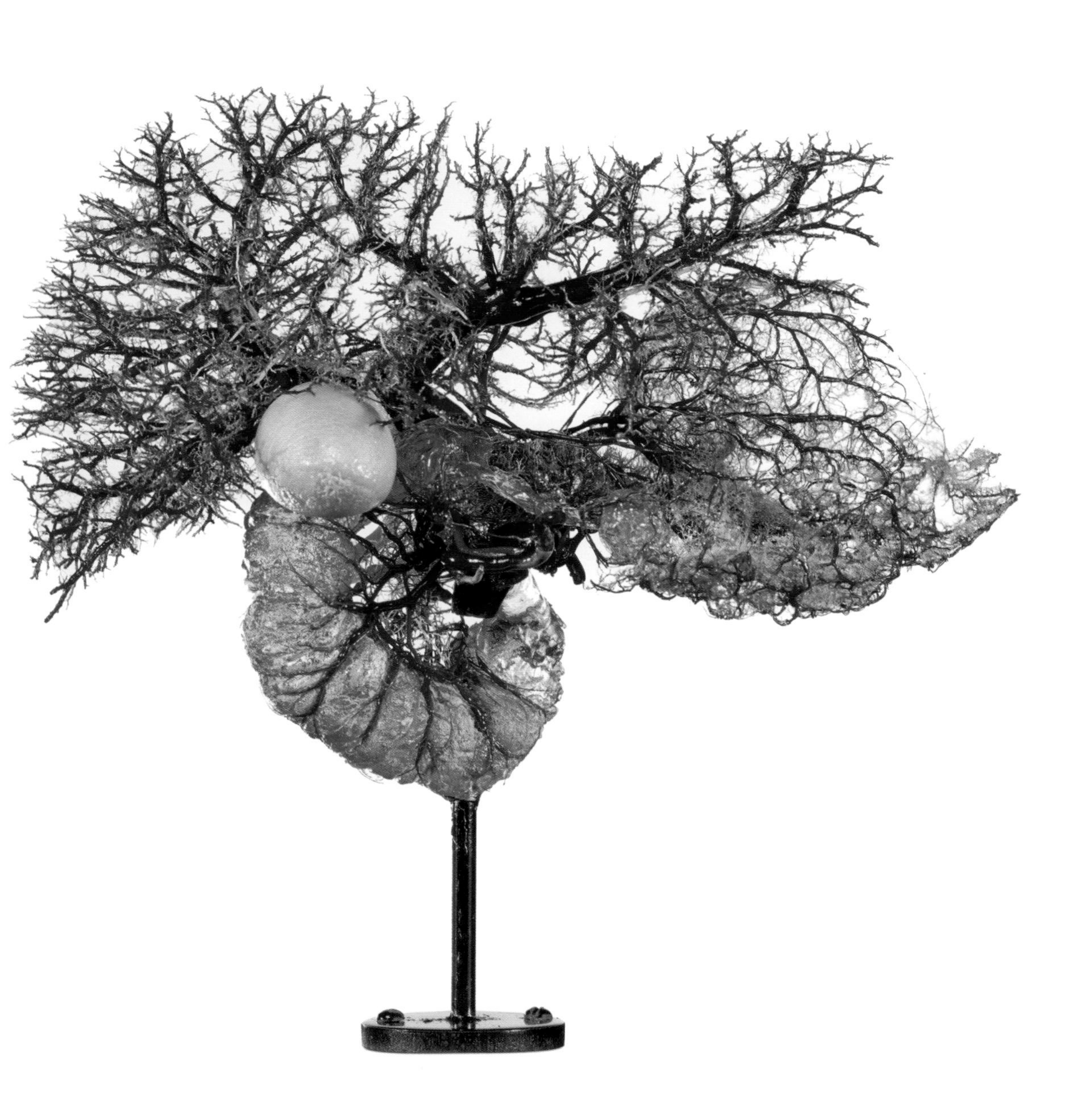

CATALOGUE 33
David Hugh Tompsett
Corrosion cast of vessels in the liver and gallbladder (yellow) (display stand removed), 1950s-60s, resin, 18 x 25 x 15 cm.
RCSAC/278h.
Photograph by Michael Frank.

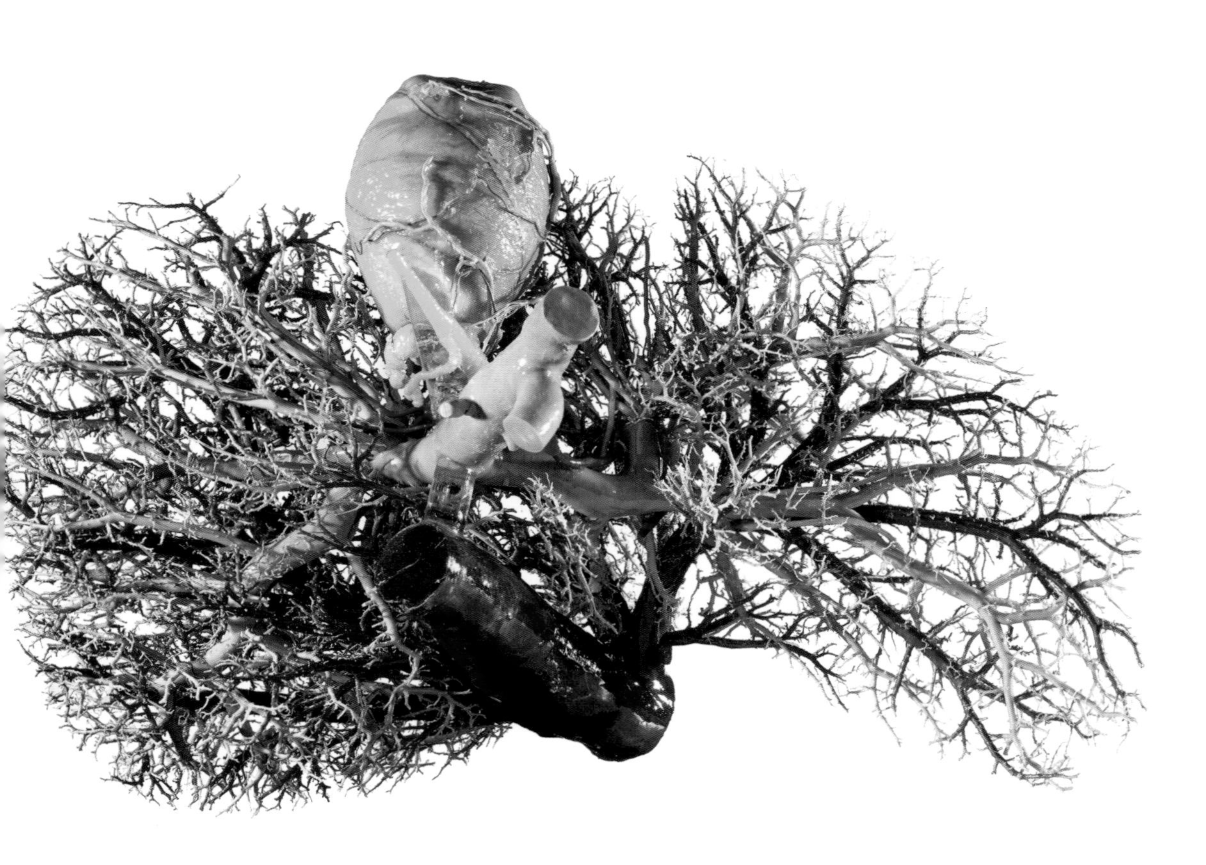

CATALOGUE 34
David Hugh Tompsett
Corrosion cast of the liver after injection of the portal vein (light blue), hepatic artery (red), biliary tract and gallbladder (yellow), and inferior vena cava (dark blue), 1968, resin, 16 x 25 x 10 cm.
RCSAC/278g.
Photograph by Michael Frank.

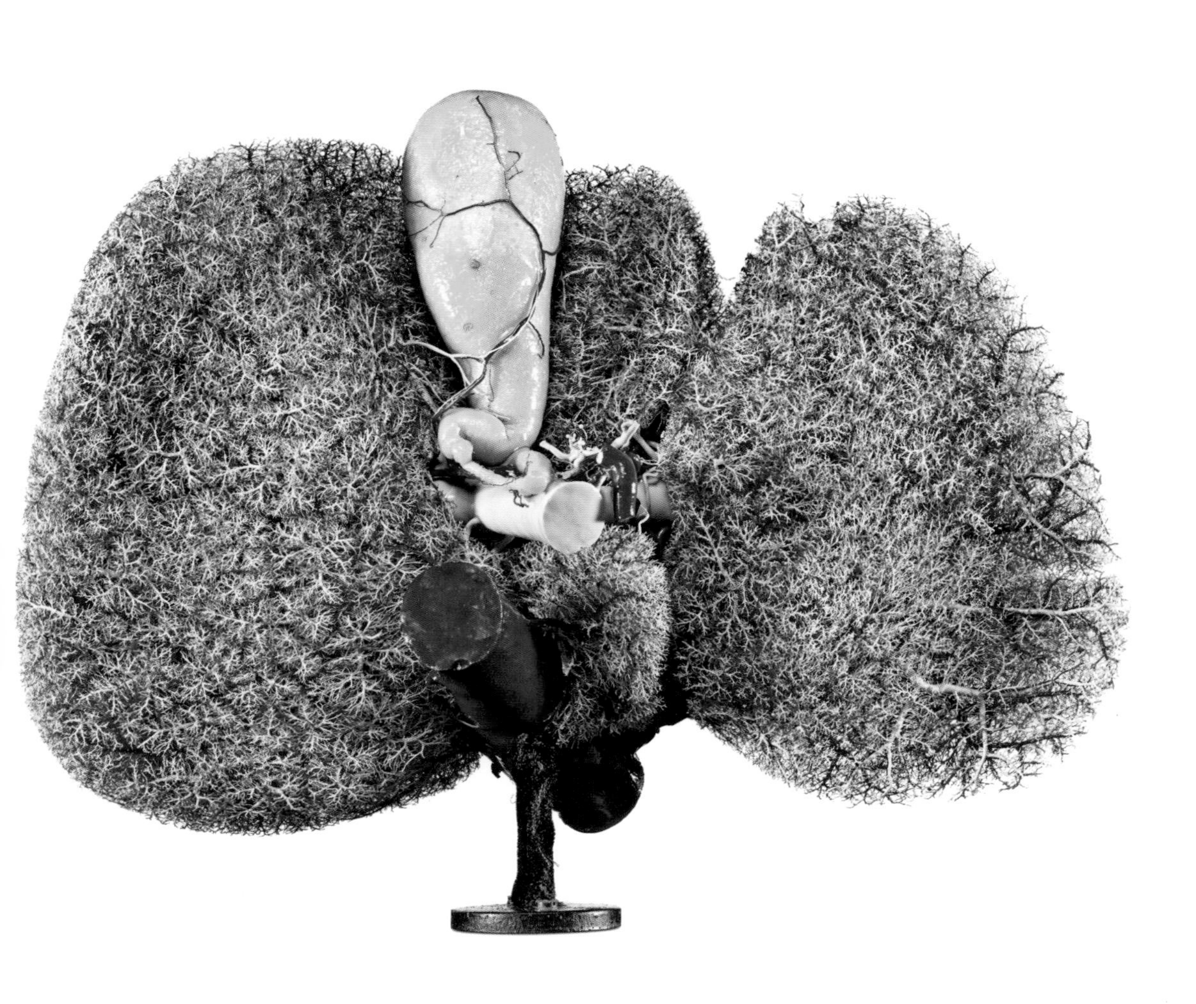

CATALOGUE 35
David Hugh Tompsett
Corrosion cast of vessels in the liver, stomach, spleen, pancreas and small intestine, 1950s–60s, resin, 34 x 22.5 x 17 cm.
RCSAC/281.
Photograph by Michael Frank.

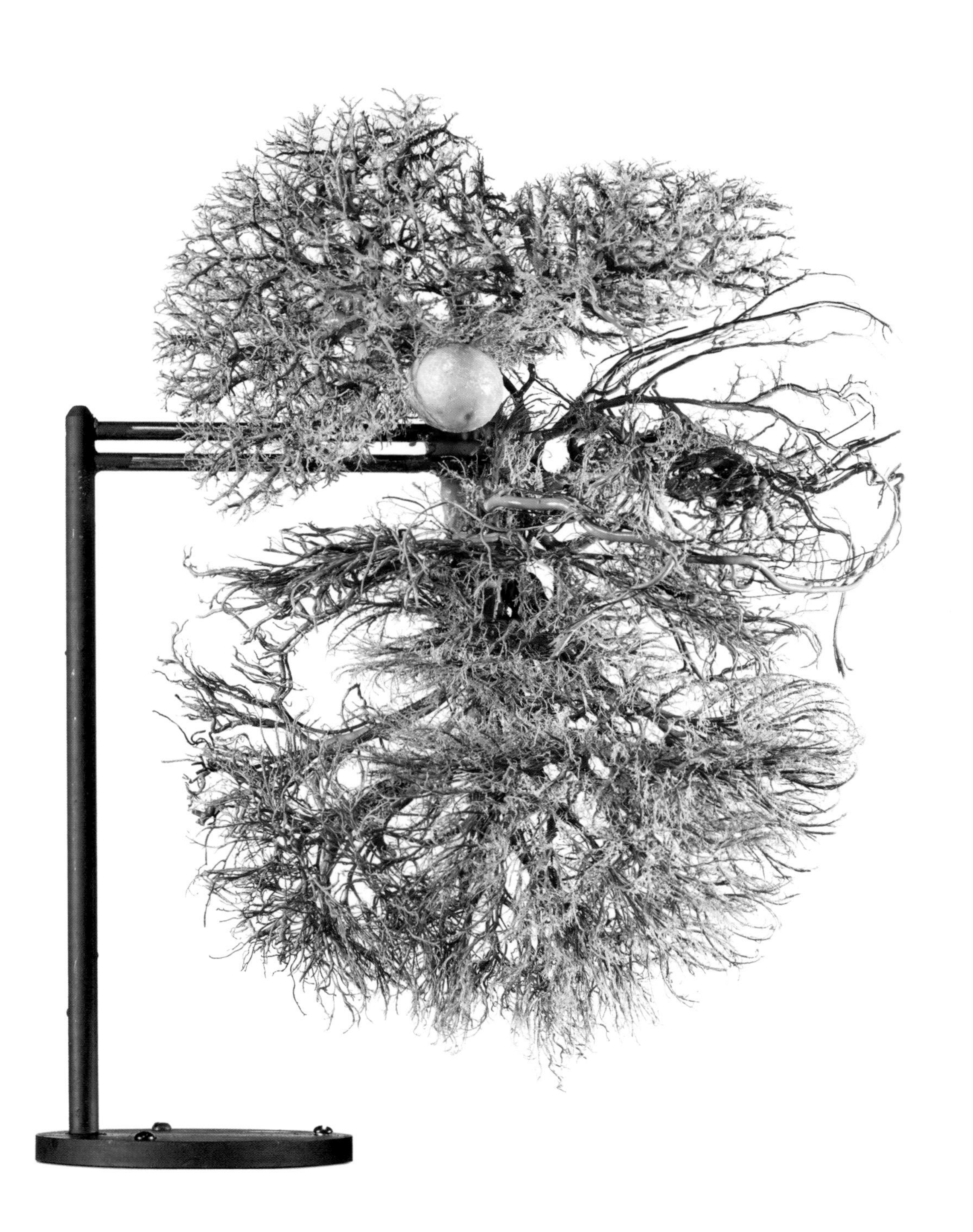

CATALOGUE 36
David Hugh Tompsett
Corrosion cast of vessels in the viscera in the thorax and abdomen, including the heart, lungs, liver, gallbladder, stomach and kidneys (from a male aged 14 years), 1965, resin, 37 x 20 x 17 cm.
RCSAC/276.
Photograph by Michael Frank.

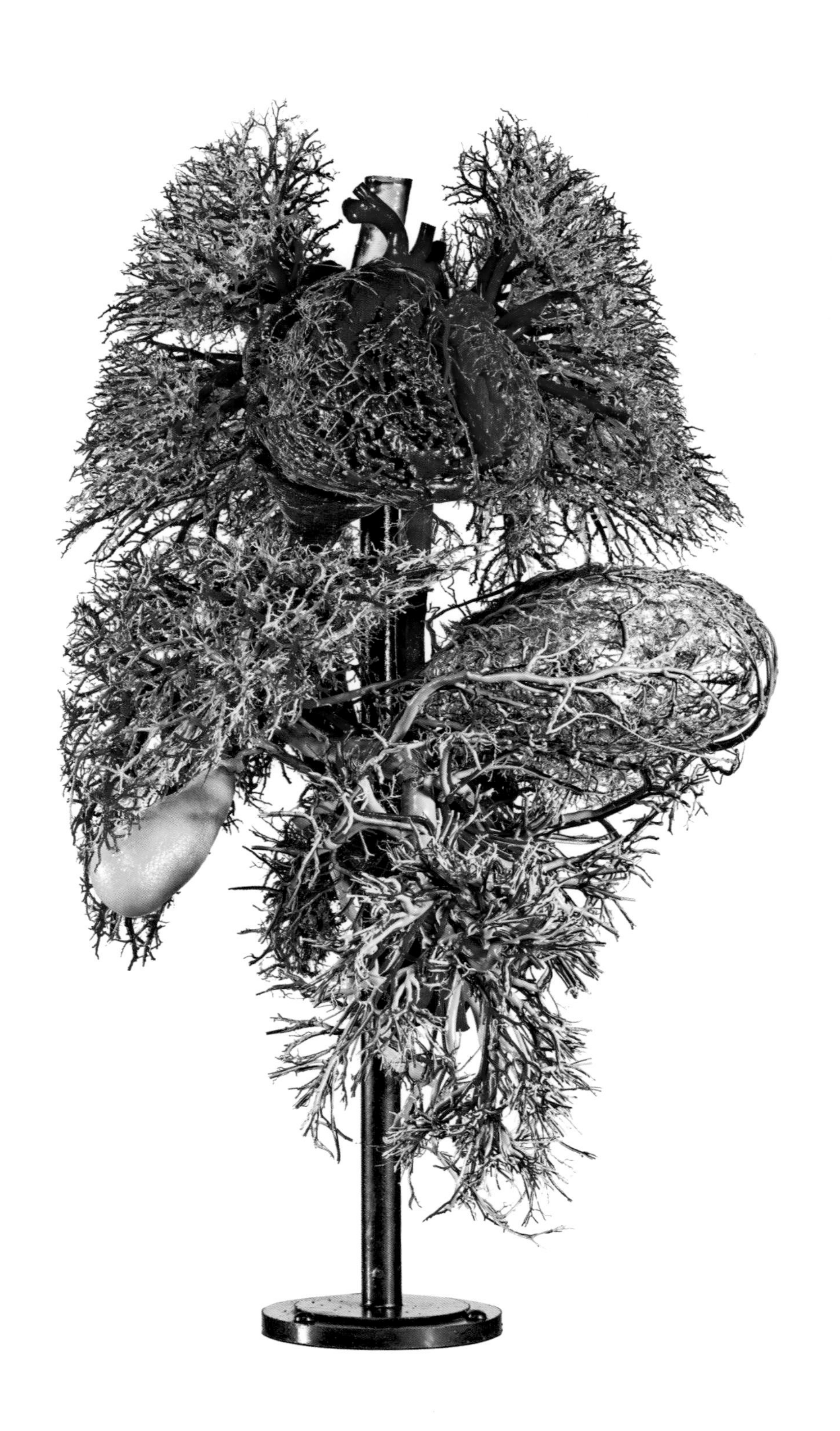

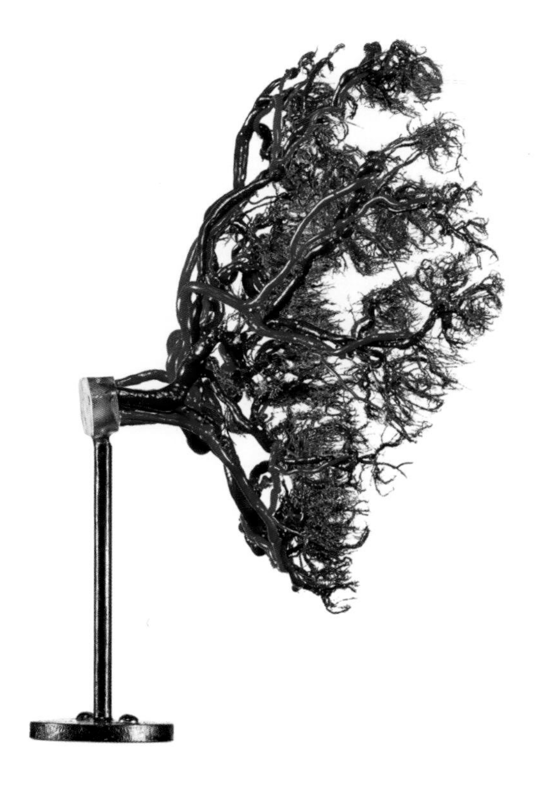

CATALOGUE 37
David Hugh Tompsett
Corrosion casts of the blood vessels supplying the placenta, front view (right), side view (left), 1963, resin, 16 x 18.5 x 7.5 cm.
RCSHM/3658b.
Photographs by Michael Frank.

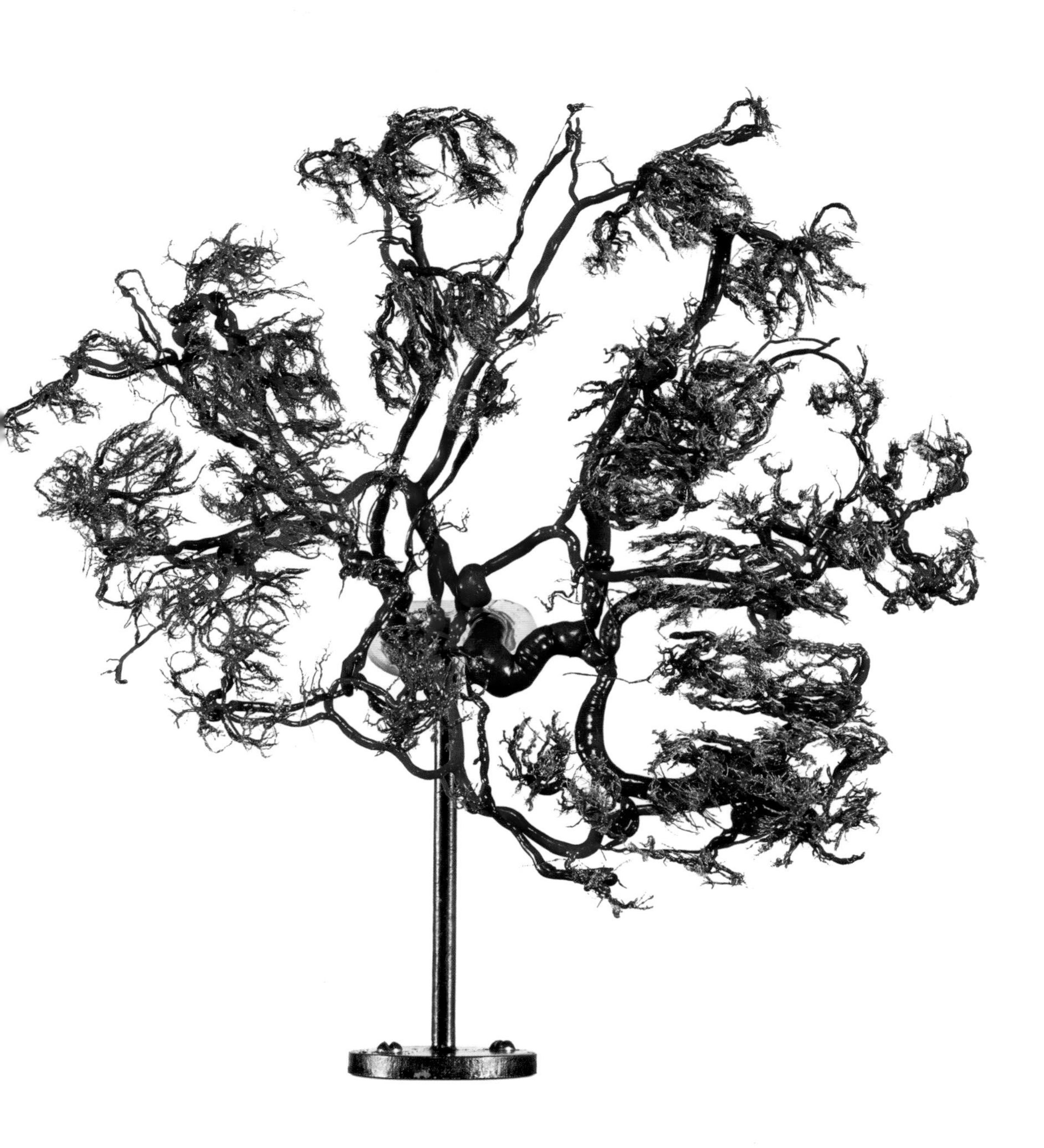

CATALOGUE 38
David Hugh Tompsett
Corrosion cast of the blood vessels supplying the placenta of identical twins, 1963, resin, 16 x 18.5 x 7.5 cm.
RCSHM/3658b.
Photograph by Michael Frank.

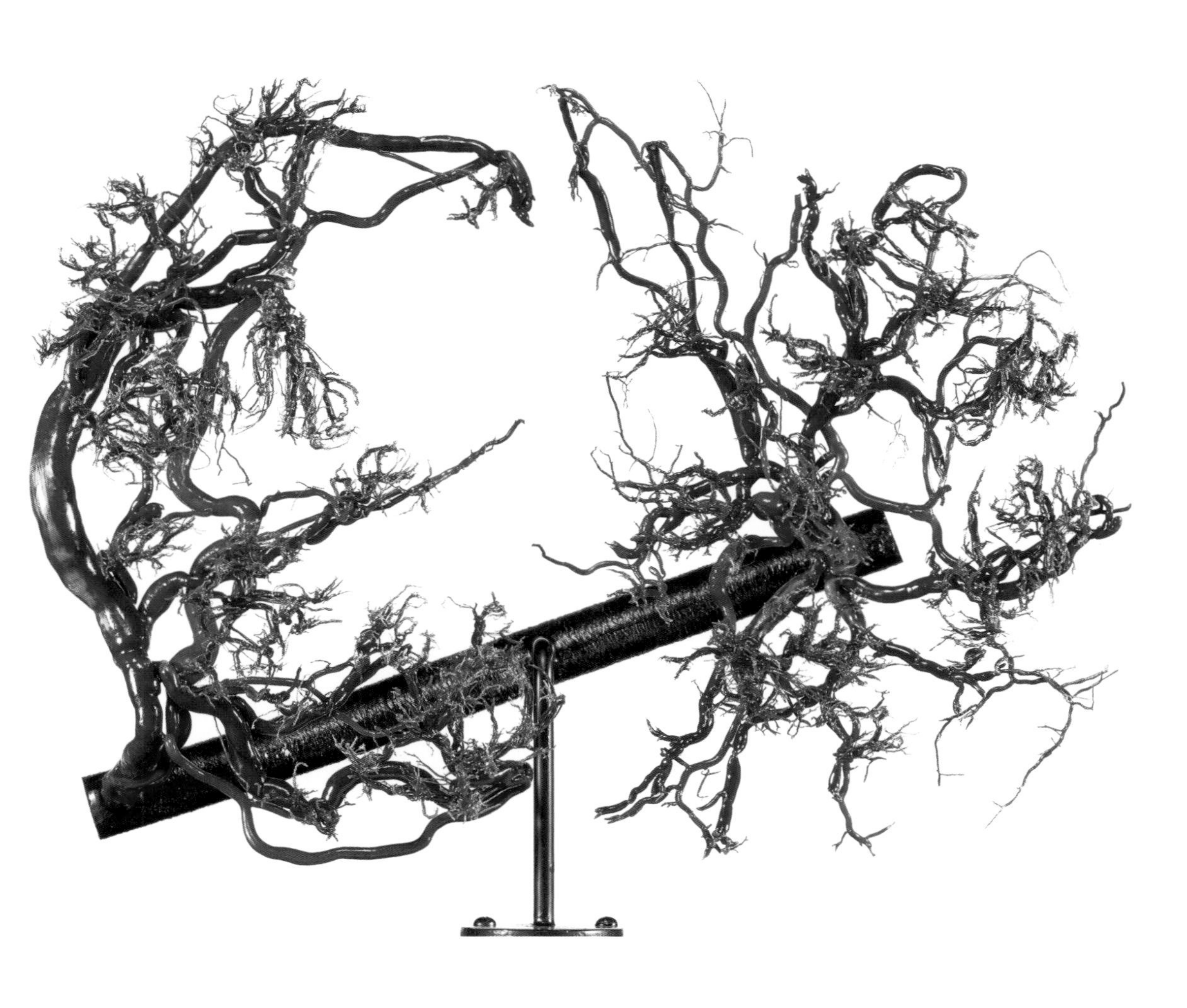

CATALOGUE 39
David Hugh Tompsett
Corrosion cast of the arteries of a male at birth, 1962, resin, 50 x 25 x 14 cm.
RCSHM/K 427.2.
Photograph by Michael Frank.

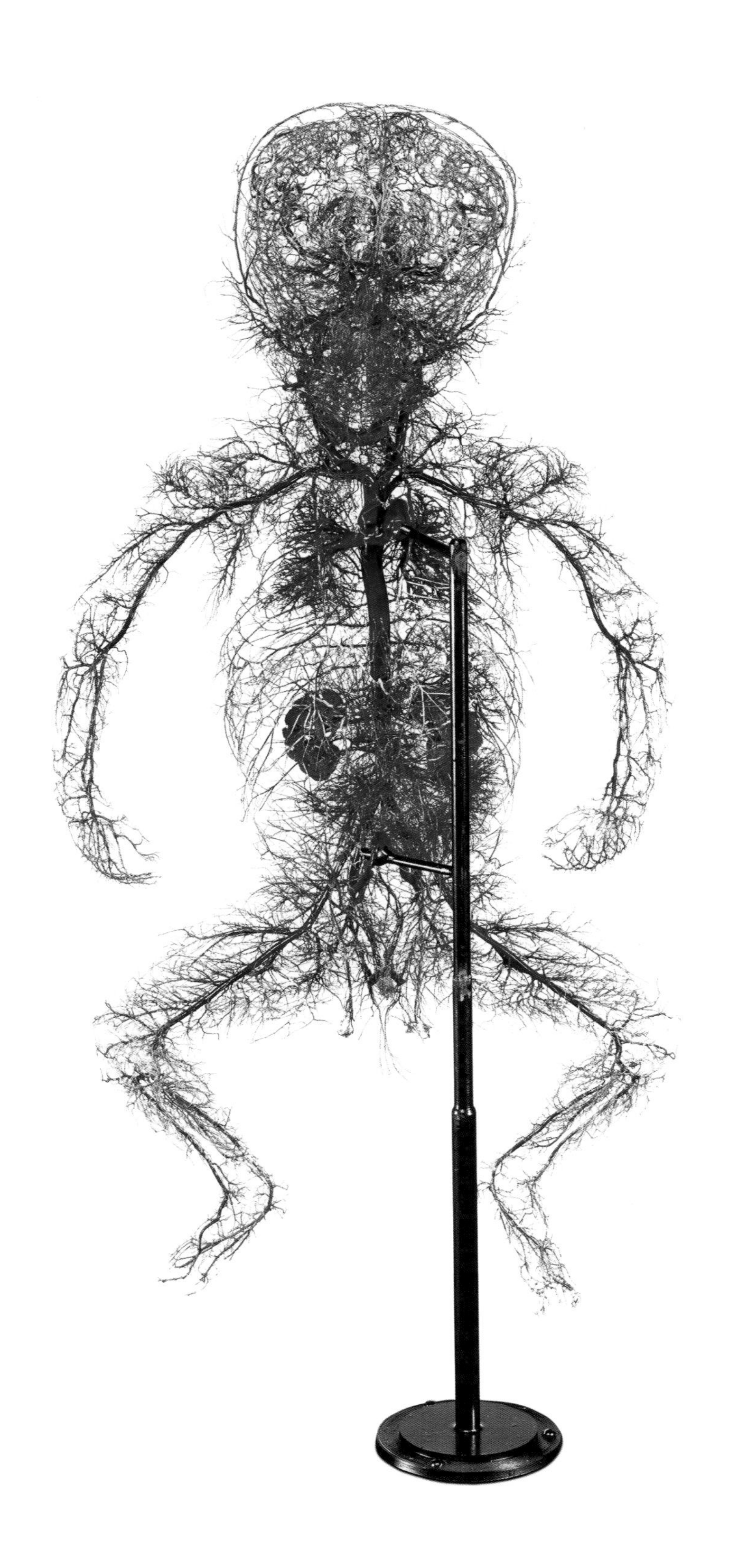

CATALOGUE 40
David Hugh Tompsett
Corrosion cast of the arteries (red) and veins (blue) of a female at birth, 1960s, resin, 49 x 23 x 14 cm.
RCSAC/603.
Photograph by Michael Frank.

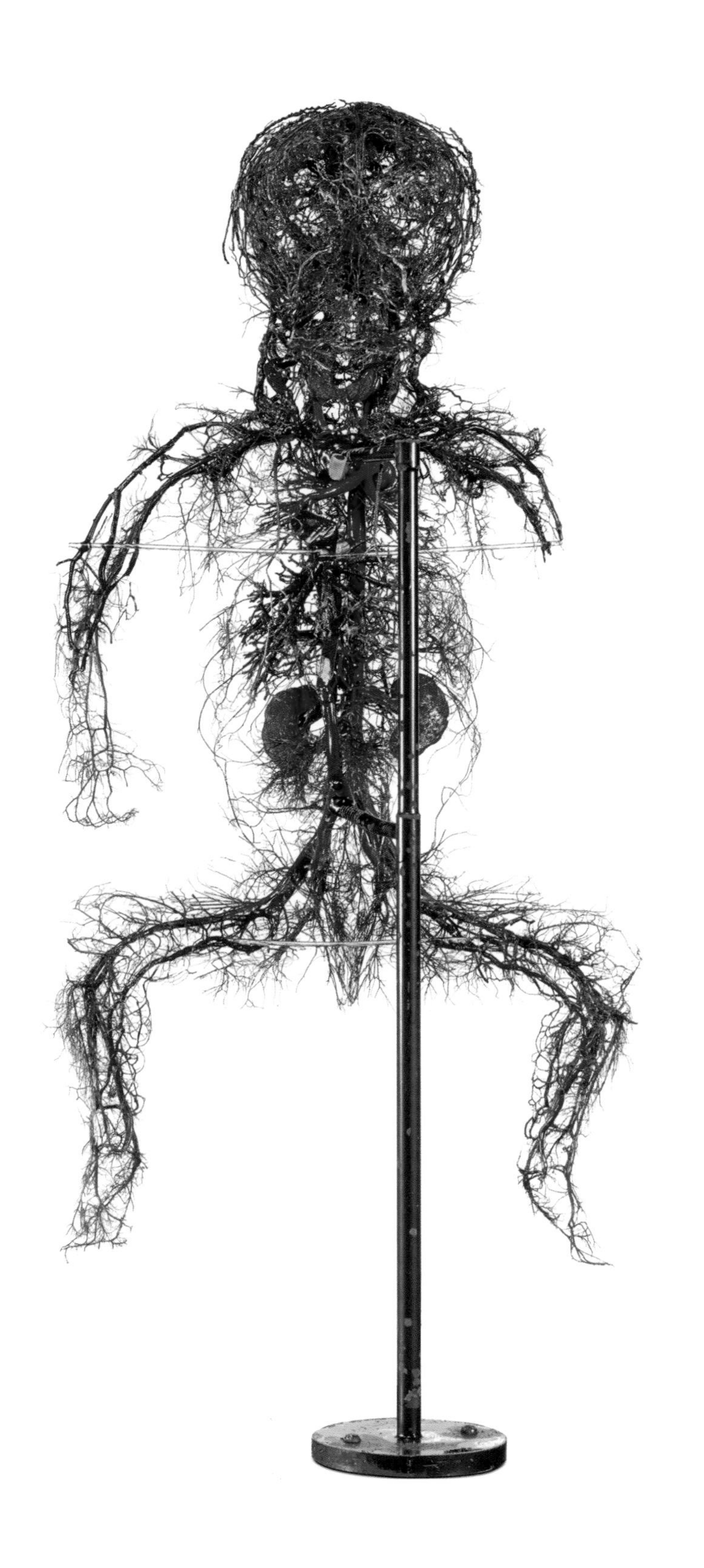

CATALOGUE 41
David Hugh Tompsett
Corrosion cast of the blood vessels of the left arm (from a male aged 62 years), 1966, resin, 68 x 18 x 11 cm.
RCSAC/150d.
Photograph by Michael Frank.

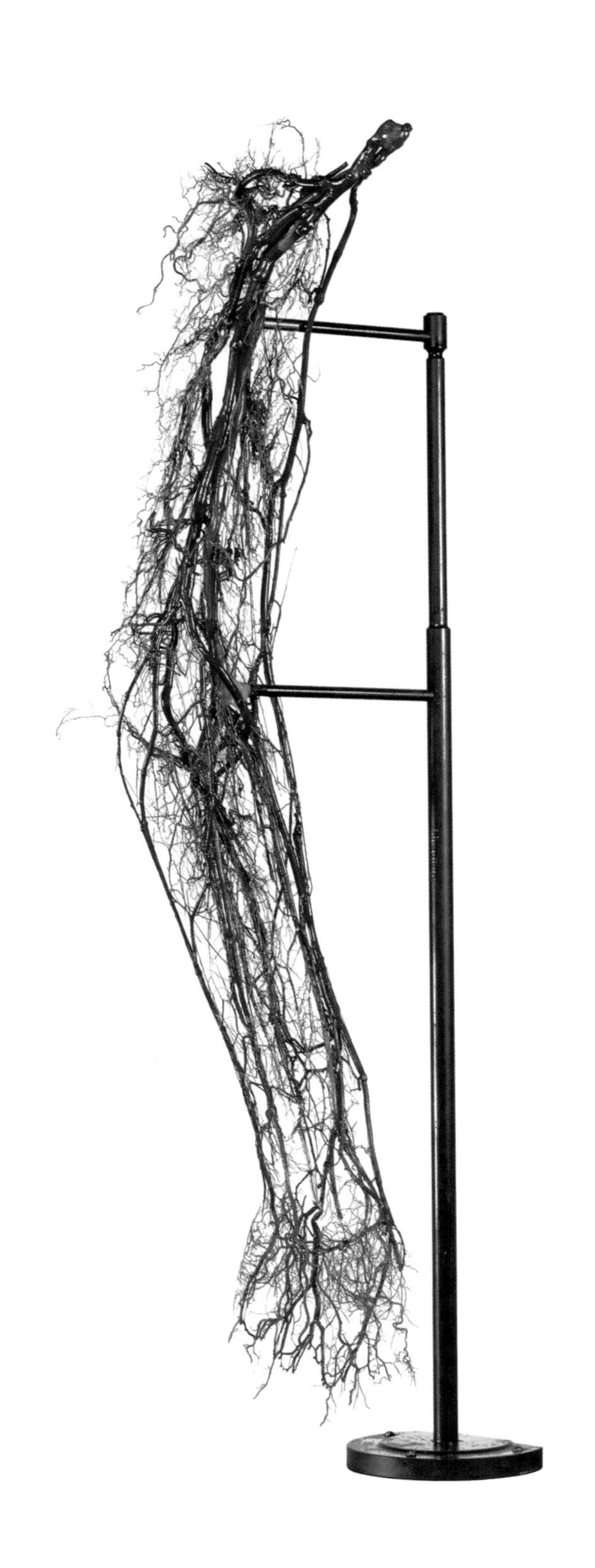

CATALOGUE 42
David Hugh Tompsett
Corrosion cast of the vessels of the right leg (from a male aged 62 years), 1964, resin, 96 x 10 x 10 cm.
RCSAC/150.1.
Photograph by Michael Frank.

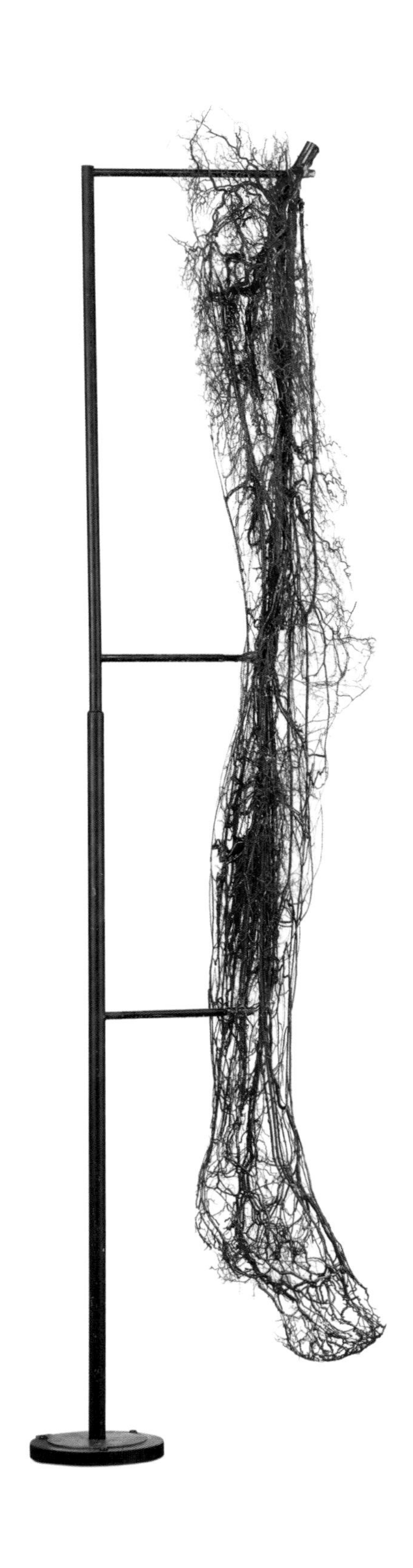

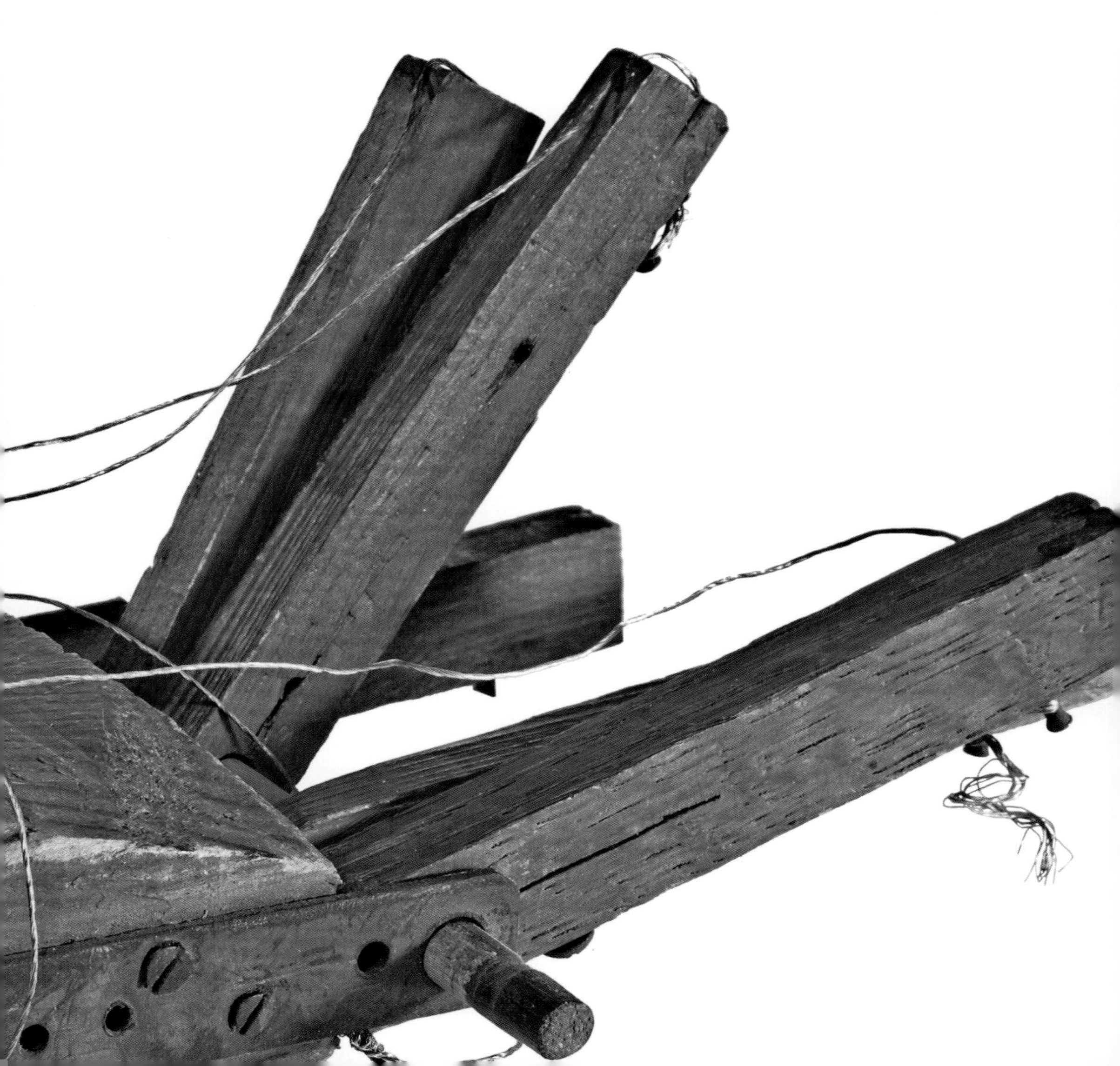

Model limbs: John Herbert Hicks

CATALOGUE 43
John Herbert Hicks
Model of the leg and foot for demonstrating movement, 1950s, wood with metal fixings, 31 x 6.5 x 17.5 cm.
RCSIC/Z 74.
Photograph by Michael Frank.

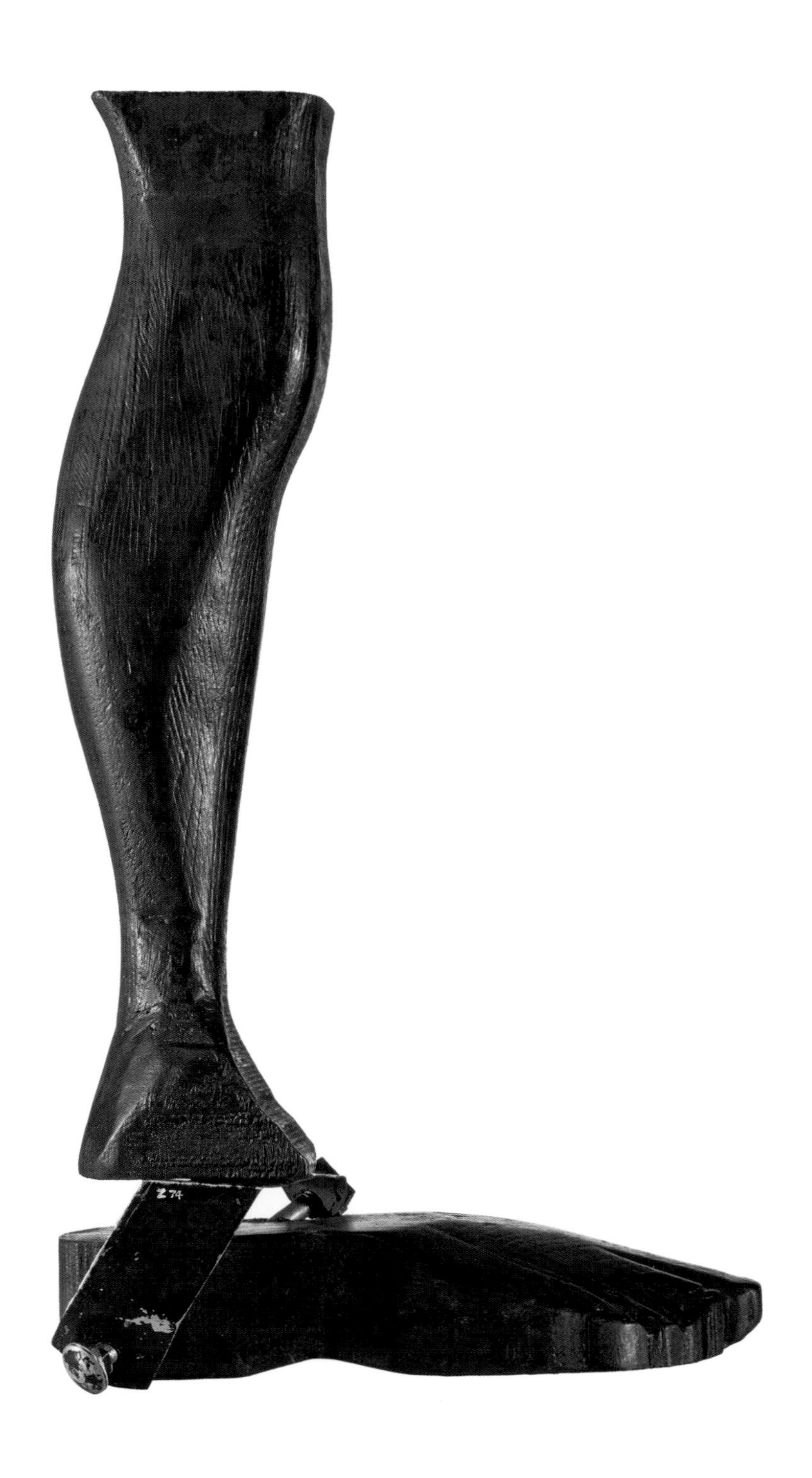
Z 74

CATALOGUE 44
John Herbert Hicks
Model of the leg and foot for demonstrating movement, 1950s, wood with metal fixings, 30 x 8 x 13 cm.
RCSIC/Z 74.1.
Photograph by Michael Frank.

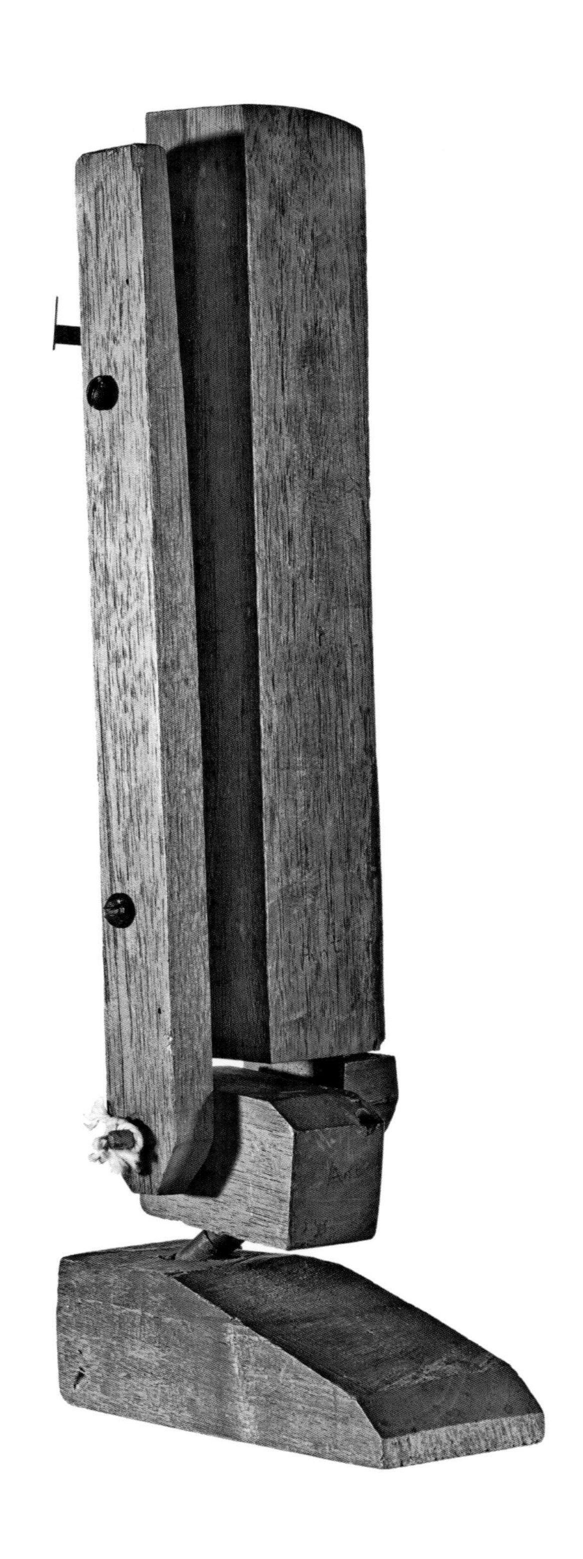

CATALOGUE 45
John Herbert Hicks
Model of the leg and foot for demonstrating movement at the talocalcaneonavicular joint, 1950s, wood with metal fixings, 22 x 3.5 x 9.6 cm.
RCSIC/Z 74.2.
Photograph by Michael Frank.

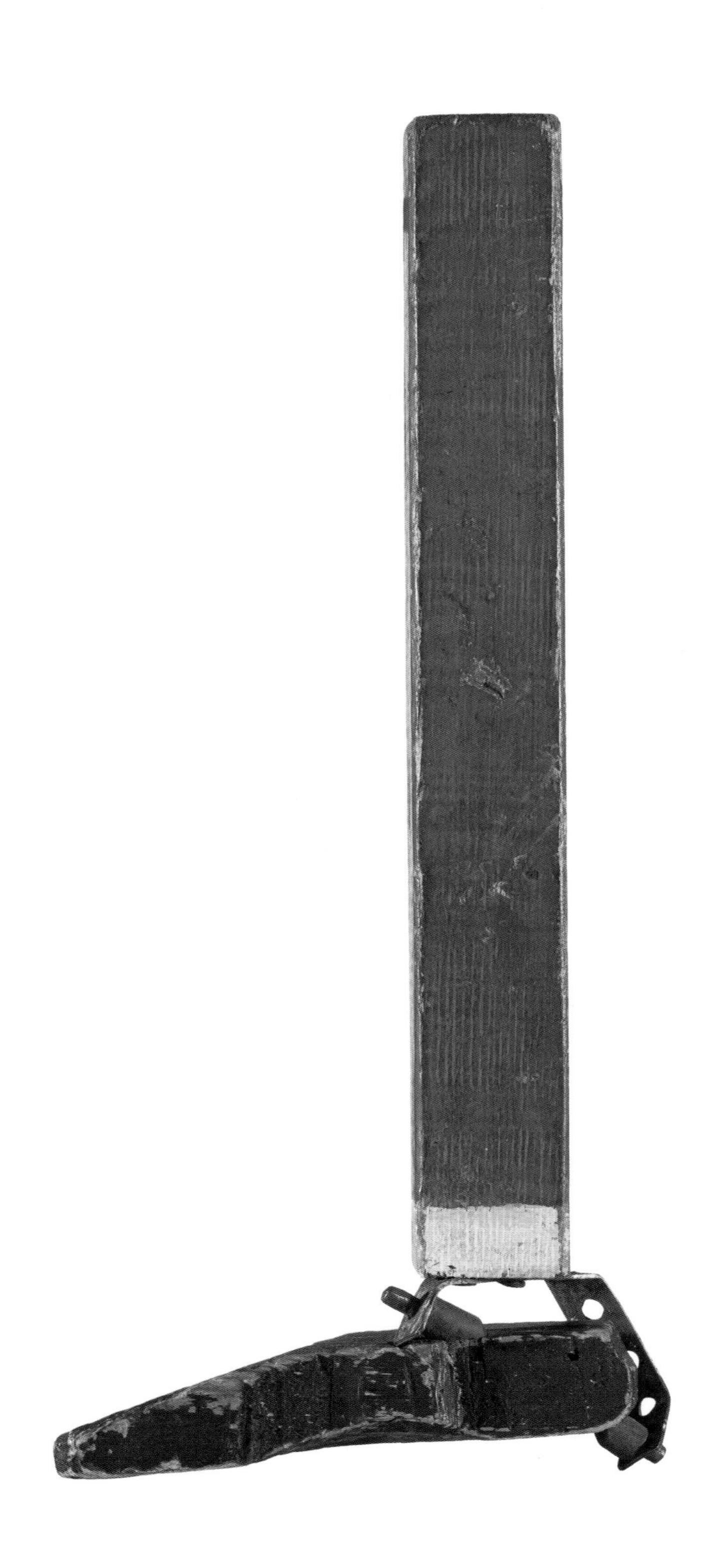

CATALOGUE 46
John Herbert Hicks
Model of the leg and foot showing the mechanism of the Achilles tendon, 1950s, wood with metal fixings, 15.2 x 7.3 x 2 cm.
RCSIC/Z 74.4.
Photograph by Michael Frank.

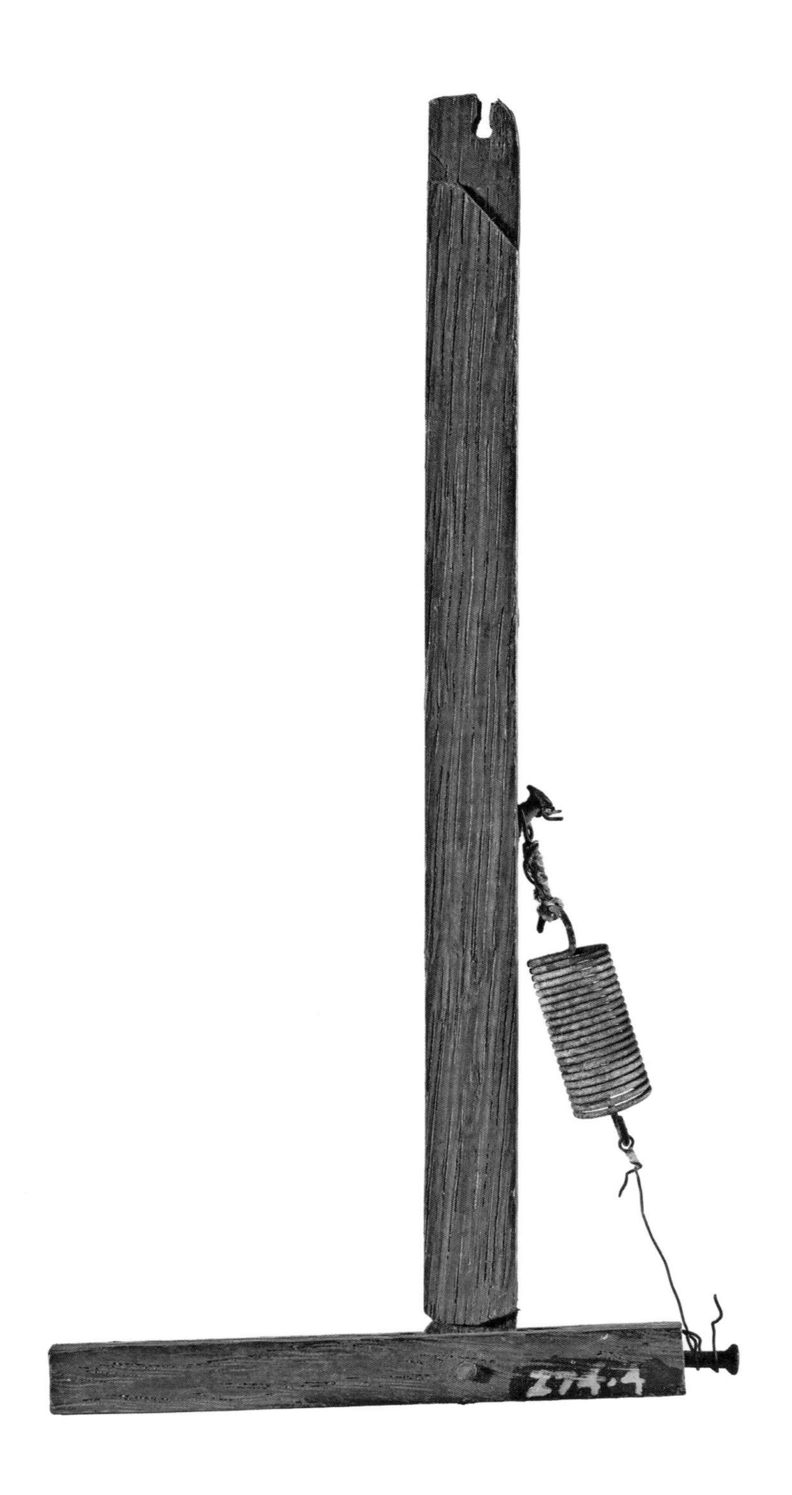

CATALOGUE 47
John Herbert Hicks
Model of the foot including tarsal and metatarsal bones, view from above (top) and view showing the bottom of the foot model (bottom), 1950s, wood with metal fixings, 8 x 8 x 19 cm.
RCSIC/Z 74.3.
Photographs by Michael Frank.

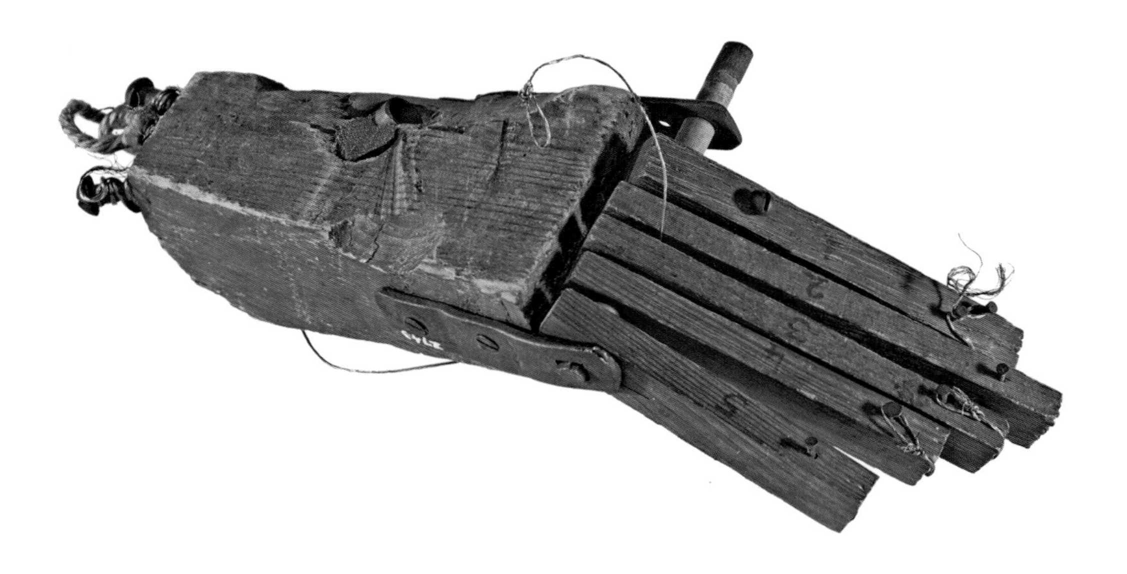

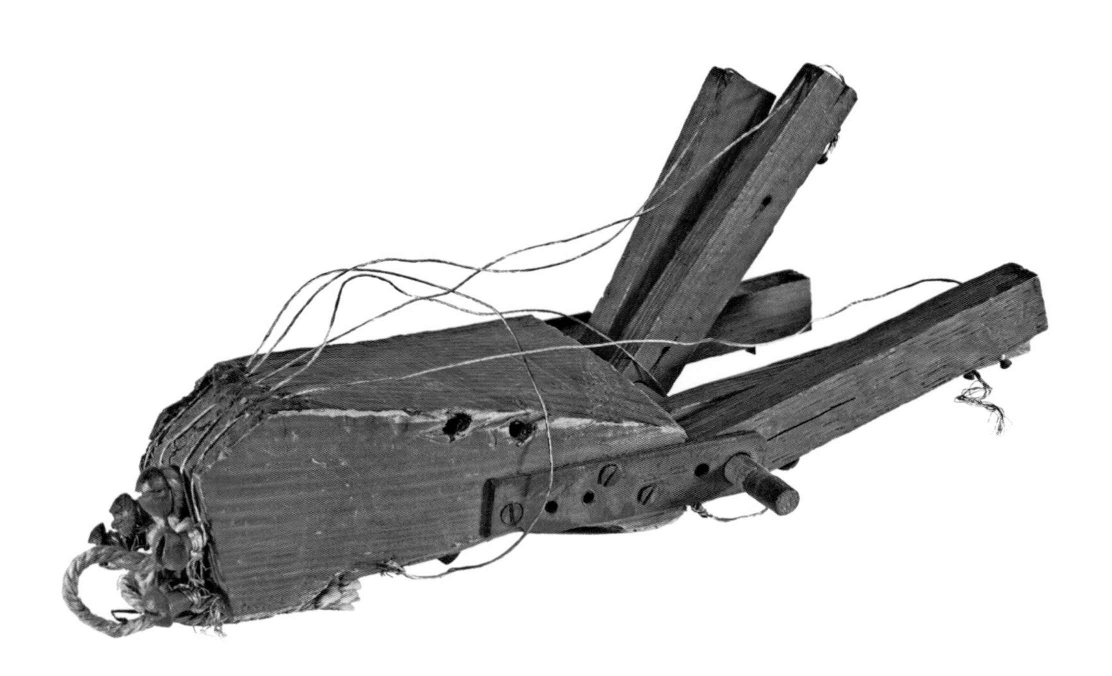

CATALOGUE 48
John Herbert Hicks
Model of the foot including tarsal and metatarsal bones, 1950s, wood with metal fixings, 7 x 7.5 x 19.5 cm.
RCSIC/Z 74.5.
Photograph by Michael Frank.

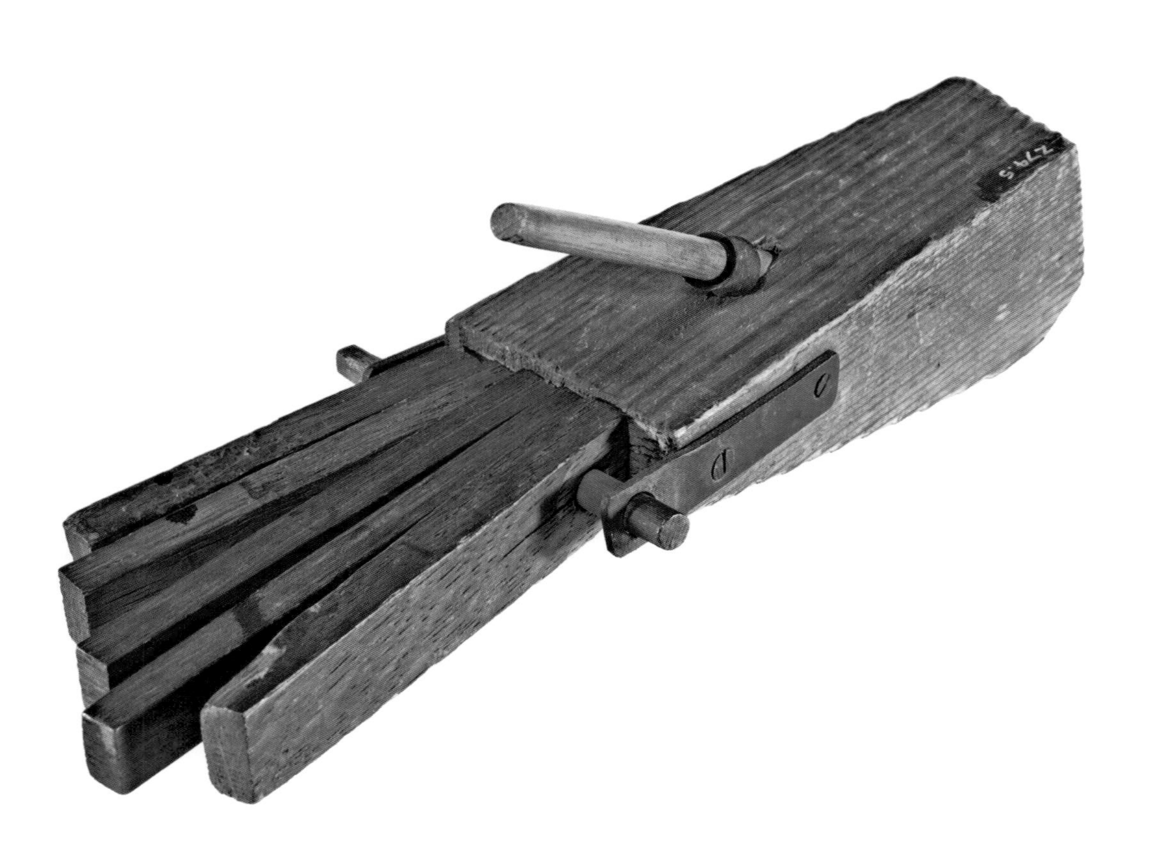

CATALOGUE 49
John Herbert Hicks
Model of the foot including tarsal and metatarsal bones, 1950s, wood with metal fixings, 15.3 x 15 x 32 cm.
RCSIC/Z 74.6.
Photograph by Michael Frank.

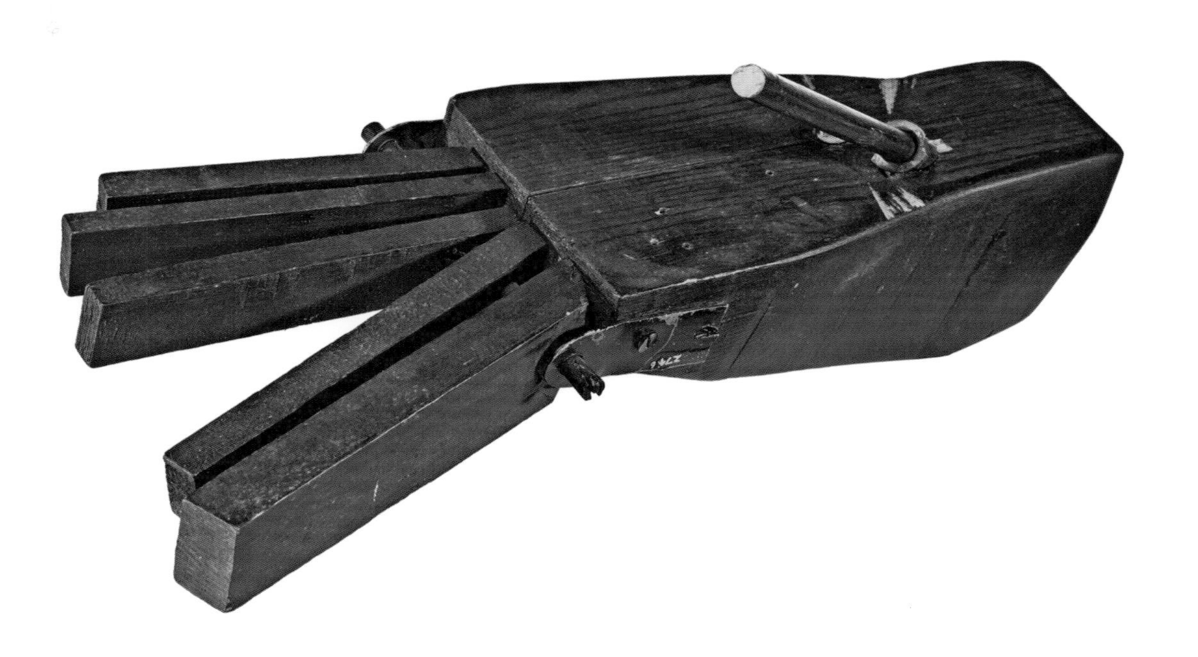

CATALOGUE 50
John Herbert Hicks
Model of the foot, for demonstrating the movements of the 1st and 5th metatarsals, 1950s, wood with metal fixings, 6 x 9 x 16.5 cm.
RCSIC/Z 74.8.
Photograph by Michael Frank.

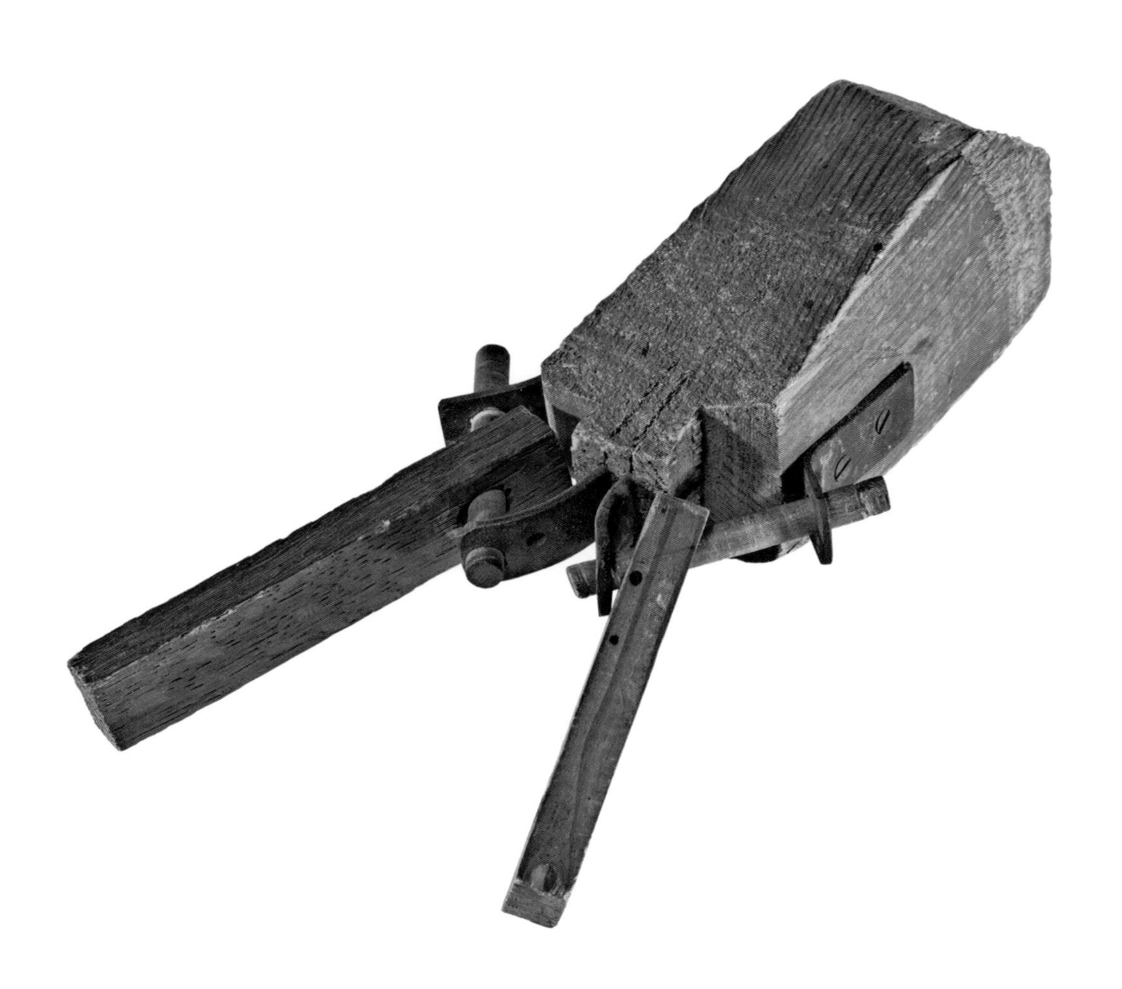

CATALOGUE 51
John Herbert Hicks
Model of the foot made to demonstrate oblique (diagonal) hinge movement. The model is assembled from three pieces, discovered 2015 in Hicks' papers at the RCS archive. The original 1950s model by Hicks had a fourth piece, the heel, which is no longer extant. Cardboard and ink, 7 x 4 x 10 cm.
RCS Archives MS0186/3/29.
Photograph by Michael Frank.

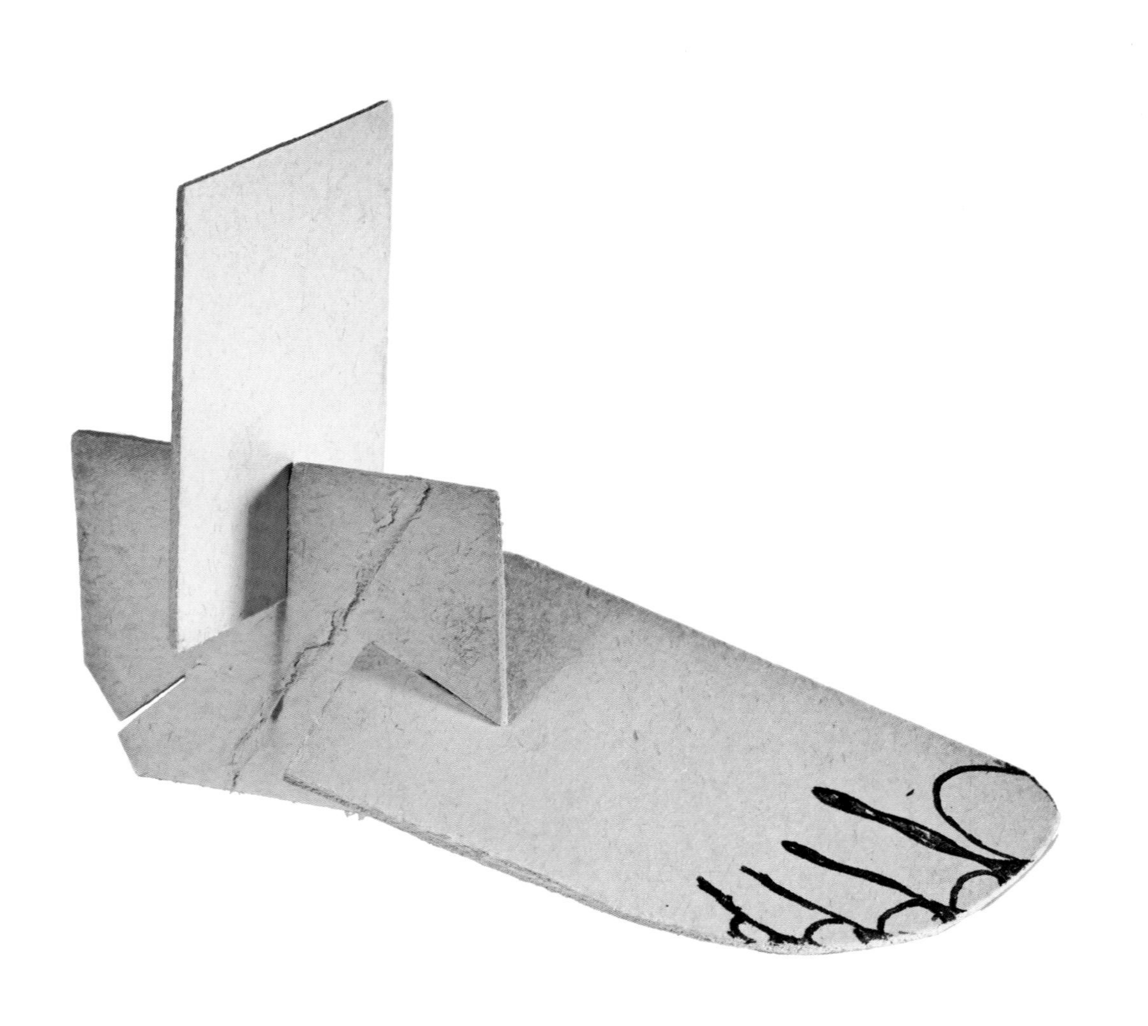

CATALOGUE 52
John Herbert Hicks
Model showing the linkage between the tarsal and metatarsal bones in the foot, 1950s, wood and plastic tape, 1.5 x 5.4 x 17.3 cm.
RCSIC/Z 74.11.
Photograph by Michael Frank.

CATALOGUE 53
John Herbert Hicks
Model showing the linkage between the tarsal and metatarsal bones in the foot, 1950s, wood and leatherette tape, 1.5 x 10 x 33 cm.
RCSIC/Z 74.12.
Photograph by Michael Frank.

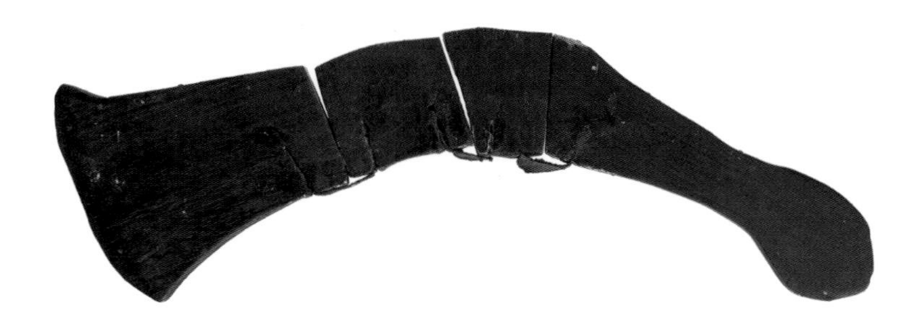

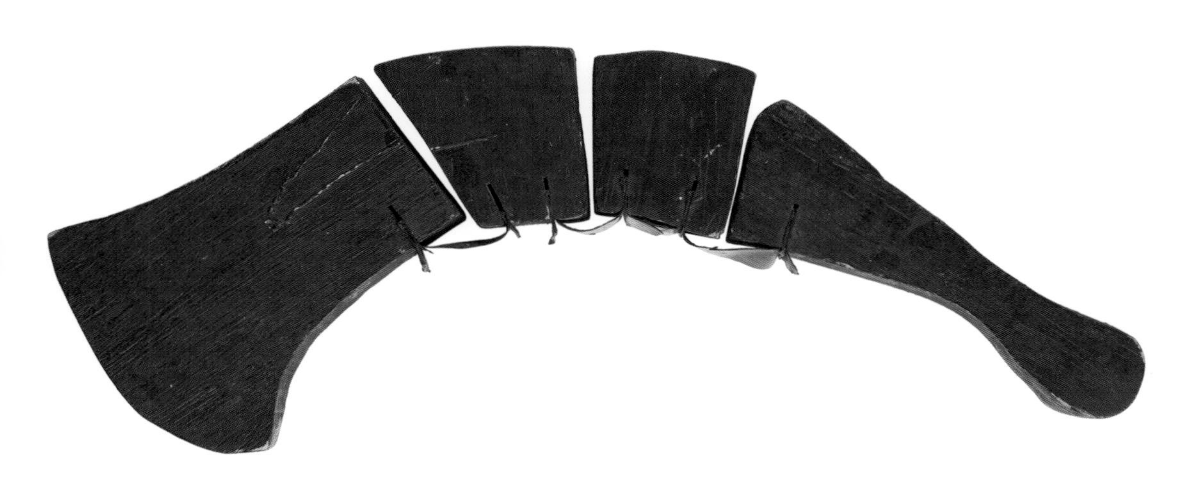

CATALOGUE 54
John Herbert Hicks
Model of the arch of the foot and the fascia (fibrous tissue) underneath it, used to demonstrate the windlass mechanism, where tension increases in the fascia and the arch rises, 1950s, wood, metal fixings and ribbon, 0.9 x 5.5 x 20.8 cm.
RCSIC/Z 74.9.
Photograph by Michael Frank.

CATALOGUE 55
John Herbert Hicks
Model of the arch of the foot and the fascia (fibrous tissue) underneath it, used to demonstrate the windlass mechanism, where tension increases in the fascia and the arch rises, 1950s, wood, metal fixings and leatherette, 1.5 x 15.7 x 38 cm.
RCSIC/Z 74.10.
Photograph by Michael Frank.

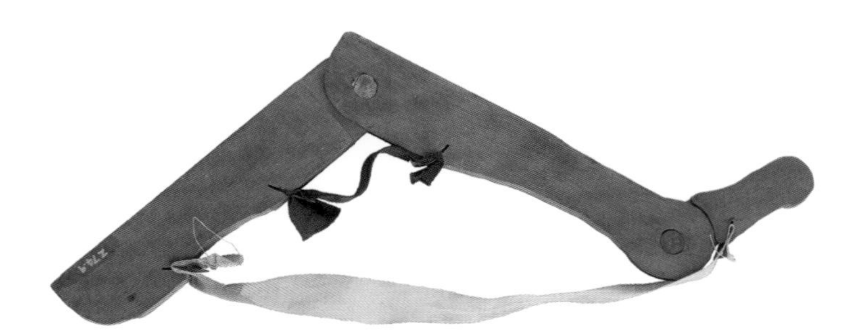

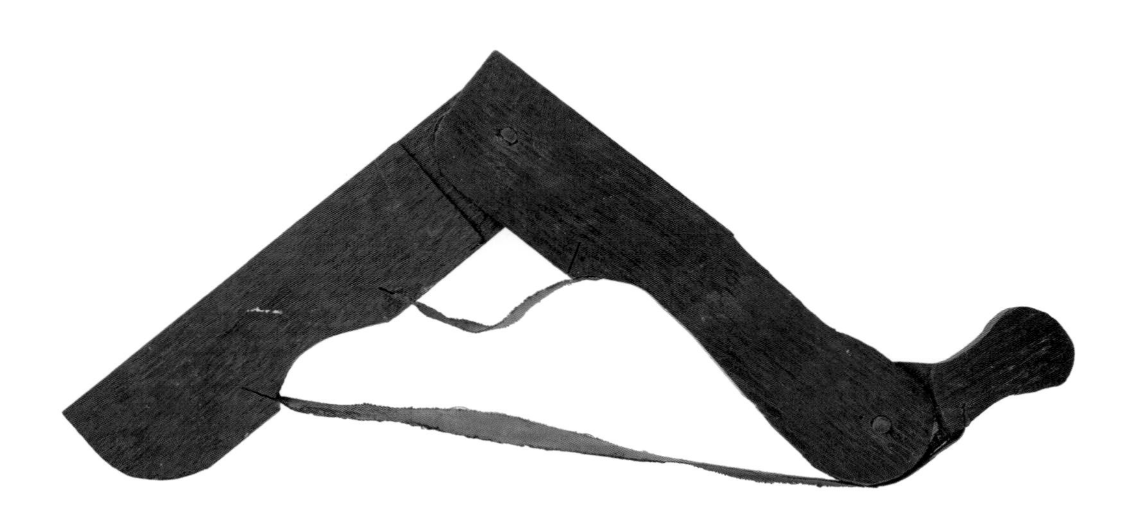

CATALOGUE 56
John Herbert Hicks
Model to demonstrate the windlass mechanism in the foot, where the fascia (fibrous tissue) tightens and loosens with movement, 1950s, wood, metal fixings and ribbon, 10.5 x 4.4 x 14.5 cm.
RCSIC/Z 74.7.
Photograph by Michael Frank.

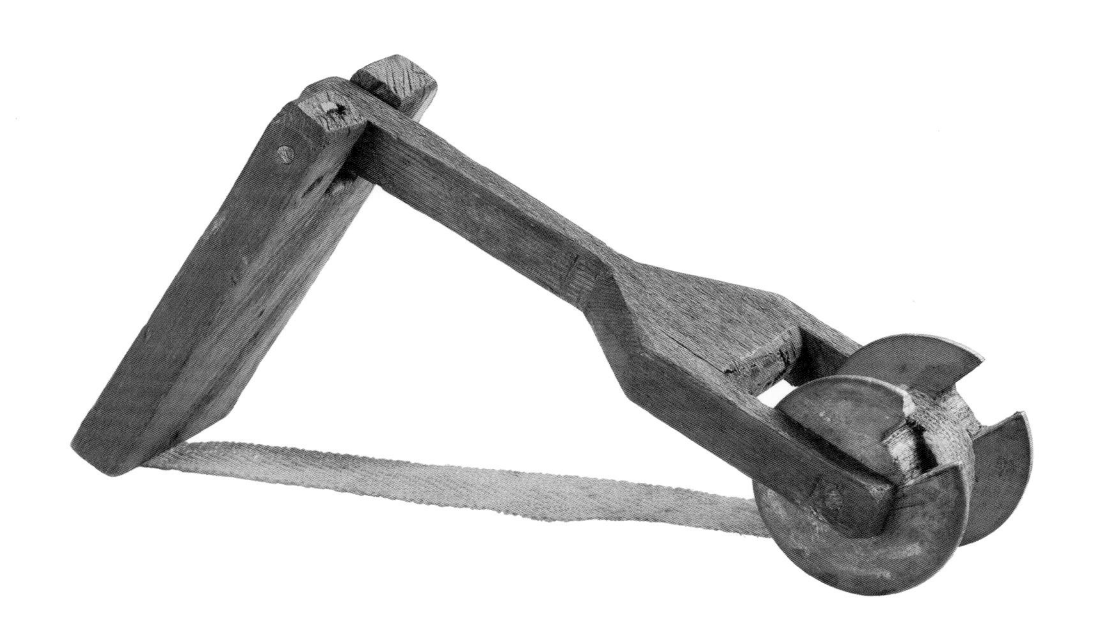

CATALOGUE 57
John Herbert Hicks
Four fracture plates to aid healing in forearm fractures, mounted on models of fractured bones, labelled 'relatively effective fixation', 1965–1975, wood and metal, 22.5 x 1.5 cm.
RCSIC/M 31.10 parts 3, 4, 1 and 2.
Photographs by Michael Frank.

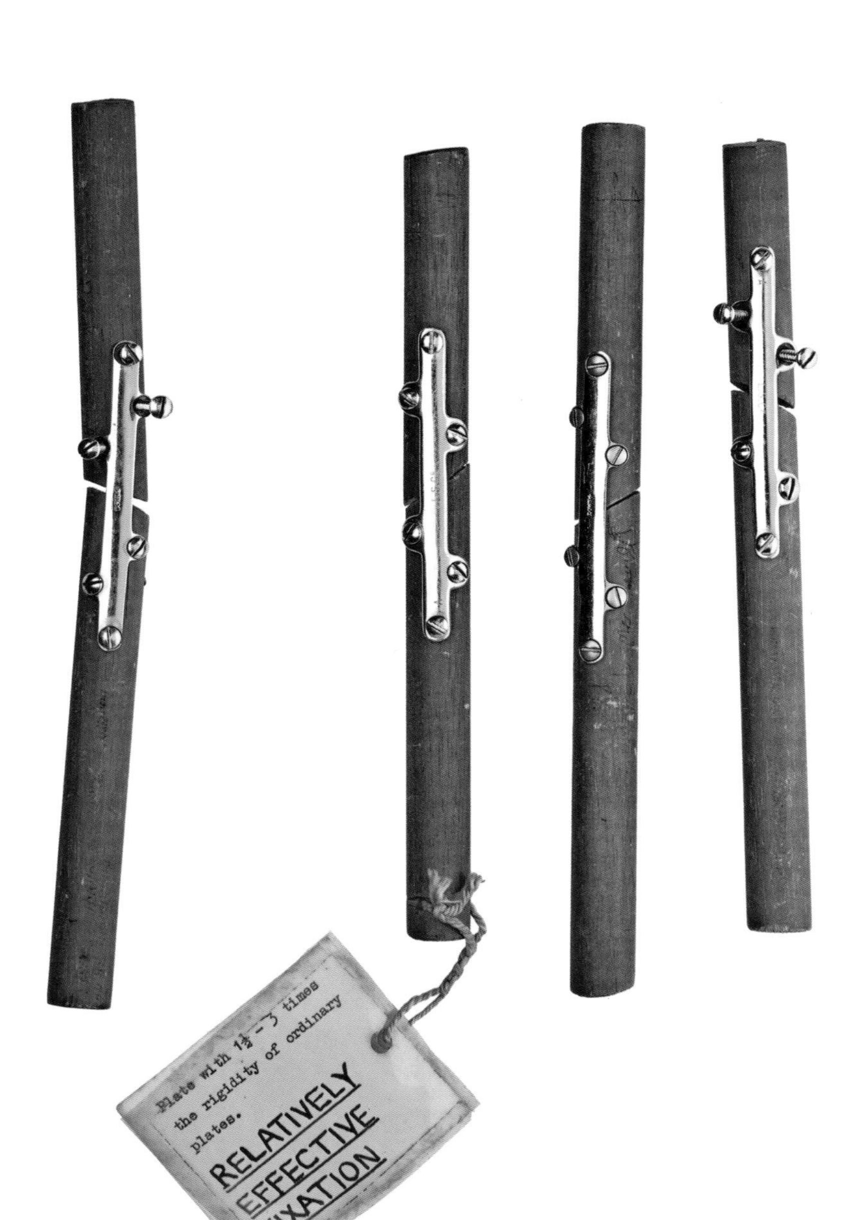
Plate with 1½ - 3 times
the rigidity of ordinary
plates.
RELATIVELY
EFFECTIVE
FIXATION

CATALOGUE 58
John Herbert Hicks
Six fracture plates to aid healing in fractures of the femur and tibia in the leg, mounted on models of fractured bones, labelled 'effective fixation' and 'relatively effective fixation', 1965–1975, wood and metal, 25.5 x 3 cm.
RCSIC/M 31.10 parts 9, 7, 10, 12, 14 and 5.
Photographs by Michael Frank.

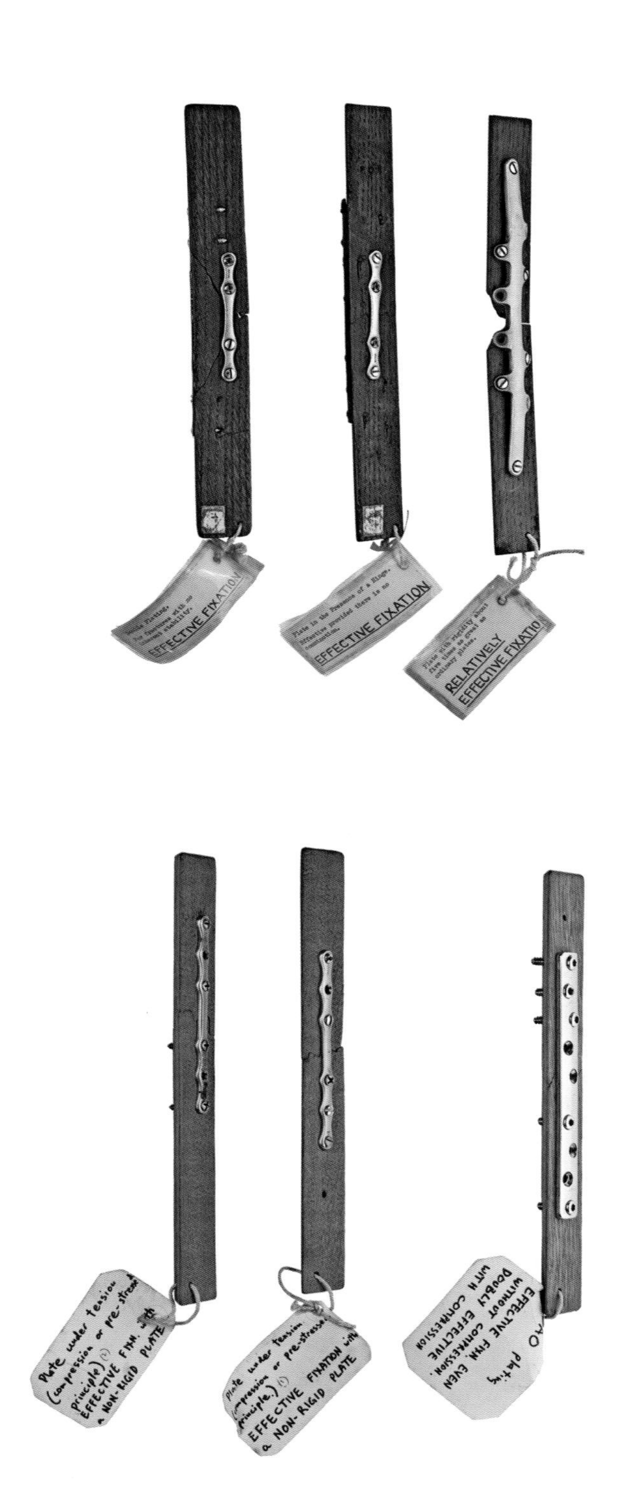
EFFECTIVE FIXATION
EFFECTIVE FIXATION
RELATIVELY
EFFECTIVE FIXATIO
Plate under tension
(compression or pre-stress
principle)
EFFECTIVE FIXN.
a NON-RIGID PLATE
Plate under tension
principle.)
EFFECTIVE FIXATION
a NON-RIGID PLATE
AO plating
EFFECTIVE FIXN. EVEN
WITHOUT COMPRESSION.
DOUBLY EFFECTIVE
WITH COMPRESSION

CATALOGUE 59
John Herbert Hicks
Four fracture plates to aid healing in fractures of the tibia in the leg, mounted on models of fractured bones, labelled 'ineffective fixation', 1965–1975, wood and metal, 25.5 x 3 cm.
RCSIC/M 31.10 parts 13, 11, 8 and 6.
Photographs by Michael Frank.

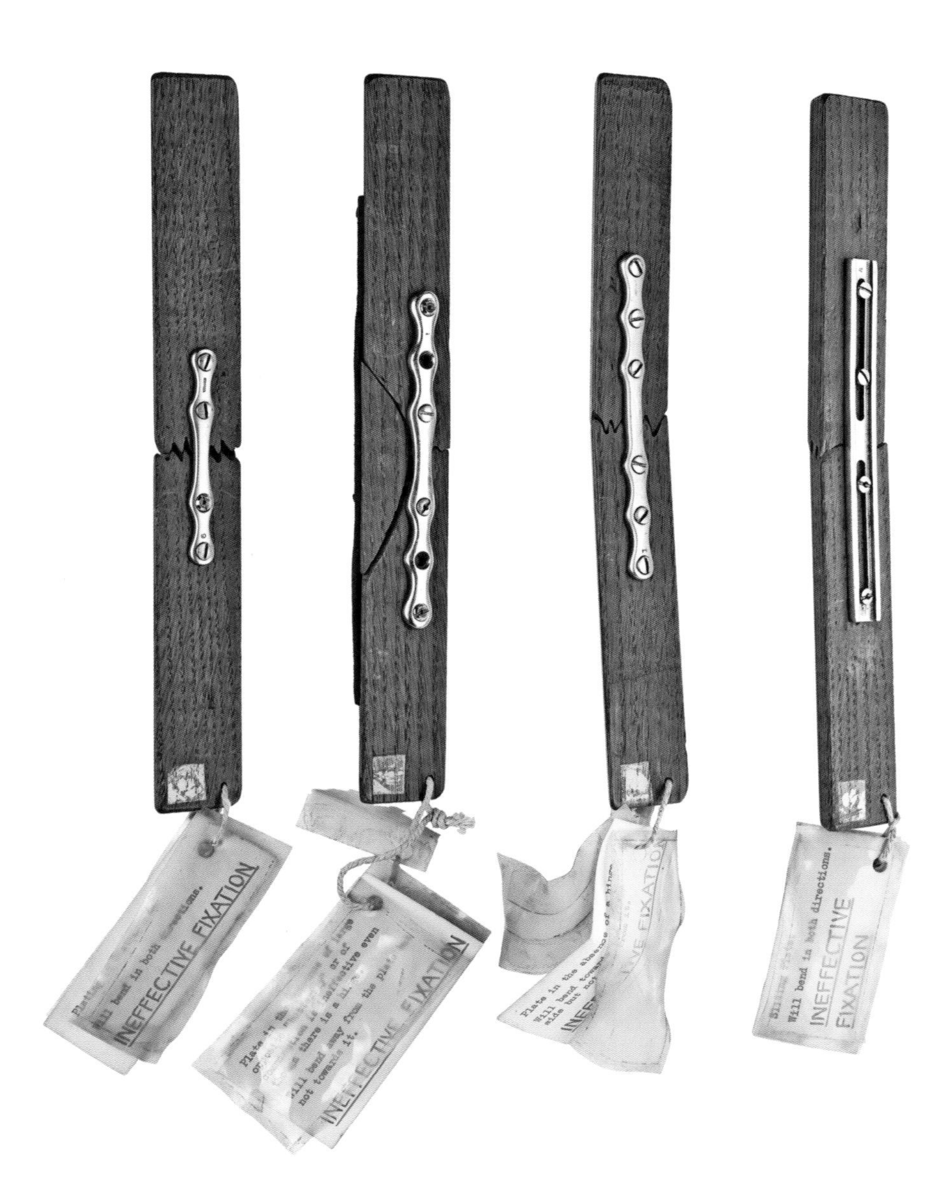
INEFFECTIVE FIXATION
INEFFECTIVE FIXATION
not towards it.
INEFFECTIVE FIXATION
Will bend in both directions.
INEFFECTIVE
FIXATION

CATALOGUE 60
John Herbert Hicks
Device to demonstrate external fixation of a fractured long bone, 1955–1965, wood, copper and brass, 44 x 19 cm.
RCSIC/P 2.2.
Photograph by Michael Frank.

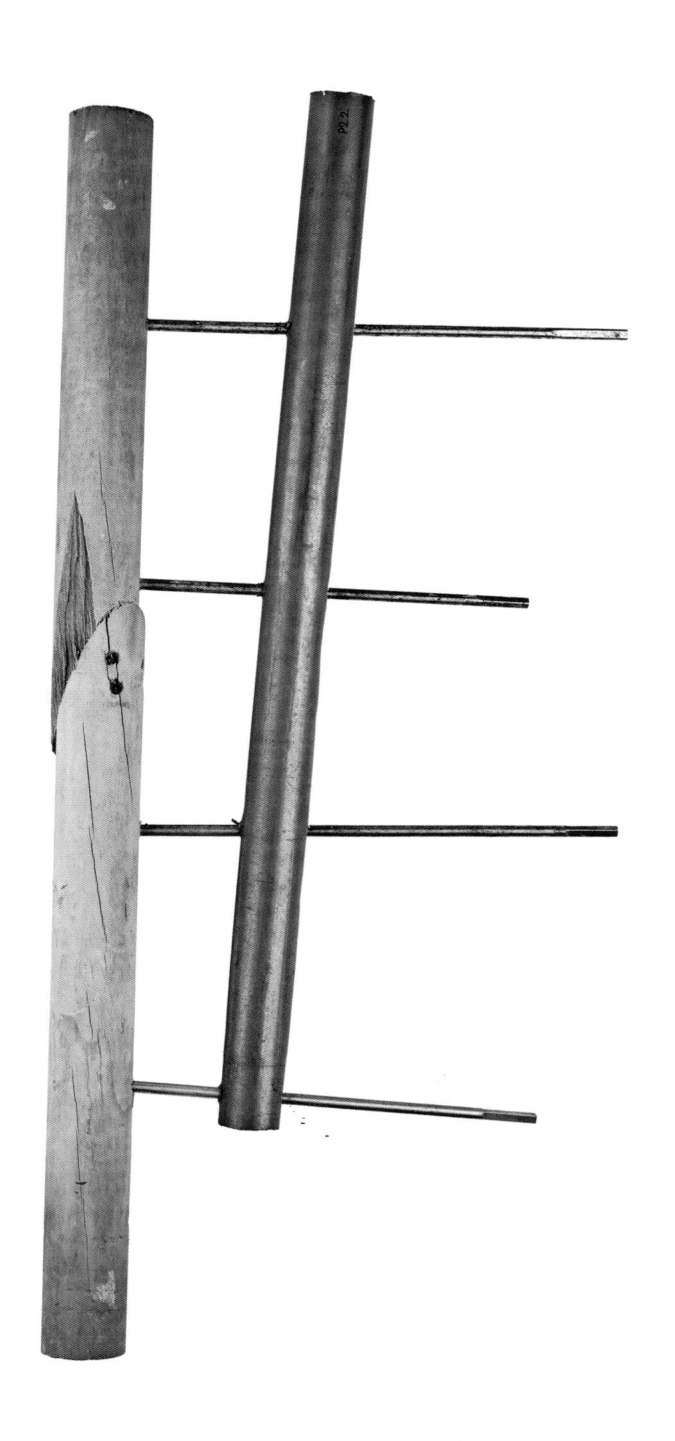
P2.2

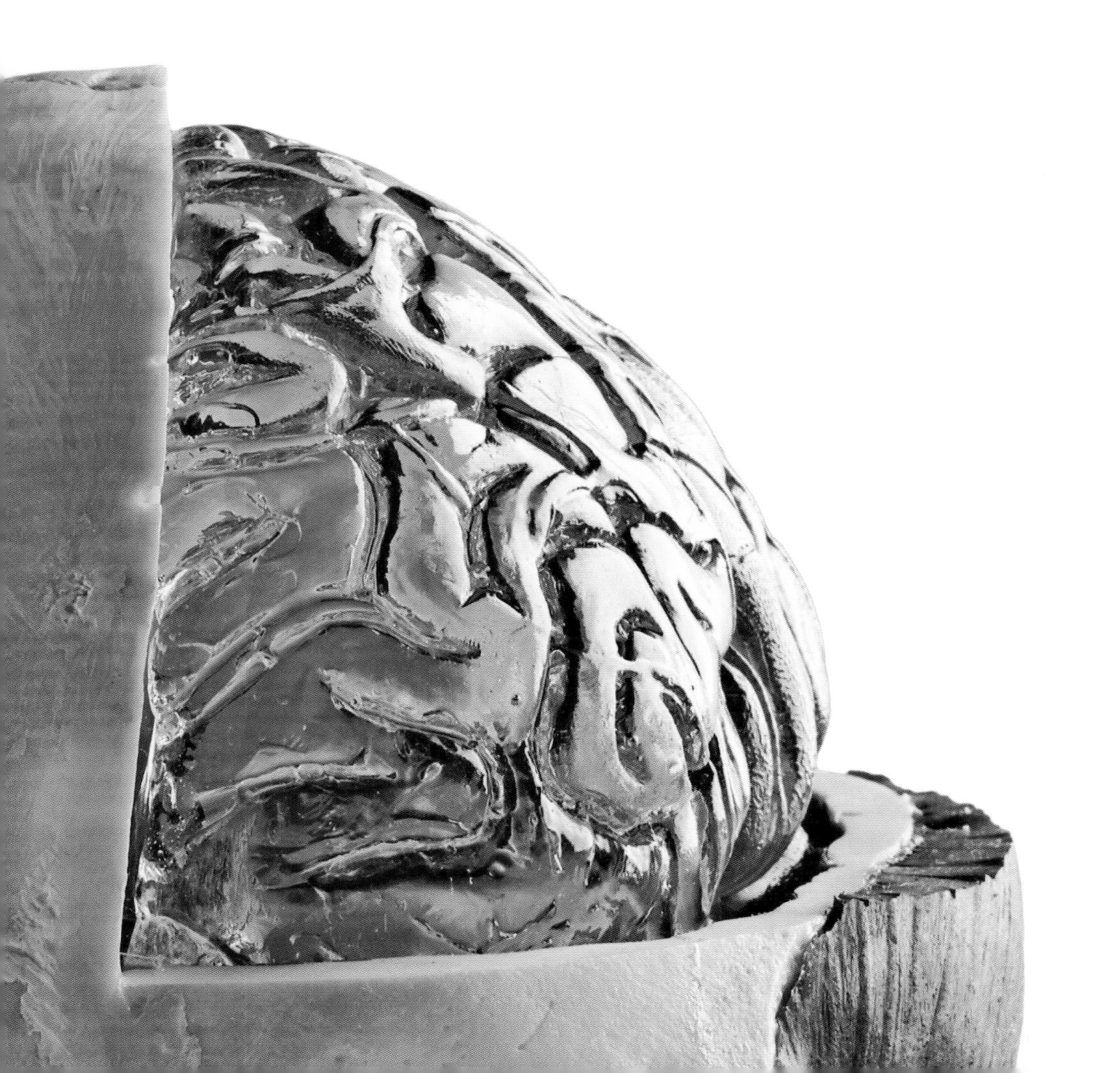

Modelled Anatomical Replica for Training Young Neurosurgeons (MARTYN)

CATALOGUE 61
Martyn Cooke
Modelled Anatomical Replica for Training Young Neurosurgeons, MARTYN, 2011 – present, polyurethane, latex and gelatine, 28 x 18 x 20 cm.
Photograph by Michael Frank.

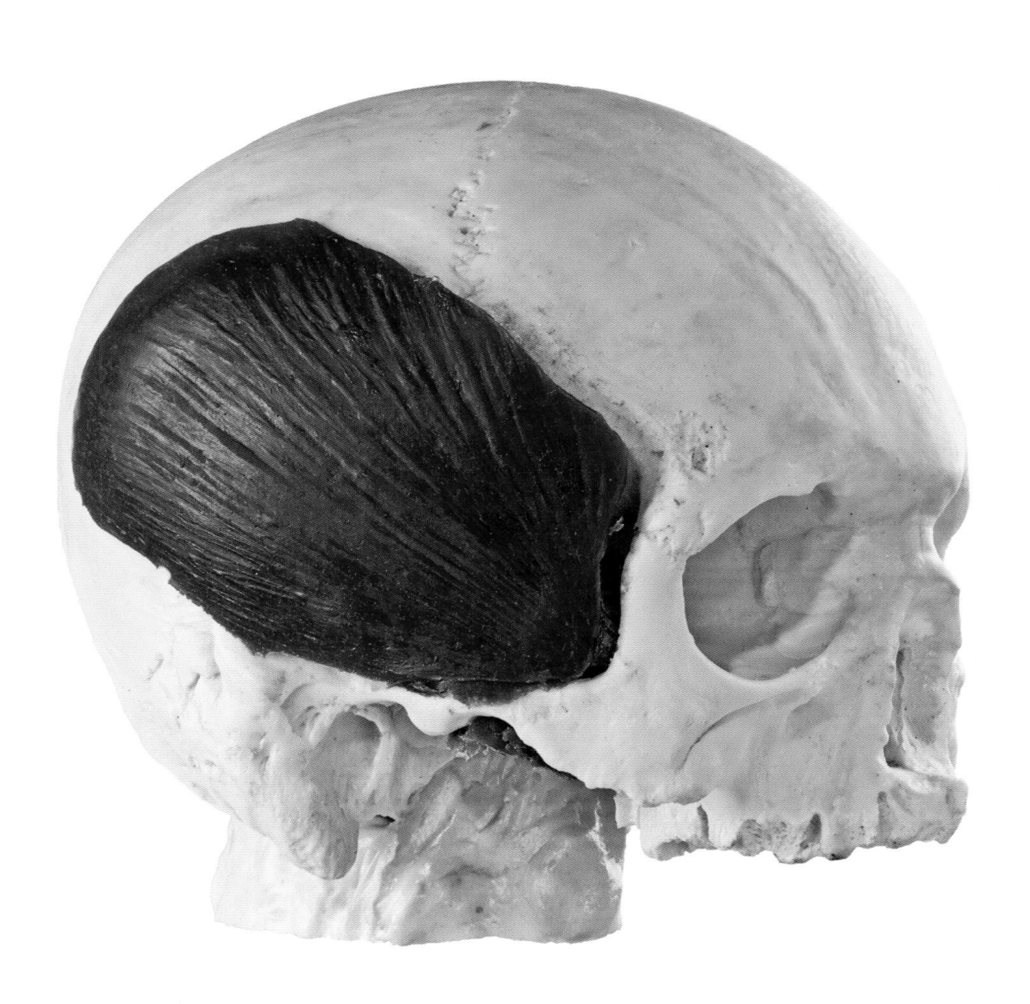

CATALOGUE 62
Martyn Cooke
Display model of MARTYN, cut away to show the brain inside the skull, 2012, polyurethane, latex and silicone, 28 x 18 x 20 cm.
Photograph by Michael Frank.

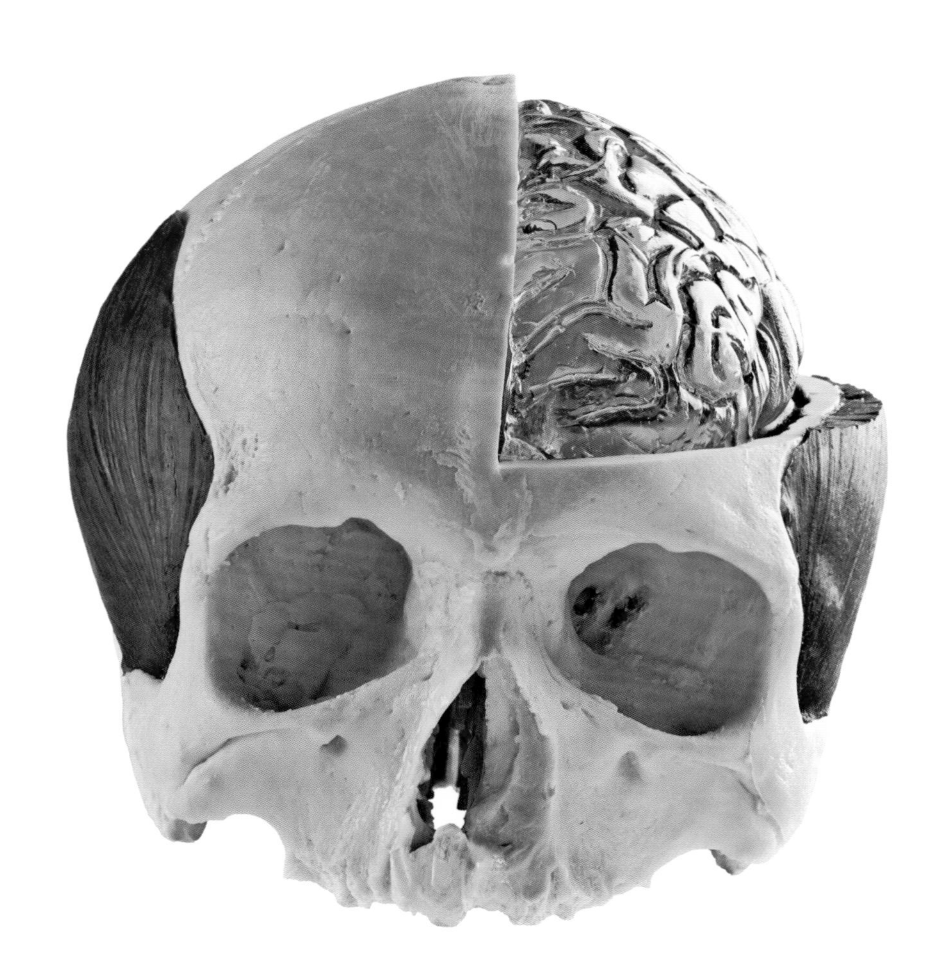

CATALOGUE 63
Martyn Cooke
MARTYN prototype, showing the first test of the surgical procedure for accessing the brain through the skull, 2011, polyurethane, latex and gelatine, 28 x 18 x 20 cm.
Photograph by Michael Frank.

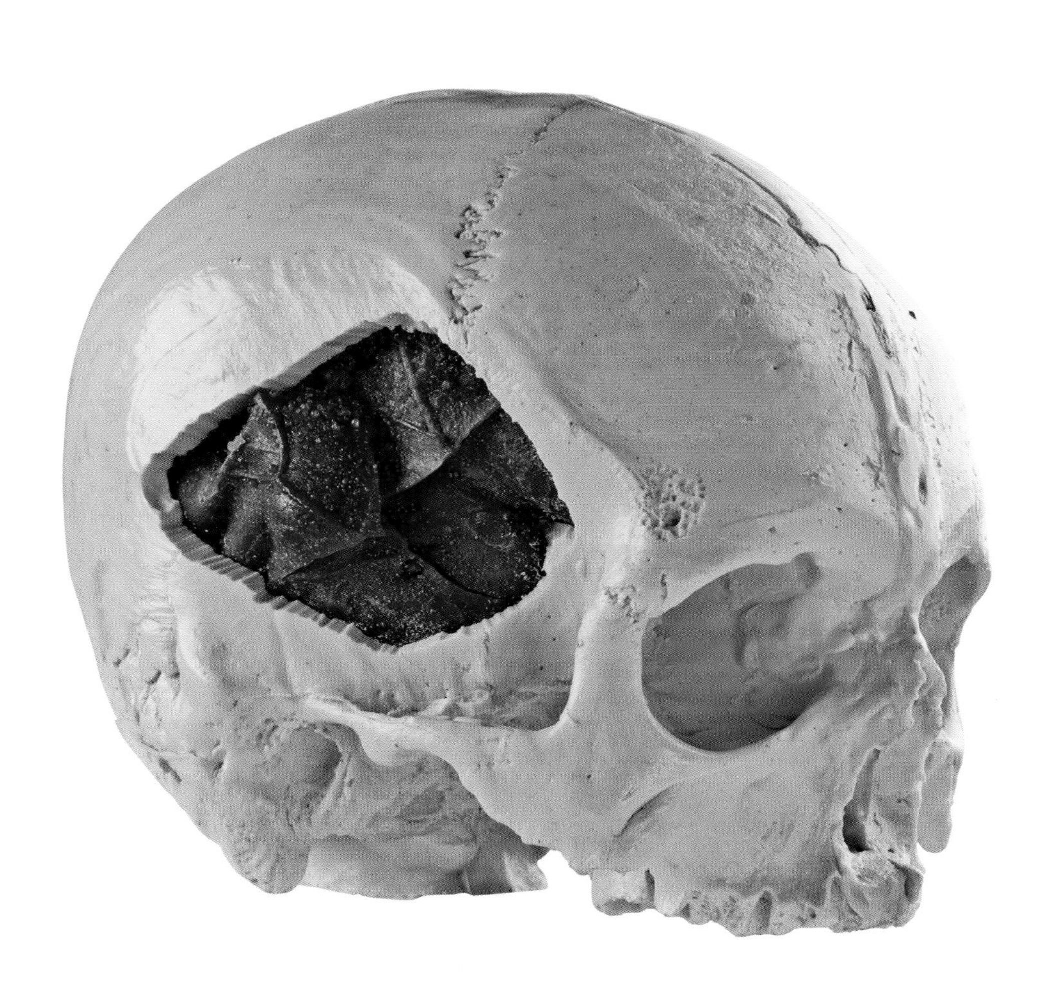

CATALOGUE 64
Martyn Cooke
MARTYN after use in surgical training sessions on cutting into the skull to access the brain, 2012, polyurethane, 28 x 18 x 20 cm.
Photograph by Michael Frank.

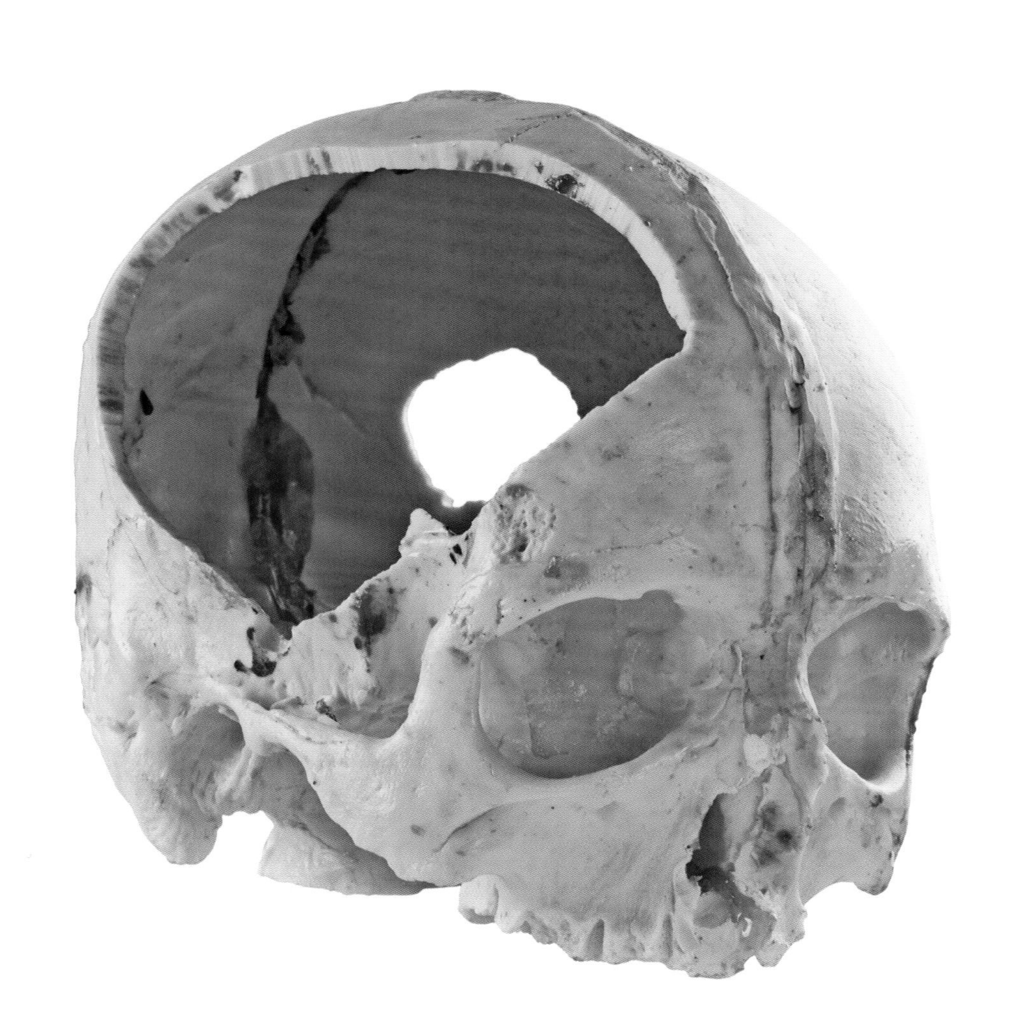

CATALOGUE 65
Martyn Cooke
MARTYN after use in surgical training sessions on cutting into the skull to access the brain, replacing the removed bone and fixing with metal attachments, 2012, polyurethane, 28 x 18 x 20 cm.
Photograph by Michael Frank.

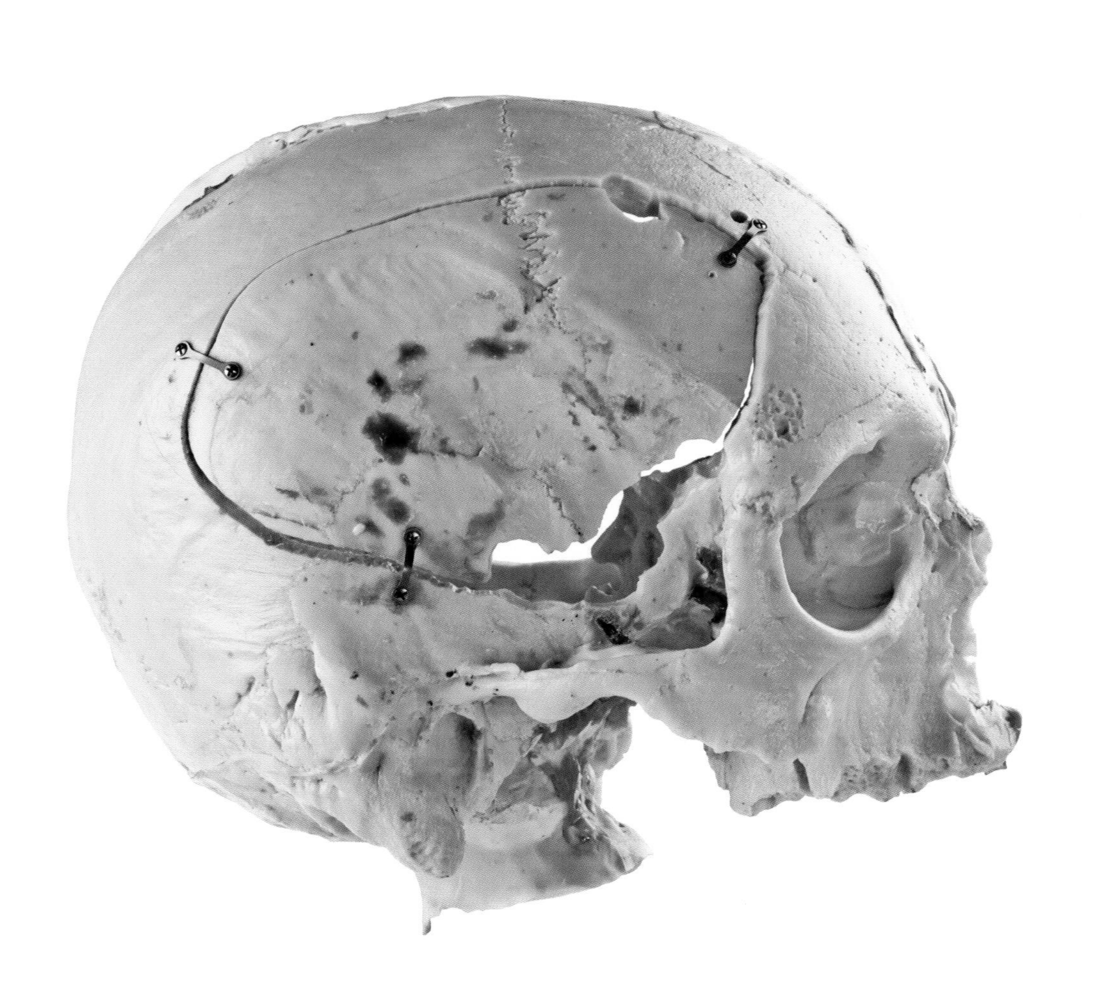

CATALOGUE 66
Martyn Cooke
MARTYN after use in surgical training sessions on cutting into the skull and with pen markings relating to future plans to develop the model for training in surgical procedures to treat acoustic tumours, 2012, polyurethane and ink, 28 x 18 x 20 cm.
Photograph by Michael Frank.

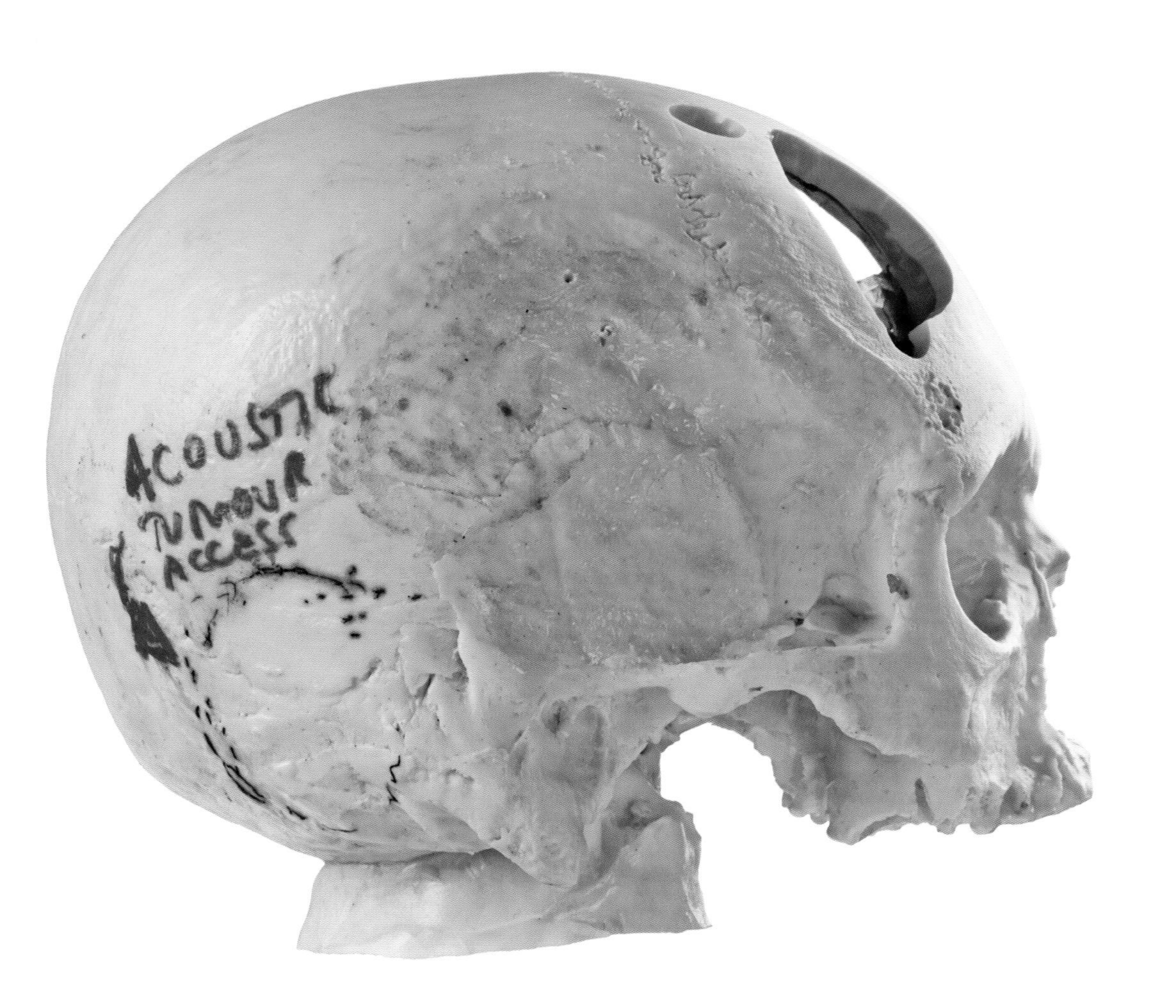
ACOUSTIC
TUMOUR
ACCESS

CATALOGUE 67
Martyn Cooke
MARTYN brain, which trainees access inside the modelled skull, 2011, gelatine, 10.5 x 16.5 x 5 cm.
Photograph by Michael Frank.

CATALOGUE 68
Martyn Cooke
MARTYN brain covered with the *dura mater* (membrane) and a haemorrhage, 2013, latex and gelatine, 10.5 x 16.5 x 5 cm.
Photograph by Michael Frank.

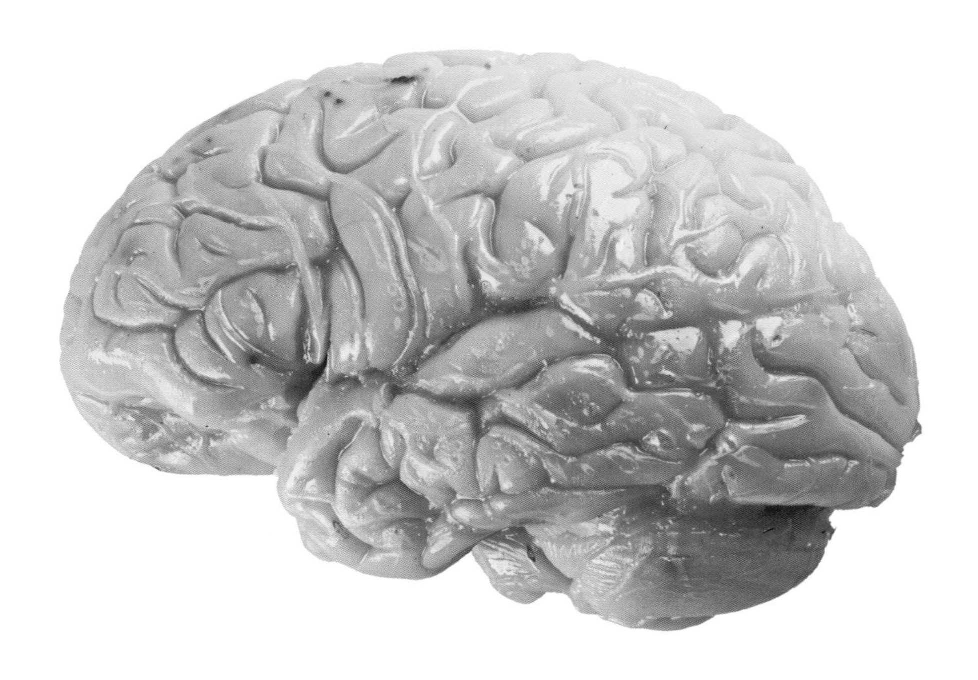

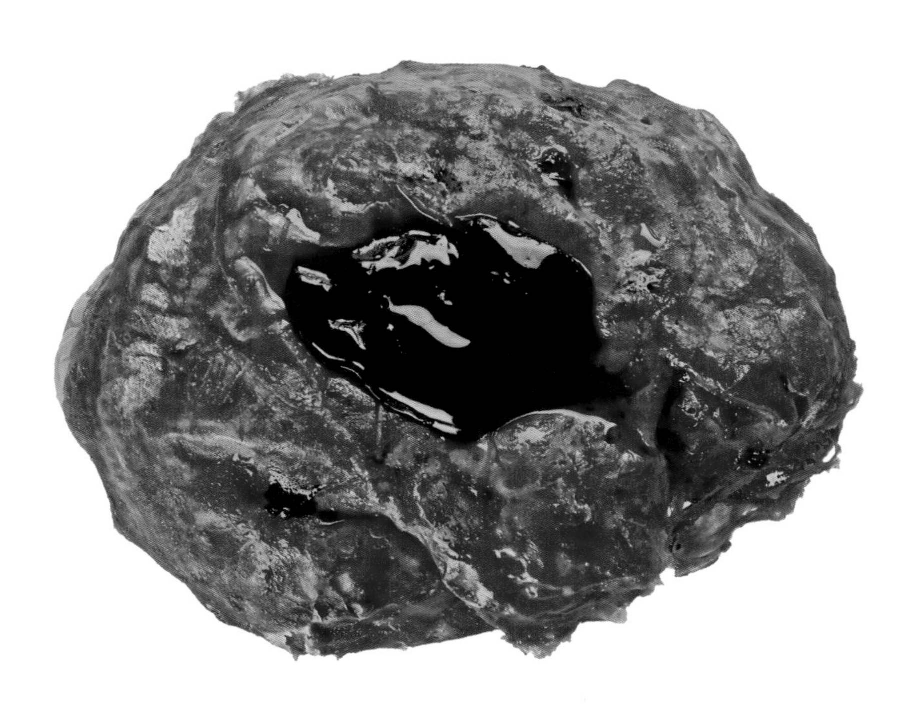

CATALOGUE 69
Martyn Cooke
MARTYN cut vertically to show the modelled ventricles and hemorrhages (rear view), 2015, polyurethane, latex, gelatine, liquid paraffin to simulate cerebrospinal fluid, 18.5 x 14 x 11 cm.
Photograph by Michael Frank.

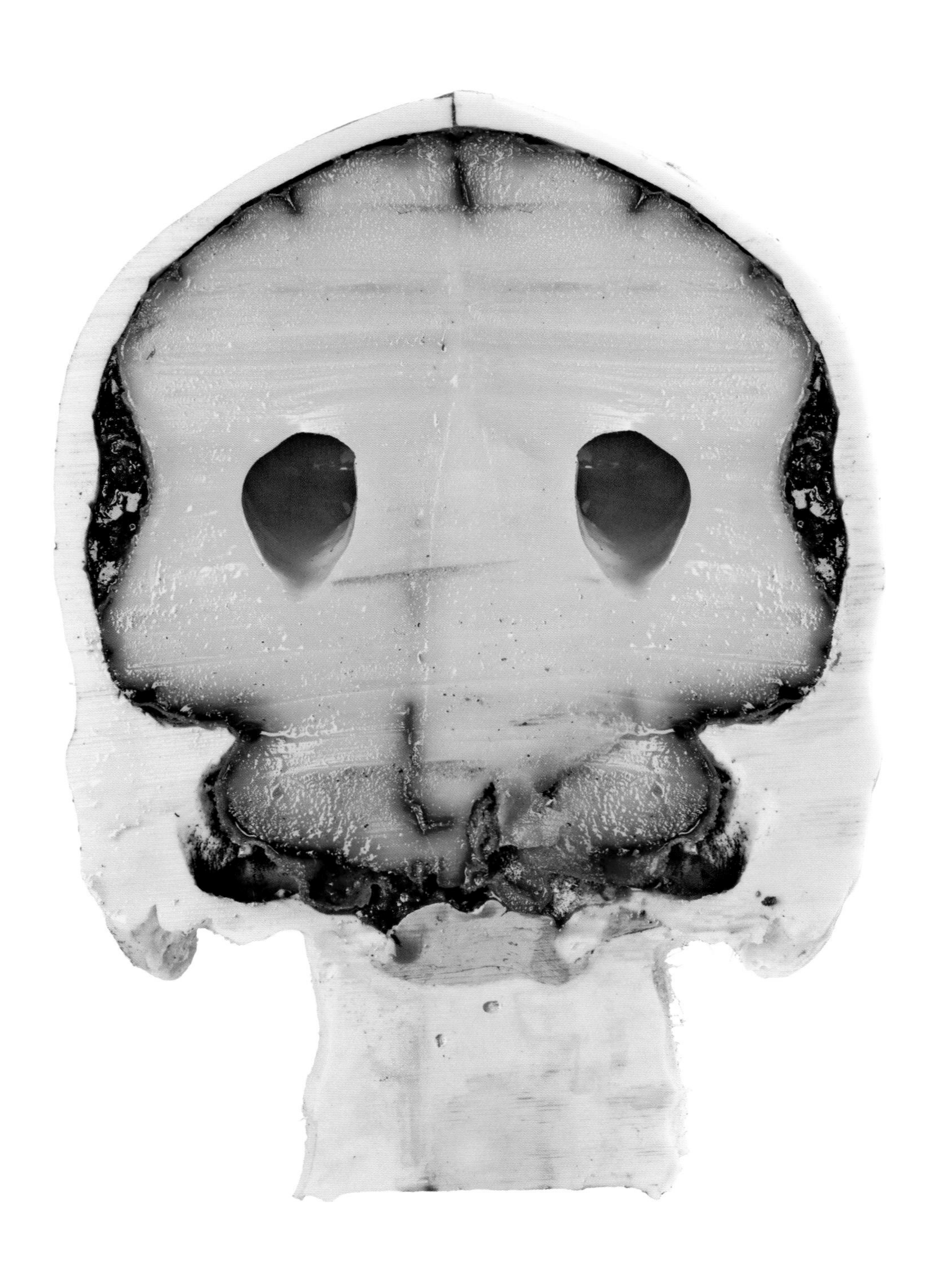

CATALOGUE 70
Martyn Cooke
Models of aneurysms in the circle of Willis (blood vessels at the base of the brain), developed for inclusion in MARTYN. The wire model (left) was constructed and used to cast the latex models (centre and right), which were then attached to the brain in MARTYN, 2014, wire, epoxy resin and latex, 11.5 x 6 x 2 cm; 10 x 4.5 x 2 cm. See diagram with Catalogue 10.
Photograph by Michael Frank.

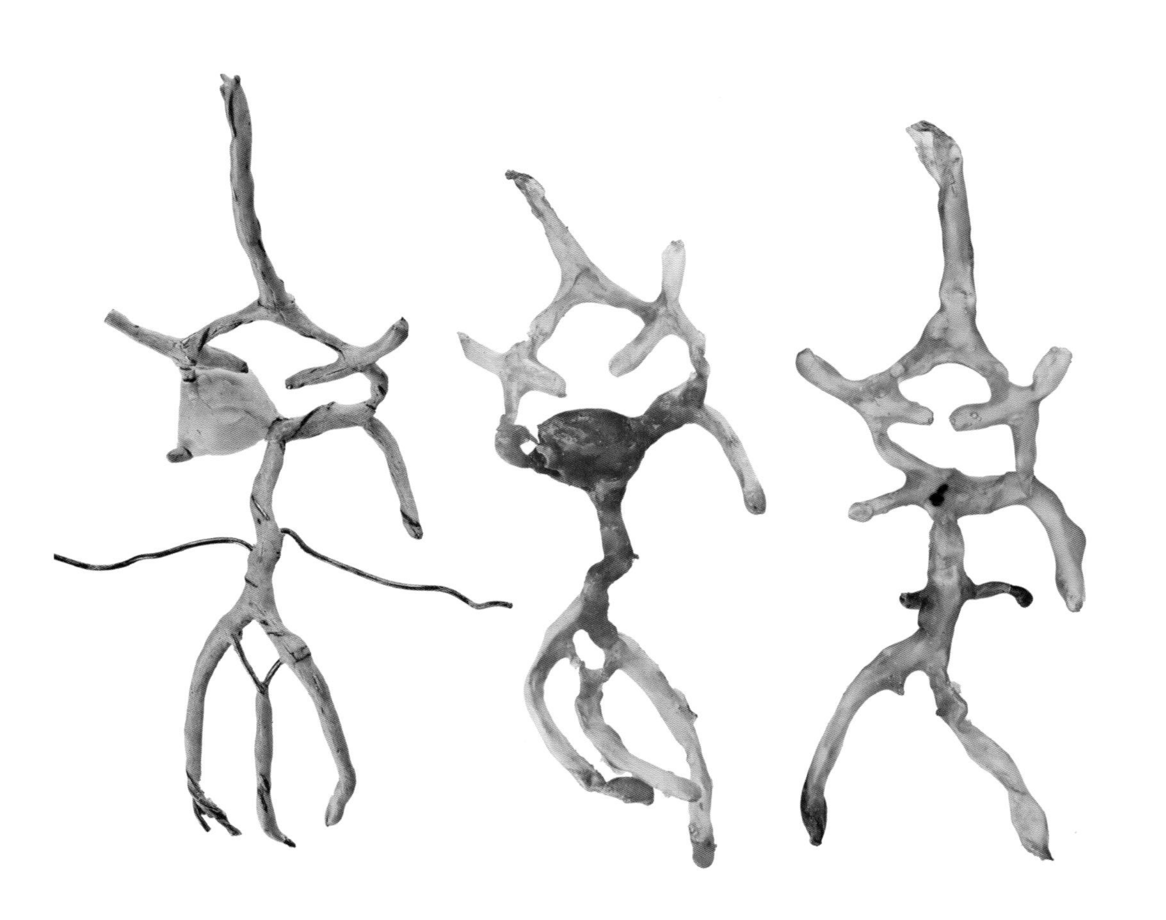

CATALOGUE 71
Clare Rangeley with Martyn Cooke
Paediatric MARTYN working prototype showing temporal muscle. The model is currently being developed to train in paediatric surgical procedures on the skull and brain. Tubes are attached to allow repeated refilling of the ventricles with fluid. 2015, polyurethane and silicone rubber, 14 x 12.5 x 15.5 cm.
Photograph by Michael Frank.

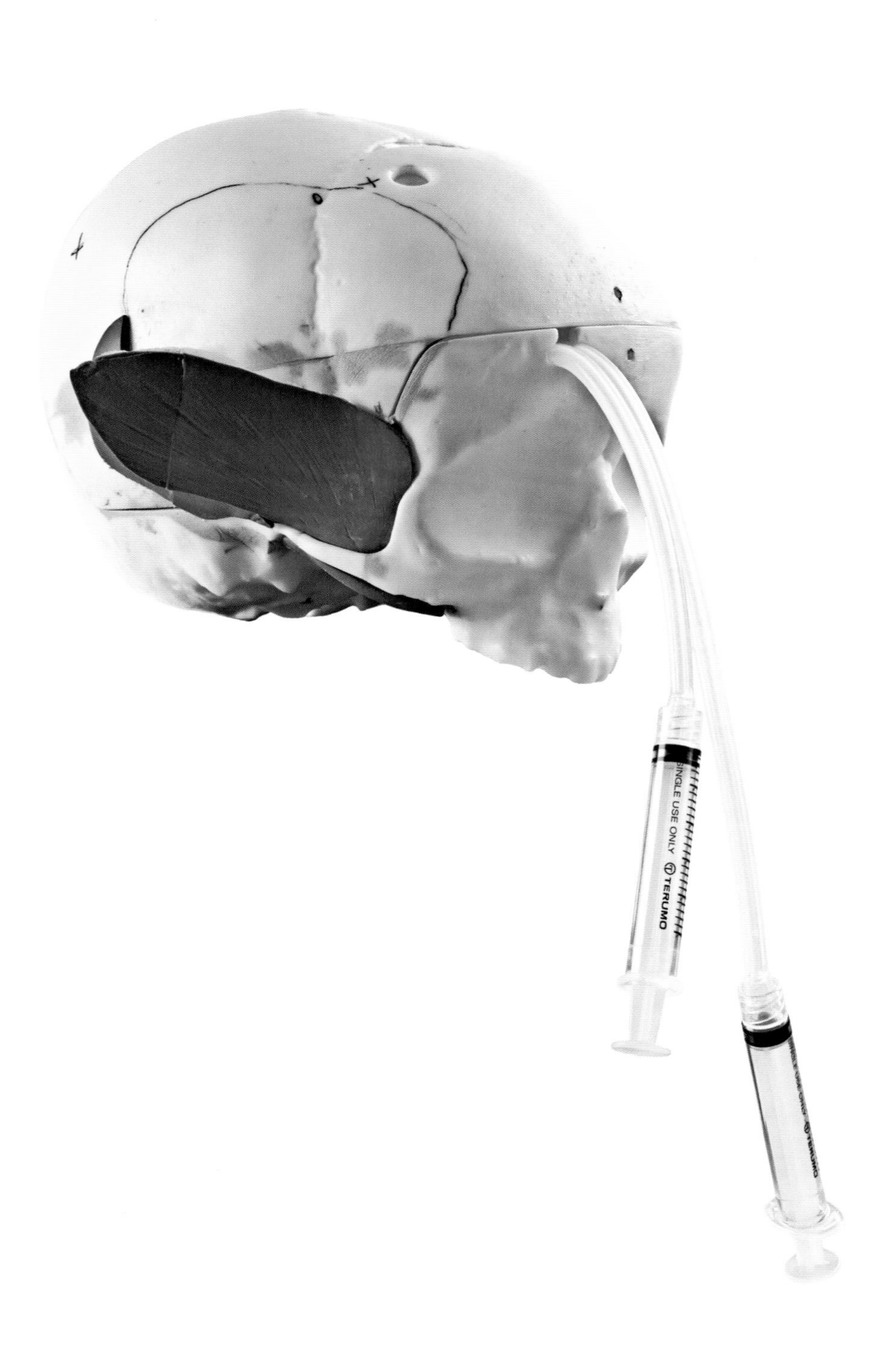
SINGLE USE ONLY
TERUMO

CATALOGUE 72
Clare Rangeley with Martyn Cooke
Paediatric MARTYN model under development, with skull cut away to show the brain, 2015, polyurethane and silicone rubber, 15.5 x 15 x 18.4 cm.
Photograph by Michael Frank.

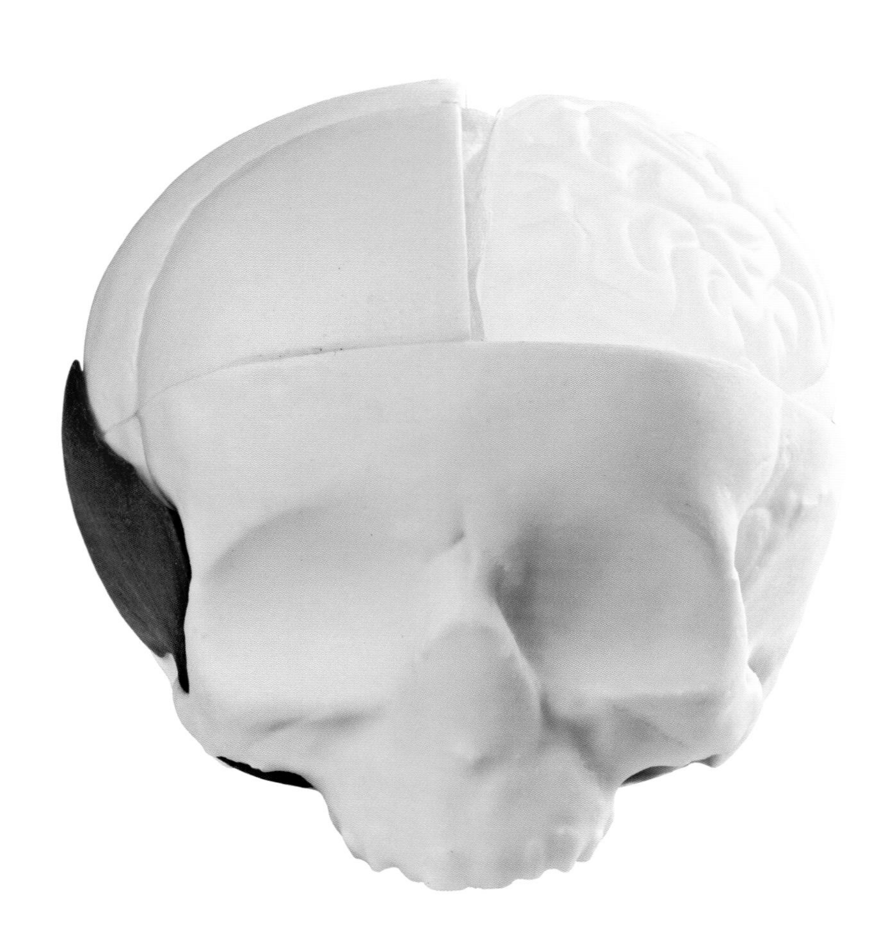

CATALOGUE 73
Clare Rangeley with Martyn Cooke
Paediatric MARTYN model under development, with skull and ***dura mater*** cut away to show the right side of the brain with enlarged ventricle inside, 2015, polyurethane, silicone rubber and plastic, 15.5 x 15 x 18.4 cm.
Photograph by Michael Frank.

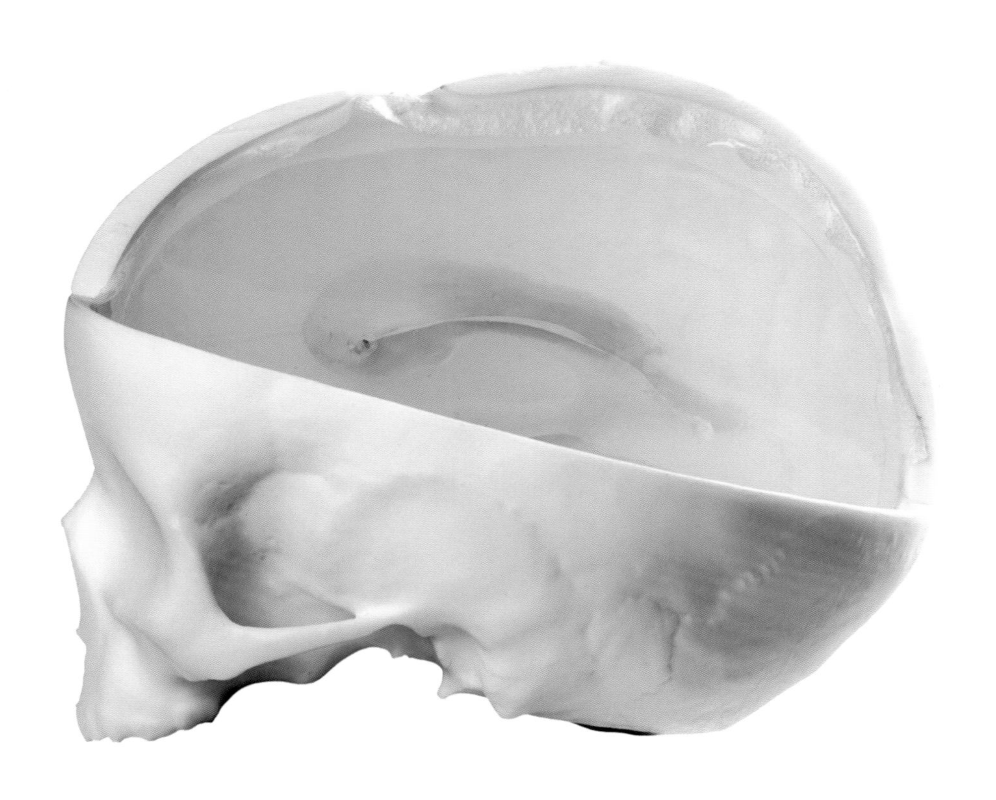

CATALOGUE 74
Clare Rangeley with Martyn Cooke
Part of Paediatric MARTYN model under development: the cerebellum, section of the spinal cord and first cervical vertebra (bottom), section of the skull (top), 2015, polyurethane, silicone rubber and plasticine, 5.7 x 16.2 x 10.9 cm.
Photographs by Michael Frank.

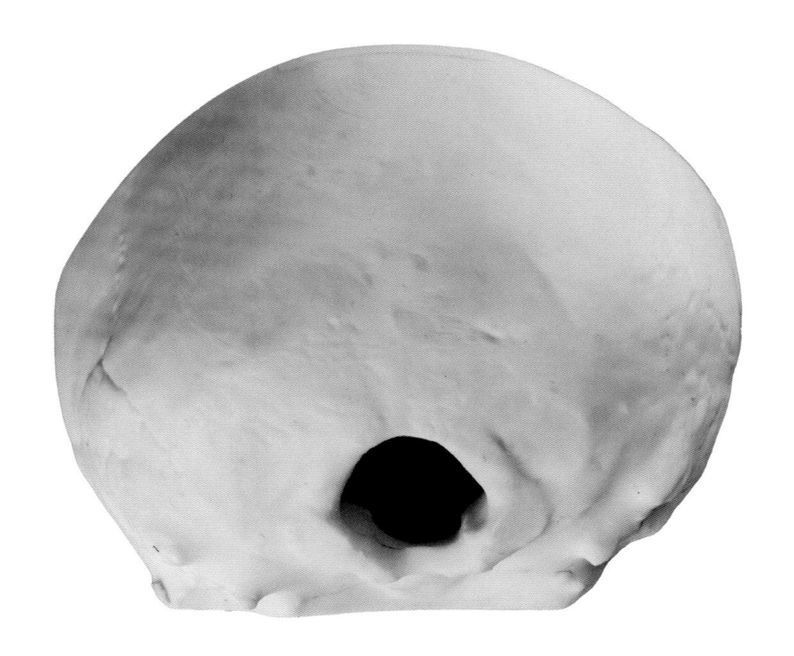

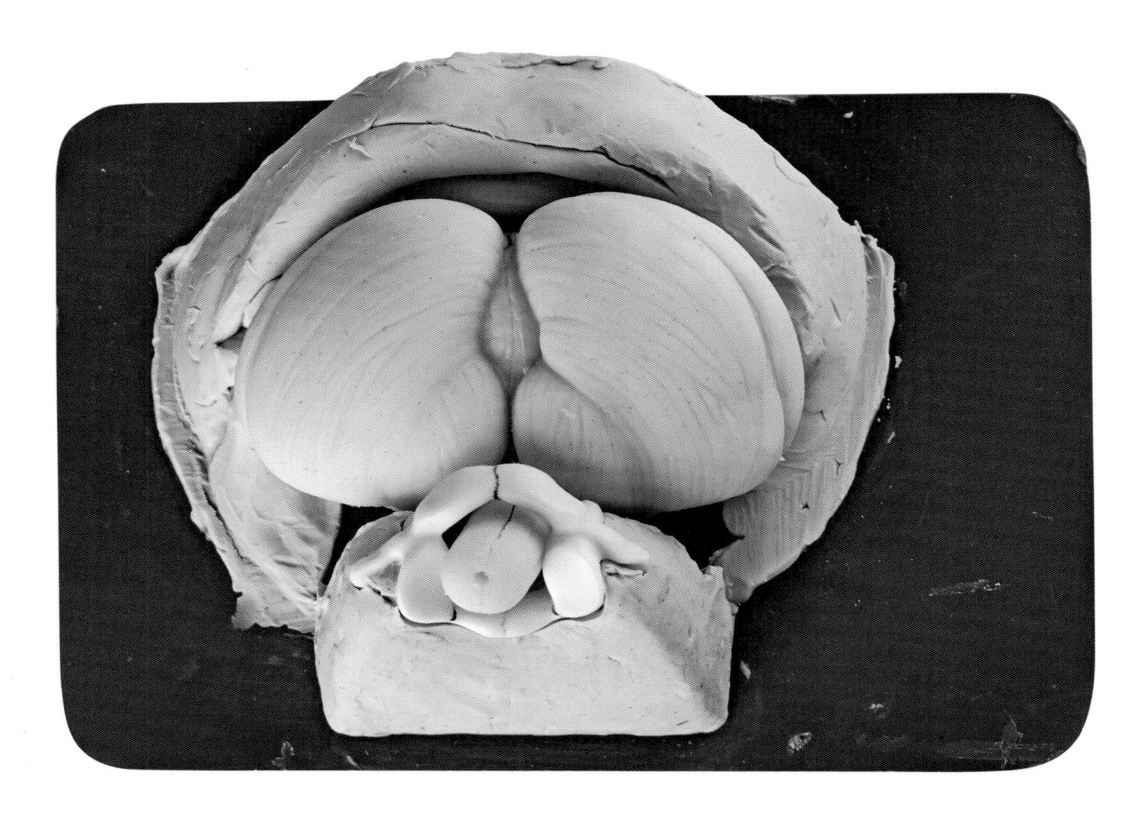

CATALOGUE 75
Clare Rangeley with Martyn Cooke
Part of Paediatric MARTYN
model under development: the
cerebellum with a tumour visible
(darker shaded area), 2015, silicone
rubber, 5.8 x 8.6 x 7.6 cm.
Photograph by Michael Frank.

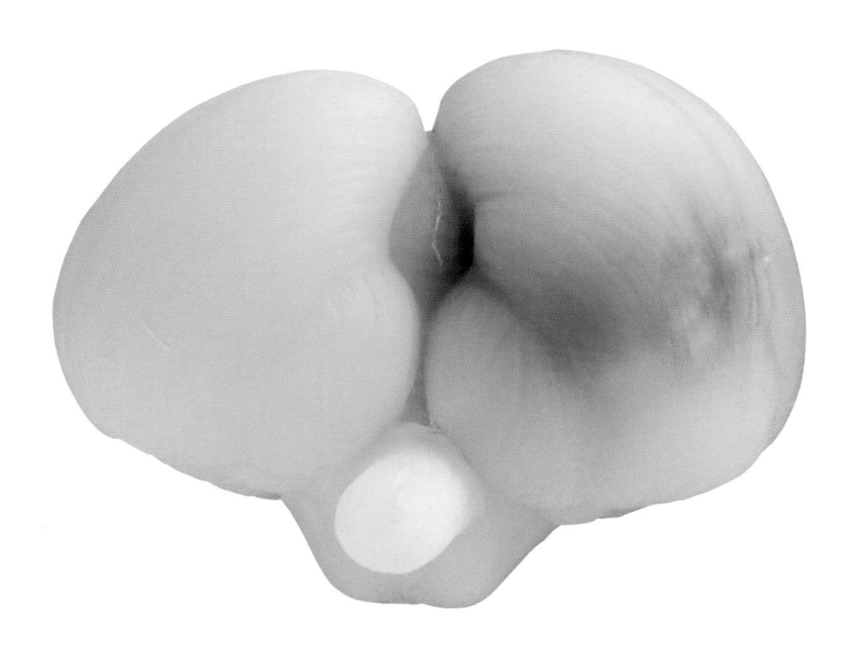

CATALOGUE 76
Clare Rangeley with Martyn Cooke
Paediatric MARTYN model under development: the cerebellum (hollowed out) and section of the spinal cord cut in half to show the modelled 4th ventricle (in white). The model ventricle was then used to cast the cerebellum, 2015, polyurethane, wax and steel. 7.2 x 9.6 x 11.4 cm.
Photograph by Michael Frank.

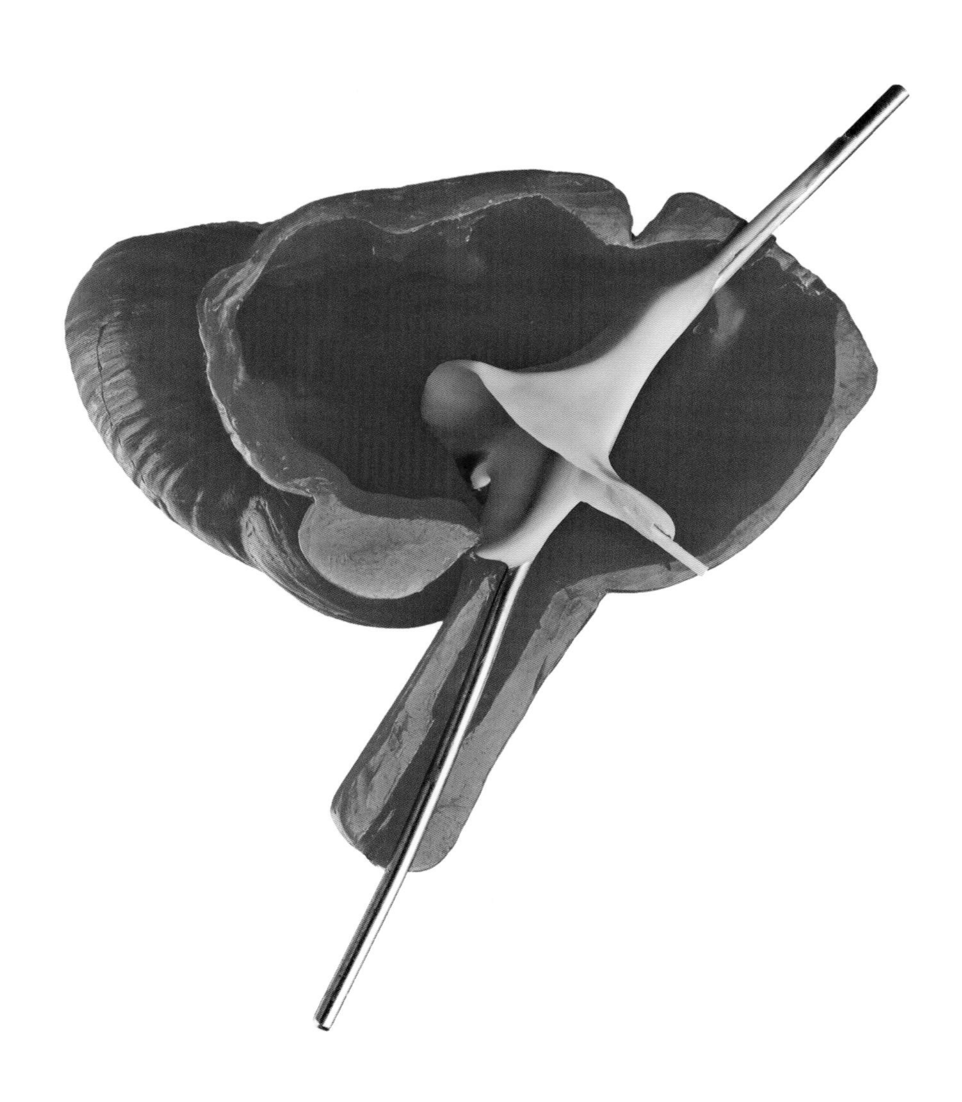

Further reading

Alberti, Samuel JMM, *Morbid Curiosities: Medical Museums in Nineteenth-Century Britain* (Oxford: Oxford University Press, 2011).

Alberti, Samuel JMM, and Elizabeth **Hallam**, eds, *Medical Museums: Past, Present, Future* (London: Royal College of Surgeons of England, 2013).

de Chadarevian, Soraya, and Nick **Hopwood**, eds, *Models: The Third Dimension of Science* (Stanford: Stanford University Press, 2004).

Coopmans, Catelijne, et al., eds, *Representation in Scientific Practice Revisited* (Cambridge, MA: MIT Press, 2014).

Dudley, Sandra, ed., *Museum Materialities: Objects, Engagements, Interpretations* (London: Routledge, 2010).

Fisher, Tom, 'A World of Colour and Bright Shining Surfaces: Experiences of Plastics after the Second World War', *Journal of Design History*, 26 (2013), 285–303.

Gabrys, Jennifer, Gay **Hawkins** and Mike **Michael**, eds, *Accumulation: The Material Politics of Plastic* (London: Routledge, 2013).

Gunn, Wendy, Ton **Otto** and Rachel Charlotte **Smith**, eds, *Design Anthropology: Theory and Practice* (London: Bloomsbury, 2013).

Hallam, Elizabeth, *Anatomy Museum: Death and the Body Displayed* (London: Reaktion, 2016).

Harvey, Penny, et al., eds, *Objects and Materials: A Routledge Companion* (London: Routledge, 2014).

Hansen, Julie V, and Suzanne **Porter**, eds, *The Physician's Art: Representations of Art and Medicine* (Durham, NC: Duke University Museum of Art, 1999).

Hopwood, Nick, *Embryos in Wax: Models from the Ziegler Studio* (Cambridge and Bern: Whipple Museum of the History of Science, University of Cambridge; Institute of the History of Medicine, University of Bern, 2002, reprinted 2013).

Hopwood, Nick, 'Model politics', *The Lancet*, 372 (2008), 1946–47.

Ingold, Tim, *Making: Anthropology, Archaeology, Art and Architecture* (London: Routledge, 2013).

Kemp, Martin, and Marina **Wallace**, *Spectacular Bodies: The Art and Science of the Human Body from Leonardo to Now* (London: Hayward Gallery, 2000).

Kwint, Marius, and Richard **Wingate**, *Brains: The Mind as Matter* (London: Wellcome Collection, 2012).

Maerker, Anna, *Model Experts: Wax Anatomies and Enlightenment in Florence and Vienna, 1775–1815* (Manchester: Manchester University Press, 2011).

Massbarger, Rebecca, *The Lady Anatomist: The Life and Work of Anna Morandi Manzolini* (Chicago: University of Chicago Press, 2010).

Mossman, Susan, *Fantastic Plastic: Product Design and Consumer Culture* (London: Black Dog Publishing, 2008).

Myers, William, Bio Design: Nature, Science, Creativity (London: Thames and Hudson, 2012).

Myers, William, *Bio Design: Nature, Science, Creativity* (London: Thames and Hudson, 2012).

Panzanelli, Roberta, ed., *Ephemeral Bodies: Wax Sculpture and the Human Figure* (Los Angeles: Getty Research Institute, 2008).

Patrizio, Andrew, and Dawn **Kemp**, eds, *Anatomy Acts: How We Come to Know Ourselves* (Edinburgh: Birlinn, 2006).

Pauwels, Luc, ed., *Visual Cultures of Science: Rethinking Representational Practices in Knowledge Building and Science Communication* (Hanover, NH: Dartmouth College Press, 2006).

Riva, Alessandro, et al., 'The Evolution of Anatomical Illustration and Wax Modelling in Italy from the 16th to the Early 19th Centuries', *Journal of Anatomy*, 216 (2010), 209–22.

Schnalke, Thomas, *Diseases in Wax: The History of the Medical Moulage* (Hanover Park IL: Quintessence Publishing, 1995).

Stephens, Elizabeth, *Anatomy as Spectacle: Public Exhibitions of the Body from 1700 to the Present* (Liverpool: Liverpool University Press, 2011).

Von Düring, Monika, George **Didi-Huberman** and Marta **Poggesi**, eds, *Encyclopaedia Anatomica: Museo Las Specola Florence* (Köln: Taschen, 1999).

Contributors

Samuel JMM Alberti is Director of Museums and Archives at The Royal College of Surgeons of England (including the Hunterian Museum) and Visiting Senior Research Fellow in History at King's College London. Trained in the history of science and medicine, before working at the RCS, he taught museum studies at the University of Manchester and was Research Fellow at the Manchester Museum. He has co-curated exhibitions on race, the Hunterian Museum's bicentenary and the First World War; his books include *Morbid Curiosities: Medical Museums in Nineteenth-Century Britain* (2011) and *Medical Museums: Past Present Future* (edited with Elizabeth Hallam, 2013). In 2014–15 he was James M Graham Visiting Professor at the University of Edinburgh College of Medicine and Veterinary Medicine.

Elizabeth Hallam is Senior Research Fellow at the Department of Anthropology, University of Aberdeen, and Research Associate in the School of Anthropology and Museum Ethnography, University of Oxford. She has a BA and PhD in social anthropology from the University of Kent. Prior to her affiliations in Aberdeen and Oxford, she taught anthropology at the University of Sussex. Her research and publications focus on the anthropology of the body; death and dying; material and visual cultures; histories of collecting and museums; human anatomy; 3D modelling; and mixed-media sculpture. Her recent books include *Making and Growing: Anthropological Studies of Organisms and Artefacts* (co-edited with Tim Ingold, 2014) and *Anatomy Museum: Death and the Body Displayed* (2016). During 2014–16 she is a visiting scholar at the University of Melbourne.

Anna Maerker is Senior Lecturer in History of Medicine at King's College London. She pursued undergraduate studies in physics and history of science at the University of Regensburg. She received an MPhil in history and philosophy of science from the University of Cambridge, and an MA/PhD in science and technology studies from Cornell University. Before joining King's, she held posts as a Postdoctoral Research Fellow at the Max Planck Institute for the History of Science, Berlin, and as a Senior Lecturer at Oxford Brookes University. She is the author of *Model Experts: Wax Anatomies and Enlightenment in Florence and Vienna, 1775-1815* (2011).

Visual index

David Hugh Tompsett

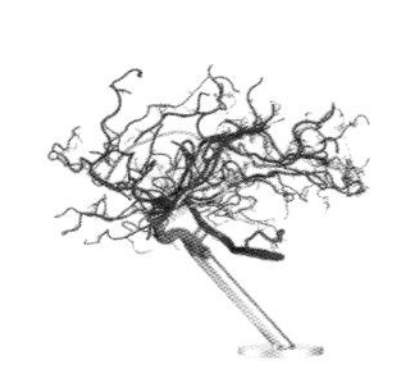
Catalogue 1
Page 83

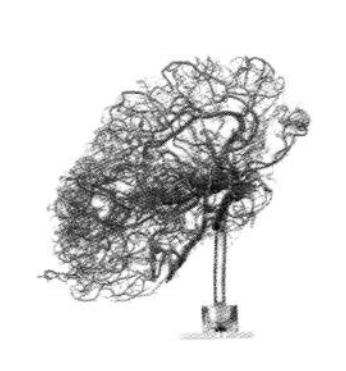
Catalogue 2
Page 85

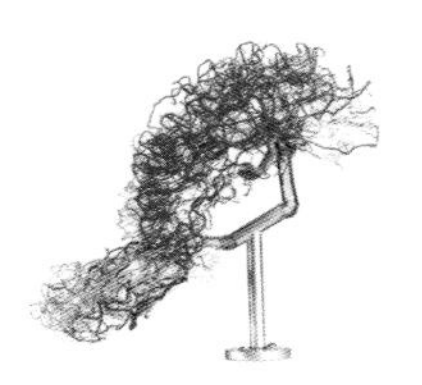
Catalogue 3
Page 87

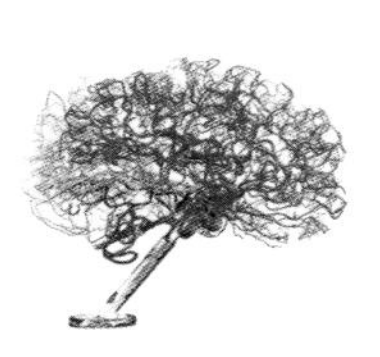
Catalogue 4
Page 89

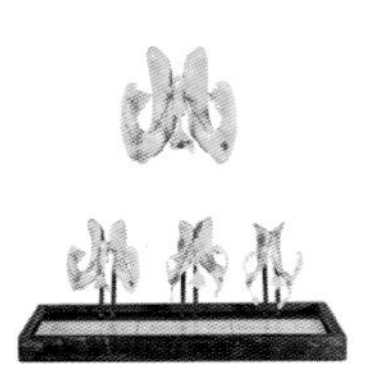
Catalogue 5
Page 91

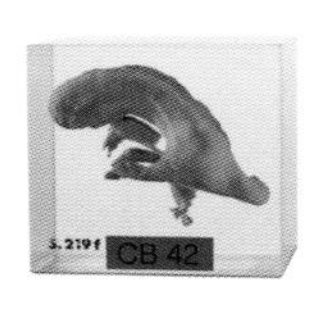

Catalogue 6
Page 93

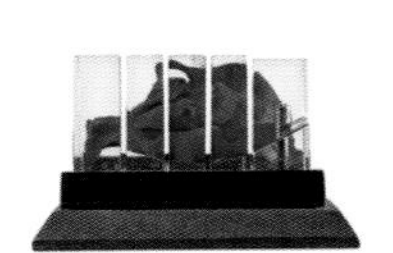
Catalogue 7
Page 95

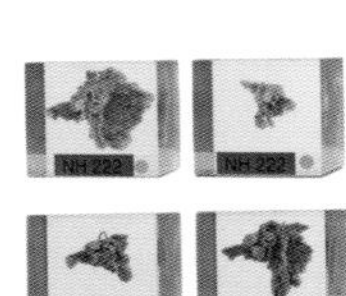

Catalogue 8
Page 97

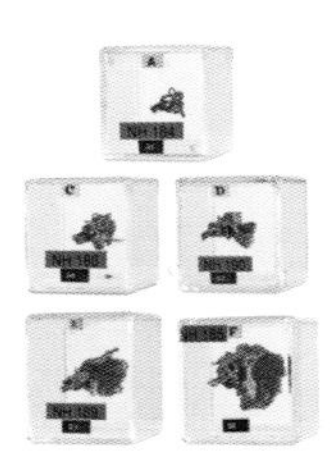
Catalogue 9
Page 99

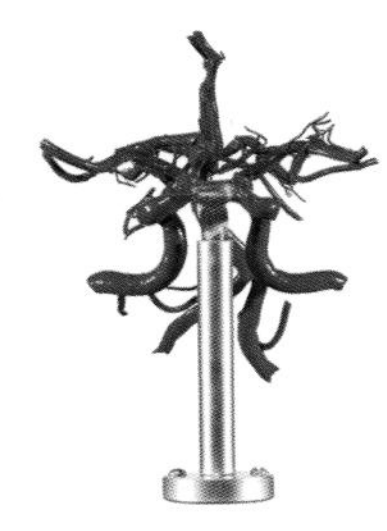
Catalogue 10
Page 101

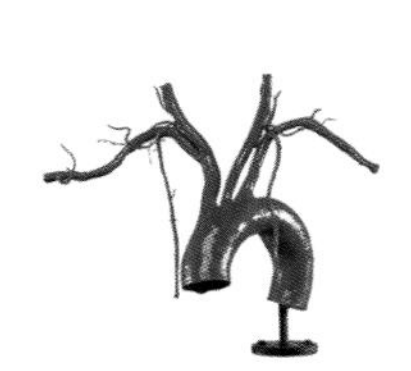
Catalogue 11
Page 103

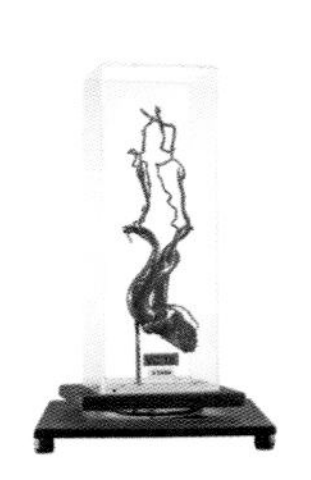
Catalogue 12
Page 105

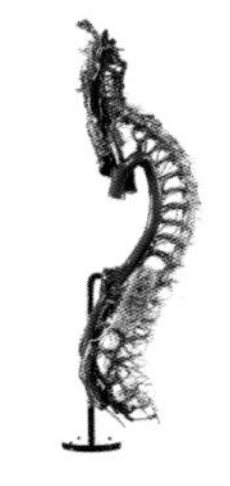
Catalogue 13
Page 107

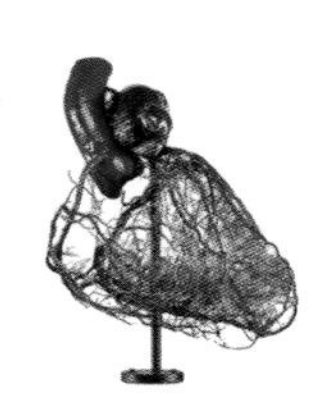
Catalogue 14
Page 109

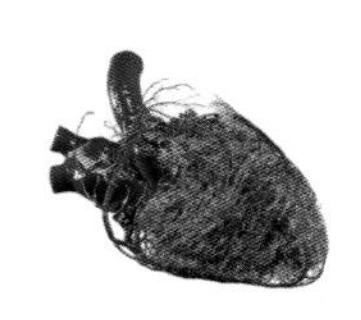
Catalogue 15
Page 111

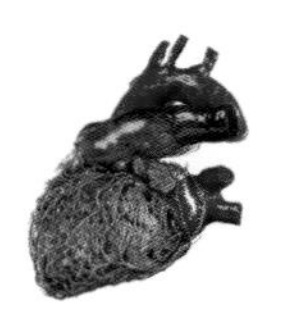
Catalogue 16
Page 113

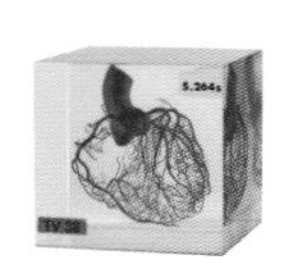
Catalogue 17
Page 115

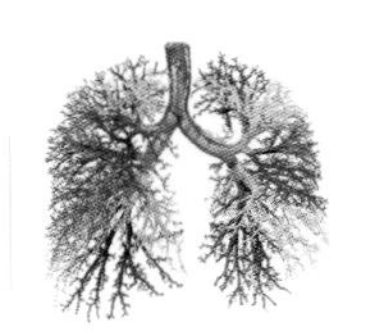
Catalogue 18
Page 117 (also features in Hallam fig 16, page 17)

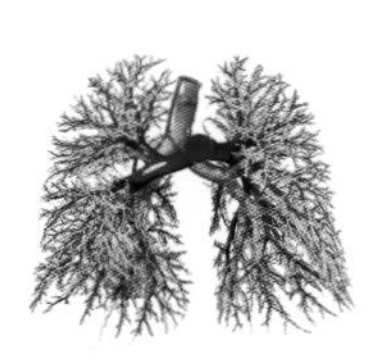
Catalogue 19
Page 119

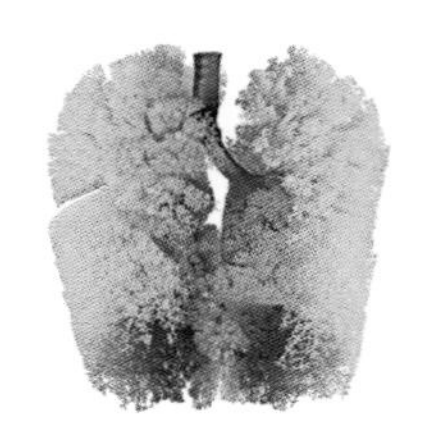
Catalogue 20
Page 121

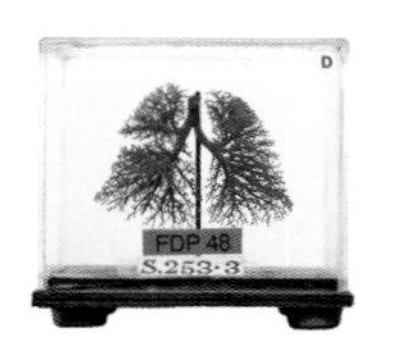

Catalogue 21
Page 123

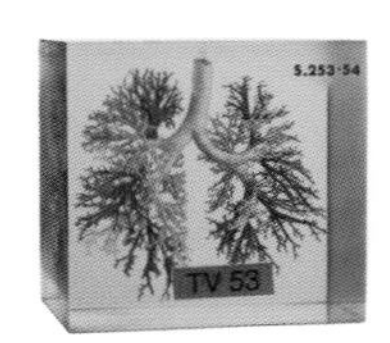

Catalogue 22
Page 125

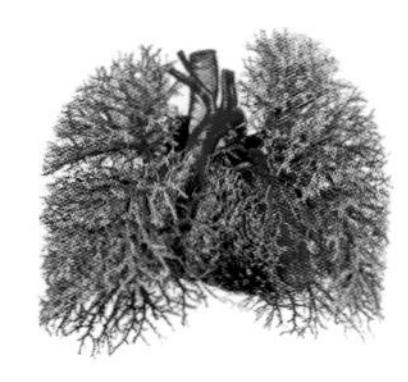
Catalogue 23
Page 127

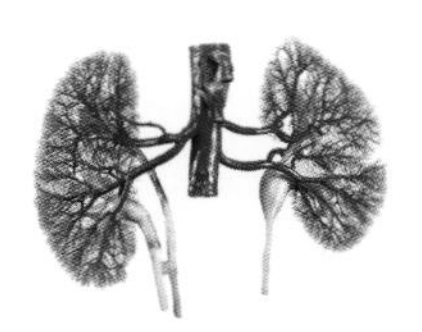
Catalogue 24
Page 129

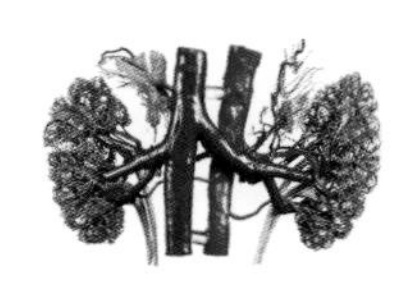
Catalogue 25
Page 131

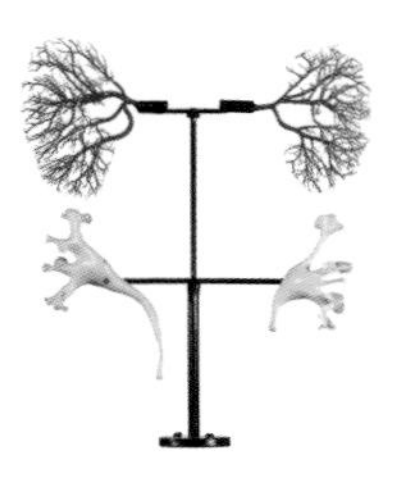
Catalogue 26
Page 133

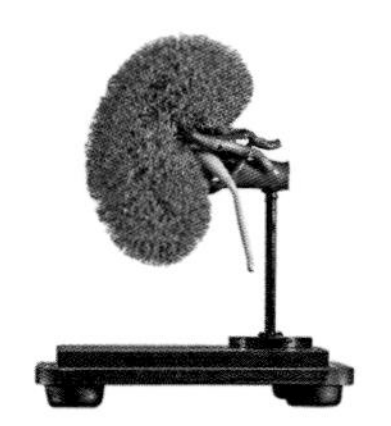
Catalogue 27
Page 135 (also features in Hallam fig 17, page 18)

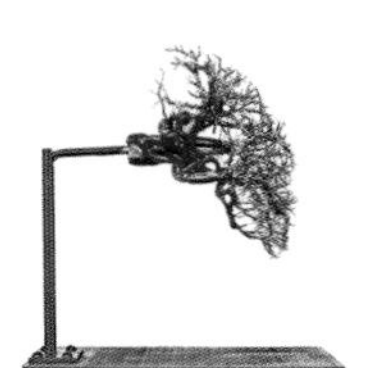
Catalogue 28
Page 137

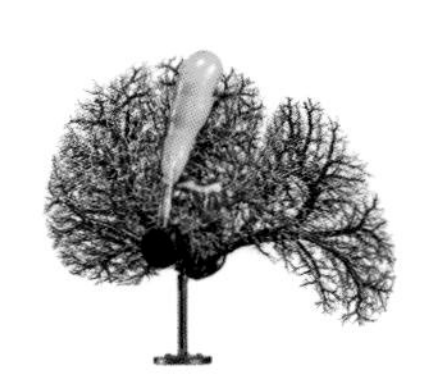
Catalogue 29
Page 139

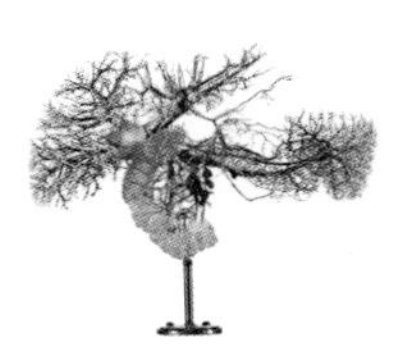
Catalogue 30
Page 141

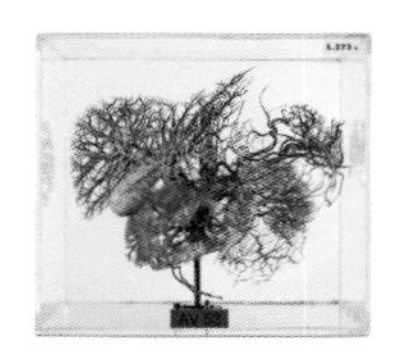
Catalogue 31
Page 143

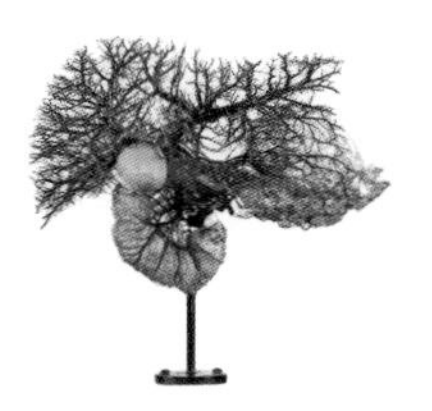
Catalogue 32
Page 145

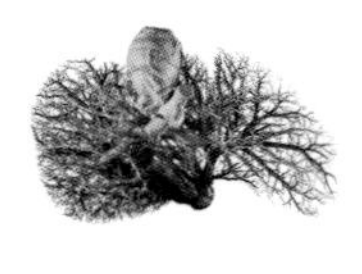
Catalogue 33
Page 147

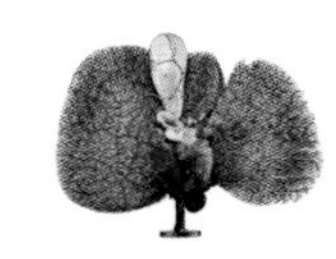
Catalogue 34
Page 149

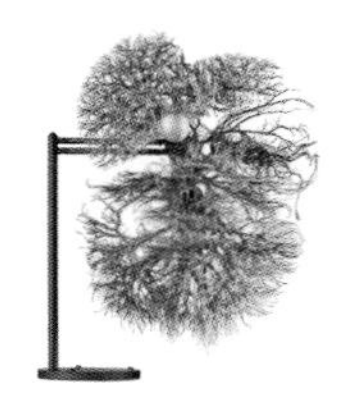
Catalogue 35
Page 151

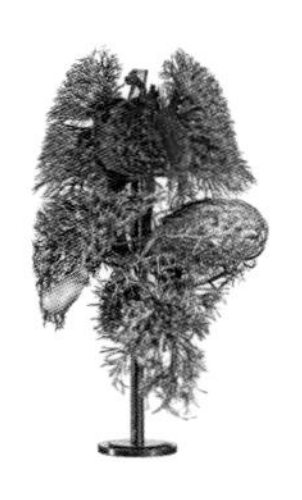

Catalogue 36
Page 153

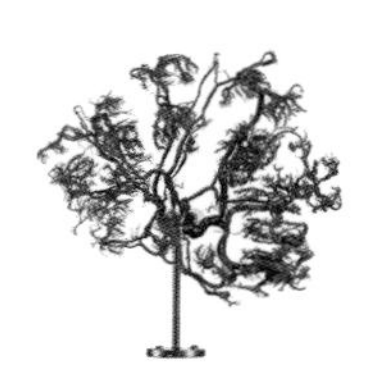

Catalogue 37
Page 155

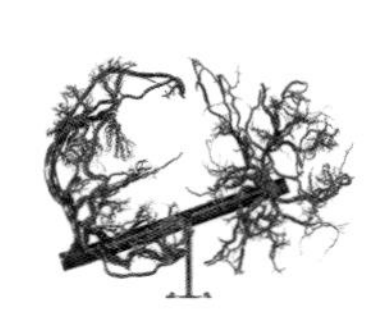

Catalogue 38
Page 157

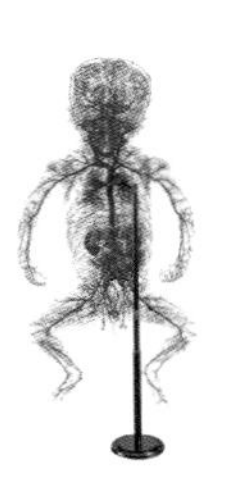

Catalogue 39
Page 159

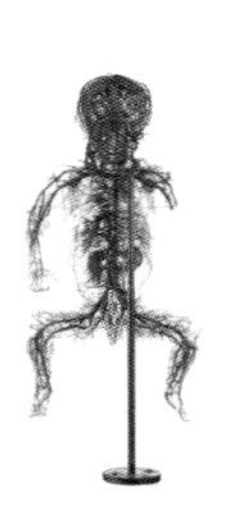

Catalogue 40
Page 161

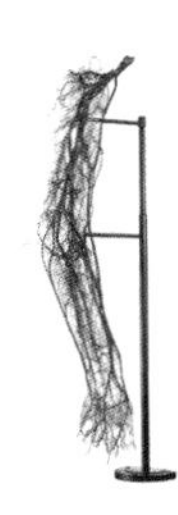

Catalogue 41
Page 163

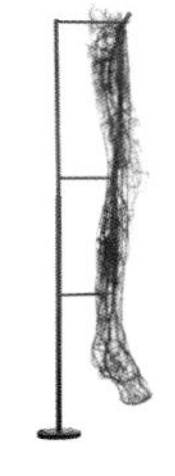

Catalogue 42
Page 165

John Herbert Hicks

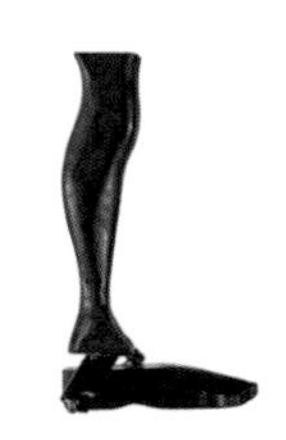

Catalogue 43
Page 169

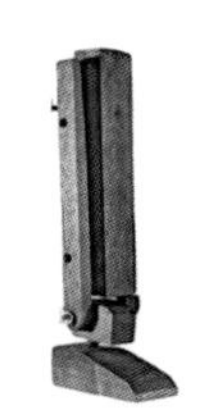

Catalogue 44
Page 171

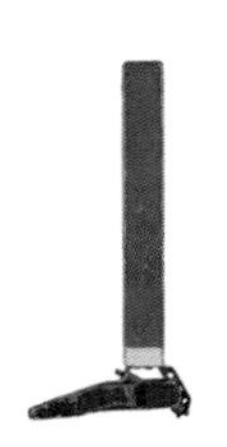

Catalogue 45
Page 173

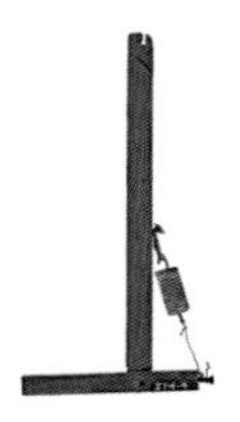

Catalogue 46
Page 175

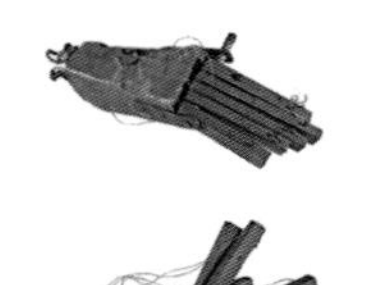

Catalogue 47
Page 177

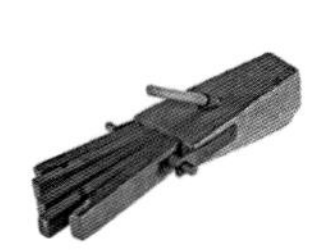

Catalogue 48
Page 179

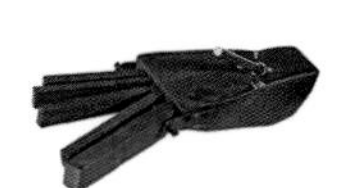

Catalogue 49
Page 181

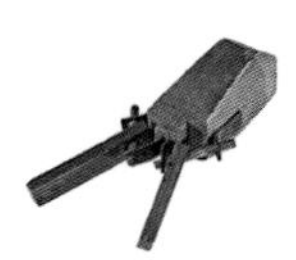

Catalogue 50
Page 183

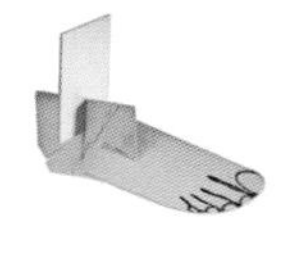

Catalogue 51
Page 185 (also features in Hallam figs 27, 28 and 29, pages 26 and 27)

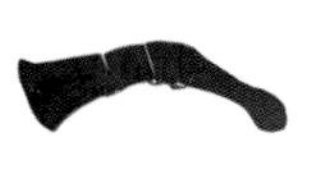

Catalogue 52
Page 187

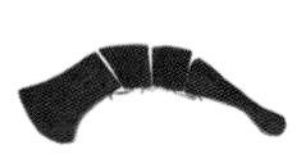

Catalogue 53
Page 187

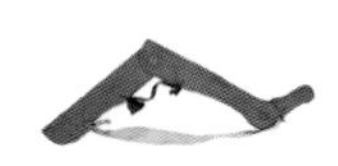

Catalogue 54
Page 189

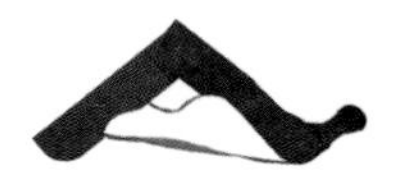

Catalogue 55
Page 189

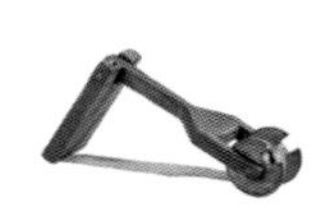

Catalogue 56
Page 191

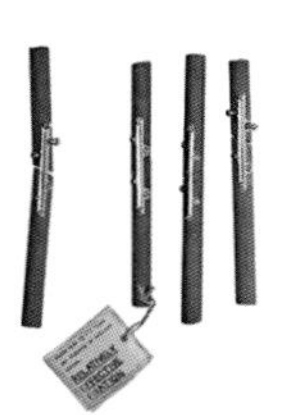

Catalogue 57
Page 193

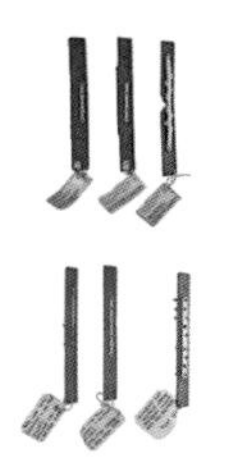

Catalogue 58
Page 195

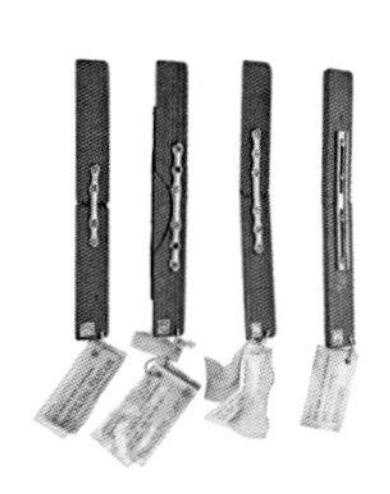

Catalogue 59
Page 197

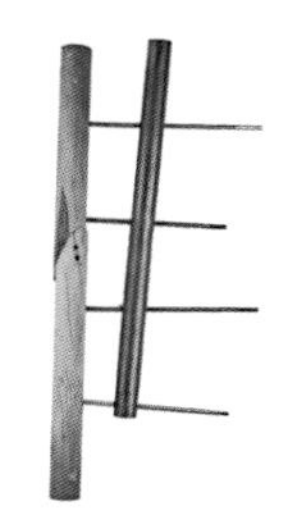

Catalogue 60
Page 199

Modelled Anatomical Replica for Training Young Neurosurgeons (MARTYN)

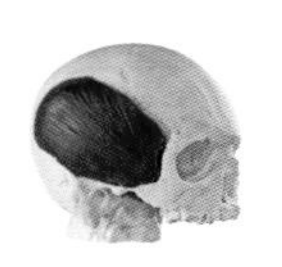

Catalogue 61
Page 203

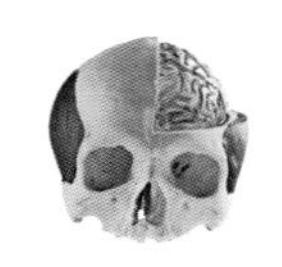

Catalogue 62
Page 205

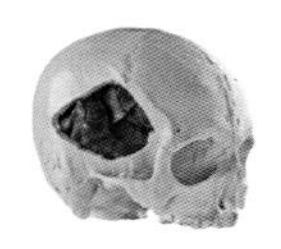

Catalogue 63
Page 207

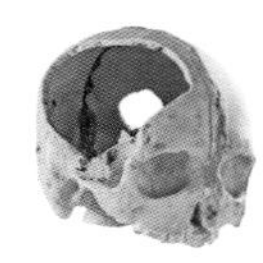

Catalogue 64
Page 209

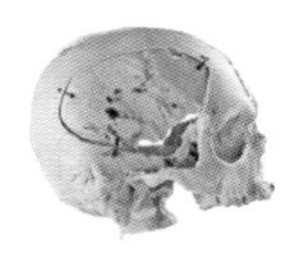

Catalogue 65
Page 211

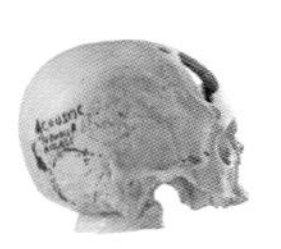

Catalogue 66
Page 213

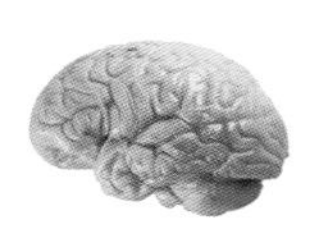

Catalogue 67
Page 215

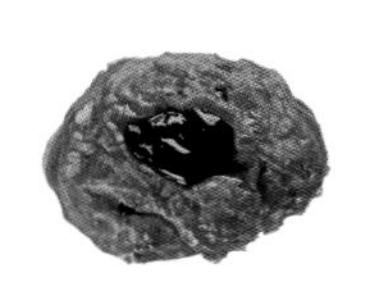

Catalogue 68
Page 215

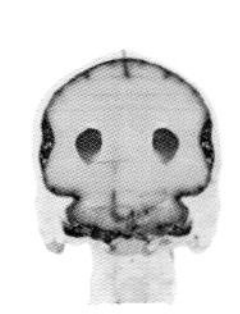

Catalogue 69
Page 217

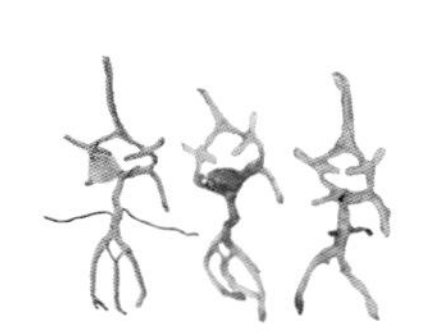

Catalogue 70
Page 219

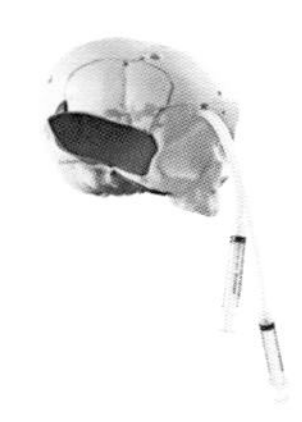

Catalogue 71
Page 221

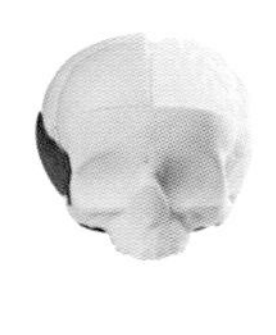

Catalogue 72
Page 223

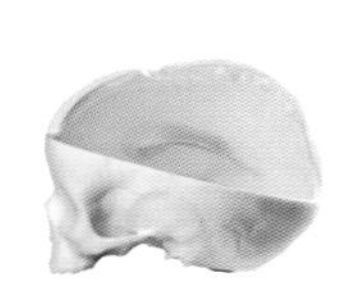

Catalogue 73
Page 225

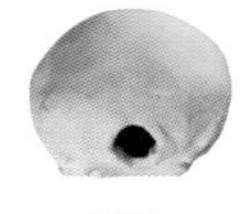

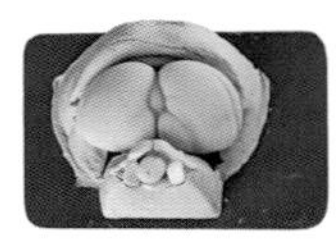

Catalogue 74
Page 227

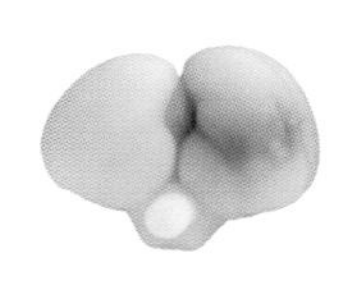

Catalogue 75
Page 229

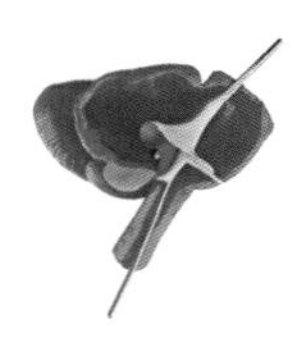

Catalogue 76
Page 231